HEALTH CARE SOCIAL WORK PRACTICE

concepts and strategies

Health care social work practice

concepts and strategies

Elfriede G. Schlesinger, Ph.D.

Rutgers—The State University of New Jersey,
School of Social Work,
New Brunswick, New Jersey

Illustrated

TIMES MIRROR/MOSBY College Publishing

ST. LOUIS · TORONTO · SANTA CLARA 1985

Editor: Diane L. Bowen
Editorial assistant: Jane E. Kozuszek
Design: Kay M. Kramer
Production: Jeanne A. Gulledge, Judith Bamert, Margaret B. Bridenbaugh

Cover art:
Point of Tranquility, Morris Louis, 1958
Hirshhorn Museum and Sculpture Garden, Smithsonian Institution
Joseph Martin/Scala

A division of The C. V. Mosby Company
11830 Westline Industrial Drive
St. Louis, Missouri 63146

Printed in the United States of America

Library of Congress Cataloging in Publication Data

Schlesinger, Elfriede G.
Health care social work practice.

Bibliography: p.
Includes index.
1. Medical social work—United States. I. Title.
[DNLM: 1. Social work. 2. Sociology, Medical.
3. Health policy—United States. 4. Social Medicine.
W 322 S342h]
HV687.5.U5S34 1984 362.1′0425′0973 83-25081
ISBN 0-8016-4380-5

TG/VH/VH 9 8 7 6 5 4 3 2 1 03/C/290

To my parents, Scheindel and Daniel Galanter, with love.

Always an inspiration, you are now becoming frail and elderly. Following a lifetime of fruitful labor you now need compassionate, comprehensive care. Because of your consistent devotion to social justice, I know you share my view that such care is also required by those individuals who are young and vulnerable, are members of minority groups, and are struggling to maintain their lives in the face of major health problems.

This book was written in the hope that it will make some small contribution to enactment of the ideals you have always conveyed to me.

Preface

Health care social workers draw on a wide range of conceptual formulations and practice modalities in their work in hospitals, primary care centers, long-term care facilities, health planning and administrative tasks, and activities designed to promote humane, equitable health care policies. Wherever they function health care social workers must integrate the basic mandates and skills of social work with their understanding of impending health problems and with the organizational, social, and psychological factors that shape the behavior of health care consumers and providers. To effectively integrate these factors they need continually to identify and synthesize those elements of social work values, concepts, and skill that have particular bearing and importance in the health field. This book was written with the objective of facilitating that task.

Intended as a comprehensive text for health care social work practice, this book draws on diverse analyses of the nature and origin of prevailing health problems, insight from the behavioral sciences, and the rich literature on health care social work practice.

A number of basic themes are contained within this work. One relates to the conviction that effective practice must be based on thorough grounding in health problems, their historical roots, and their major dimensions. A second theme focuses on the importance of understanding major health policies and the pluralistic character of the American health care delivery system. Another theme derives from the view that insights from the sociology of health make a significant contribution to the social worker's efforts to understand how people respond to and manage illness.

Of major importance are those developments in social work theory and practice that can guide social workers in thinking about and acting on the health problems with which they deal in their daily work. These developments in turn require adaptation to meet the particular needs of health care consumers.

Using these perspectives, I present a number of principles for health care social work practice. They are derived from core social work values, the knowledge of human behavior considered essential for all social work practice, and a specialized body of knowledge focused on health and illness. A basic principle revolves around the view of social work as a problem-solving endeavor that aims to facilitate the release of coping capacities, even in those individuals facing the most severe insults to soma and psyche that come in the wake of many health problems. Reviewing current health problems and assessing developments in social work practice generated a major principle stressed throughout this book. That principle is that most practice in the health field calls for simultaneous attention to the difficulties experienced by individuals and to the environmental and systemic factors that can enhance health, or trigger health problems.

This book is divided into two parts. Part I consists of six chapters. Chapter 1, The Health Problems Before Us, reviews the prevailing health problems in contemporary American society and traces their historical origins. Contributions of medical technology, increases in the standard of living, and public health measures in reducing certain problems are assessed, as is the emergence of chronic health difficulties as a major health concern. The needs of those populations particularly at risk for health problems and those requiring special attention (the elderly, the young and vulnerable, and the minority groups) are considered.

Chapter 2, Health Policy, Costs and Financing, Delivery Systems, and Providers, presents an overview of the mix of financing, organizational mechanisms, and providers that constitutes the American health care delivery system. Major policies governing Medicare, Medicaid, and private health insurance are summarized, and the inequities inherent in the present financing structure are considered. The roles of physicians, nurses, and social workers as health care providers are reviewed.

Chapter 3, Health, Disease and Illness: Social Work, Sociological and Medical Perspectives, reviews various definitions of health, disease, and illness and presents a definition of health consonant with social work perspectives. Chapter 4, Variations in Response to Health and Illness, presents a number of sociological conceptions of health and illness behavior, and their application to social work practice is considered. Special attention is paid to the relationships between ethnicity, social class, gender, age, and health and illness behavior.

Chapter 5, Conceptual Formulations for Health Care Social Work Practice, presents a number of conceptual formulations for health care social work practice. These formulations include a public health perspective, the concept of "person-environment fit," the continuum from care to cure, and the "illness careers." A typology of caring conceptualizing social work tasks in the health field is also presented. Chapter 6, Principles for Health Care Social Work Practice, considers in detail the principles for health care social work practice introduced in Chapter 5.

Part II focuses on practice. Chapter 7, Strategies and Skills for Health Care

Social Work Practice, outlines a series of strategies and skills for health care social work practice. The stages of the problem-solving process are delineated, and necessary adaptations for health practice are presented.

Chapter 8, Interdisciplinary Practice, reviews key concepts and strategies in health practice. These are necessary because interdisciplinary endeavors are an integral part of all health practice. Chapter 9, Social Work in Hospitals, focuses on hospital social work, which has been and continues to be a major arena in which health care social work is carried out. The organizational context of the hospital is analyzed, and special attention is paid to the development of high-risk screening and discharge planning. Examples from work in medical/surgical services, dialysis, and neonatal intensive care are presented as illustrative of the range and diversity of hospital social work practice.

The movement toward deinstitutionalization has generated a number of innovative approaches to providing care for people with long-term care needs. Chapter 10, Social Work Practice in Long-Term Care, concentrates on developments in this arena and on social work's role in long-term care. Primary care has captured the attention of many in the hope that this approach to the provision of health services can minimize fragmented, depersonalized care. Chapter 11, Social Work Practice in Primary Care, considers the potential for social work's contribution to primary care.

Research on health care and approaches to quality assurance have accelerated. Chapter 12, Research and Quality Assurance in Health Care Social Work Practice, discusses some key perspectives of this research, emphasizing how social work practitioners can use these perspectives in their daily work.

Several appendixes are included. Appendix A presents an approach to guide social workers in acquiring the medical information they need in their daily work. Appendix B outlines some principles of recording health practice data. Appendix C lists current criteria used in identifying people at risk for illness-related psychosocial crises. Appendix D outlines how to develop a profile of the community in which the health agency is located to help social workers understand the community where they work and the available health and social service delivery mechanisms.

Clearly there are areas of health practice where social workers function that have not been discussed in separate chapters. No one book can do justice to all areas. It is hoped that people working in specialized areas not explicitly addressed here will nevertheless find that the knowledge base, conceptual formulations, and practice principles presented can help to guide their work.

This book is intended for social work educators, students needing in-depth knowledge of practice in the health field, and health care social work practitioners. It can be used in a number of ways. Schools of social work having a specialized health curriculum will find that the book can be used for a number of courses: those presenting fundamental knowledge concerning health problems and policy, financing, and health and illness behavior, and those dealing with health practice. Individuals using the book in courses devoted to direct health care practice may want to use supplemental materials in such areas as crisis intervention or other specific modalities of intervention. People using the book in courses focused on community organization and health care planning and administration may with to use supplemental, specialized material to highlight and specify the material presented here. The book can be used by social work educators who organize their courses to cover a number of substantive areas. It can also serve as a useful reference in continuing education efforts.

The help and insight of many people must be acknowledged. Foremost are my present and former colleagues in the School of Social Work at Rutgers—The State University of New Jersey with whom I worked for many years in joint efforts to develop a health curriculum, namely David Antebi, Yetta Appel, Eileen Corrigan, Nancy Humphreys, Greta Stanton, and Kay Wood. Special thanks are due Miriam Dinerman and Anne Adams. Some of the perspectives on social work and practice in the health field presented here are an outgrowth of many hours of discussion and collaborative teaching efforts. I hope I have not misrepresented these individuals' insightful and penetrating contributions. Isabel Wolock, colleague and fellow health care researcher, also deserves special mention.

Not to be neglected are the students who have been in my various classes. Their reflections on practice and on the practice principles presented have been most helpful. Special thanks go to those who took the trouble to read earlier, unedited versions of the manuscript. Field instructors who have worked hard to educate students in keeping with some of the principles presented here are too numerous to mention.

Pat Costante, a former student and a most competent health care social worker, helped with the literature review and contributed many key ideas. Diane Bowen, editor at The C.V. Mosby Company, and Jane Kozuszek, editorial assistant, deserve thanks for their unending patience and help.

A number of reviewers who carefully read and critiqued the first draft of the manuscript also merit special mention. They are Rita Black of the Columbia University School of Social Work; Joyce Brengarth of the University of Pittsburgh School of Social Work; Karen Holmes of the Graduate School of Social Work, Central Campus, University of Houston; Lynne Riehman of the School of Social Work, San Diego State University; and Kristine Siefert, of the Jane Addams College of Social Work, University of Illinois at Chicago. My thanks to you all for your encouraging words and especially for your penetrating insights, comments, and suggestions. I have no doubt that the final manuscript was strengthened because of your careful work.

A number of secretaries carefully typed various portions of the manuscript. Thanks go to Barbara Molnar and especially to Susan Tiller.

Thanks also go to David Antebi for his hard work and creative photography. The pictures are intended to convey the image of the health care social worker in action that is reflected in this book.

And finally, I am most grateful to my husband Richard, my daughter Adrienne, and my son David. Although comments about the family's forbearance and patience while a book is being written are legion, they are nevertheless quite accurate. To Richard, also a health care practitioner, special thanks for the many years of discussion and debate that helped shape much of my thinking.

Elfriede Schlesinger

Contents

Appendixes

Part One

Conceptual Formulations

Part One presents the conceptual formulations for health care social work. Chapter 1 focuses on the health problems before us. The contributions of medical technology and public health measures are presented and assessed, as are competing views concerning the priorities assigned to various types of health care and prevention. Chapter 2 reviews major health policies and organizational arrangements and discusses the roles of physicians, nurses, and social workers. Chapter 3 considers various views of disease, health, illness, and characteristic responses to illness. Chapter 4 examines the relationship between age, gender, ethnicity, and health and illness behaviors. Chapter 5 reviews a number of conceptual formulations for health care. Chapter 6 presents a series of practice principles for health care social work.

PEDIATRICS
ADULT MEDICINE
NEW

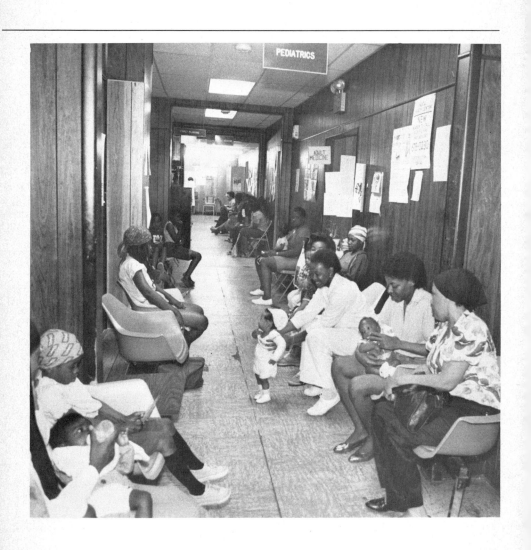

Chapter 1

The health problems before us

There are many ways of thinking about contemporary health problems. Diverse approaches have been presented for enhancing health status, changing the manner in which health care is organized, and improving the quality and accessibility of care. Disagreement abounds about which problems call for immediate attention. While demographic changes lead to increasing appropriation of resources to care for the health needs of the elderly (*Health, United States,* 1978), compelling voices point to the importance of early and preventive services for young children and their families (Children's Defense Fund, 1976). Resources required for supportive services for people afflicted with chronic mental or physical handicaps are juxtaposed with those required to finance the expensive medical technology available to treat many people who suffer from heart and kidney disease, cancer, and other illnesses. The ability to save the lives of productive individuals stricken in their middle years with heart disease through coronary bypass surgery is dramatic and welcome. Alongside such an achievement, efforts to develop and sustain services that assure continuing innoculation and routine examination to detect treatable problems of vision or hearing may appear less glamorous and dramatic. Nevertheless, governmental bodies responsible for charting public policy directions in health care have identified preventive approaches that call for a major national effort (*Health, United States,* 1980).

There is increasing deliberation about the psychological, social, and financial costs entailed in sustaining the seriously impaired. Questions are raised about the way in which care is rendered, the quality of life engendered, and the relative allocation of funds for different types of care. These questions revolve around such issues as the ways in which nursing homes, intensive care units, and home care are used. For example, as of 1978, 42% of monies paid in connection with the Medicaid program (Chapter 2) was used for care in facilities such as nursing homes. In contrast, only 1% of payments was applied to home health care (Congressional Research Service, 1981).

These comments call brief attention to the range of health problems encountered in contemporary western society in general and in the United States in particular. These and related issues confront those who provide and those who use health services. Contemporary health services must provide for the care of the young, assuming that attention to their health needs can prevent problems that retard growth and the capacity for a productive existence. Attention to those problems that are viewed as major killers (heart disease, cancer, and accidents) is essential (*Health, United States,* 1982). At the same time, the health system has an obligation to people who have benefited from recently developed techniques that prolong the lives of people with grave impairments (Gruenberg, 1977). Most important are those technological developments that generate dramatic and costly diagnostic and treatment procedures. For many people these procedures allow continuation of the capacity to work and play with minimal disruption. Other people whose lives have been saved also join the ranks of the chronically impaired. These people, those with whom they are intimately involved, and the larger community must deal with the psychological, social, and financial costs entailed in care of the chronically ill.

A major issue confronting contemporary health care delivery revolves around how to allocate limited resources to meet diverse and competing demands. Within the health care sector the needs for the varying types of care identified compete with those required for further research. Simultaneously, other sectors of the society (education, housing, welfare, and the defense industry) have an eye on financial and human resources that cannot be infinitely stretched. The decisions made concerning which of these areas are given priority have far-reaching philosophical, moral, and political implications.

The decisions made concerning financing and the relative priorities accorded to the needs of the young and old, the chronically impaired, and people benefiting from modern medical technology derive from implicit and explicit value judgments. These judgments are translated into decisions about the kinds of personnel to be trained and the type of "health work" that is to be rewarded with acclaim, prestige, and resources for development.

For many years a high proportion of federal funds was deployed for the education of highly specialized physicians. Subsequent decisions led to emphasis on the education of primary care physicians, who were expected to provide more comprehensive and continuous care (*Interim Report,* 1979). Investment in what is often described as technology intensive care is still high. Many hospitals find money to purchase equipment such as the CAT scanner* or new respirators. This investment reflects the esteem and awe with which such symbols of contemporary health care are regarded. Social work, health education, and preventive services budgets often are approved less readily. Allocation for resources that are designed to wrest and prolong life compete with those that attempt to cope with the "failures of technology" (people having daily needs for supportive services). Both efforts reflect attempts to improve the quality of life. Some of these efforts are focused on attempts to cure. Others are focused on prevention; on the provision of home care, health aides, or

* Refers to a device for performing computed axial tomography, a complex piece of costly x-ray equipment that permits taking three-dimensional x-ray films of the head and body interiors.

Meals on Wheels; and on counseling for those undergoing the agonies of illness.

There is a major way in which financing decisions have a significant effect on access to health care delivery in this country. In the United States, more than in any other western industrialized nation, access to health services is largely governed by individual financial status, the type of employment available to the head of a household, age, and financial need. The United States is the only industrialized western nation having virtually no provision for universal access to health services that is not in some way related to ability to pay. Many people incur substantial out-of-pocket costs. Those Americans who advocate the development of a national health insurance scheme analogous to that available in Great Britain and other countries have long declared that "health care is a right." To date that right has not been established in American public policy.

Closely related is the series of data pointing to the fact that those who are lower on the socio-economic ladder suffer disproportionately from acute and chronic illness and die sooner than those in more favorable economic positions (*Health Status of Minorities and Low-Income Groups;* Pear, 1984). Members of minority groups (American Indians, Blacks, and some Hispanic populations) are most seriously affected. In addition to the data on the health status of minority groups and the poor are those data suggesting that the health services available to this segment of the population are lacking in many respects. Frequently cited are problems of poor access, negative attitudes on the part of health care providers, and services organized in a manner not congruent with the particular needs of many in this population (for example, Children's Defense Fund, 1976; President's Commission on Mental Health, 1978). Analysis of the health problems confronting this nation must take into account the special and unmet needs of the millions who are poor and are members of minority groups.

A number of analysts challenge the view that health services, especially as currently structured, markedly affect health levels (for example, Blum, 1974; Fuchs, 1974). In the view of many, improvements in the level of housing, sanitation, nutrition, and income are thought to be as important a determinant of health levels as the number of physicians and medical and other health care facilities. People concerned with promoting improvements in the nation's health must be ever mindful of the living conditions of the poor and minority groups. It is not an easy task to maintain a proper balance between improving health levels related to economic status, creating health facilities that make available the best possible health care, and caring for the range of other needs generated by illness. Yet this task is a major health issue.

There are aspects of health and health care delivery that transcend the special concerns of any one population group or any particular category of health problems. Some of these aspects revolve around the tension between specialized and integrated, holistic care. Few people would dispute the contention that contemporary health care developments are extremely complex and require a core of highly trained specialists. Those who need renal dialysis, coronary bypass surgery, or drug therapy to quiet hallucinations associated with some schizophrenias want and must have care from those who have consummate skill in using these therapies and understanding their social and psychological sequellae. This group includes physicians, nurses, and social workers.

Most people, including those who are healthy, have episodic needs for health care. They use hospitals when giving birth to their children and turn to physicians to monitor the growth and development of those children. Many people also seek physicians' advice when they have tension-related headaches or backaches, marital problems (sometimes under the guise of a "nervous stomach"), and real or imagined sexual dysfunction. The resolution of many of these kinds of problems is intertwined with family relationships, love, hate, joy, and disappointment. Therefore health professionals are needed who have the training to recognize the social and psychological insults that trigger tension-related physical symptoms. These health professionals need the capacity to help people recognize and cope with the interplay of soma and psyche. Such skill requires knowledge of culture, economics, and the unique dynamics of individual and family history. When people turn themselves over to the health care system, they look not only for technical skill but also for compassion.

These and related issues form the background and context within which health care social work is practiced. They all have bearing on the way social work carries out its responsibilities in the health care system. Social work has long-standing commitments and values related to social equity and justice. Therefore social workers have a particular obligation to be knowledgeable about those aspects of health care policy that mitigate against equal distribution of services so vital to the well-being of the people they serve. Indeed, social work has a long history of actively taking part in efforts to change such policies.

Other issues are of concern because of the direct effect they have on clients and social work. For example, social workers claim no expertise about the duration or nature of training required of medical specialists. However, how those specialists organize their work and communicate with patients, families, and other members of the interdisciplinary team, including social workers, is very much a part of social work's domain. The same holds true for those decisions that are made concerning allocation of funds for specialized education and varying kinds of health care activities. These funds affect the kinds of resources available, not the least of which is the availability of social work services. Social workers must understand the source and nature of issues, as well as related conflicts. Such understanding can serve to guide social work action in its effort to bring seasoned knowledge and skill to bear on social work practice in the health field. Social work is a profession whose commitments derive from values focused on the importance of self-determination, on the intrinsic worth of the individual, and from conviction that those values can only be realized by creating environments conducive to growth and health.

Some of the issues that have been identified in a quick, bold sweep will be examined in greater detail in the rest of this chapter. Emphasis will be placed on the nature, scope, and extent of contemporary health problems and their historical origins and social roots.

THE NATURE AND SCOPE OF CONTEMPORARY HEALTH PROBLEMS

A number of developments converge to give shape to the character, nature, and scope of contemporary health problems. These include (1) major developments in public health, (2) improvements in the level of living that accompanied industrialization and urbanization, (3) control of major infectious diseases, and (4) a virtual revolution in medical technology. Many of these developments date to the nineteenth century whereas others continue to take place at an ever-accelerating pace.

Historical perspectives and current issues

The past 100 years may well be characterized as the period in history when large segments of the industrialized world made dramatic improvements in public health measures; increased the life span of all segments of the population; reduced or virtually eliminated such earlier killers as tuberculosis, diphtheria, scarlet fever, and typhoid; and substantially reduced infant mortality. Dramatic and welcome as these changes are, the expectations for general good health, a comfortable old age, and cure of the major killers have not been achieved. Although the battle against a whole group of diseases has essentially been won, methods for curing many prevailing problems have not yet been found. Modern medicine currently has the capacity to sustain or prolong life for many people without effecting total recovery. Large numbers of people now survive with varying degrees and types of disabilities. Many of these individuals require extensive medical, social, environmental, and other support to lead reasonably comfortable lives.

The long-standing struggle to understand and treat chronic, long-term mental illness has not been successful to date (Linn and Stein, 1981). Many people are directly or indirectly affected by a variety of developmental disabilities (Andrews and Wikler, 1981). The dream of cure is elusive for those who are left partially disabled following a stroke. They lose some ability to walk or care for all of their personal needs. The problems of the isolated, frail elderly, many of whom are women alone (Libow, Schecter, and Margolis, 1981), are increasingly capturing national attention.

A clear perspective of the problems presently facing social workers requires some understanding of the past and its influence on the current state of affairs. Therefore an overview of the factors that have contributed to the problems and challenges before us will prove useful in suggesting directions and thrusts for social work in health care. Emphasis is placed on those elements of social life, public health, and social work that illustrate the intricate relationships between quality of life, socioeconomic status, and community action designed to enhance health status.

Most people recall lessons learned in history classes about the crowding, high disease rates, and epidemics that took the lives of masses of people during the eighteenth and nineteenth centuries. Current problems are brought into perspective by referring to some of the statistics available from that time.

Massachusetts offers an interesting example. In 1850 the tuberculosis death rate was 300 per 100,000; the infant mortality was approximately 200 per 1,000 live births; and smallpox, scarlet fever, and typhoid were the leading causes of death (Hanlon and Pickett, 1984). Some people associated these high death rates with the "barbarism of life in the United States" (Hanlon and Pickett, 1984, p. 30), unkempt appearance of cities, and delayed development in sanitation improvements. Efforts to reduce "gross" unsanitary measures began in Massachusetts and Virginia during the late seventeenth century. However, "Protection against the dirt and filth of human aggregation which threatened the life of every man, woman, and child, had to wait upon the adequate enforcement of law and order" (Newsholme, 1925).

Other analysts also recognized the negative impact of unsanitary and crowded living conditions. Excerpts from a communication by John H. Griscom, New York City Health Officer in 1845, are well worth citing at some length. He conveys a sense of the conditions of life that prevailed in cities of that time and the degree to which those conditions were implicated in disease and death rates.

> There is an amount of sickness and death in this, as in all large cities, far beyond those of less densely peopled, more airy and open places, such as country residences. . . . The congregation of animal and vegetable matters, with their constant effluvia, which has less chance of escape from the premises, in proportion to the absence of free circulation of air, is detrimental to the health of the inhabitants.
>
> These circumstances have never yet been investigated in this city, as they should be. Our people, especially the most destitute have been allowed to live out their brief lives in tainted and unwholesome atmospheres and be subject to the silent and invisible encroachments of destructive agencies from every direction. . . . Fathers are taken from their children, husbands from their wives, 'ere they have lived out half their days,' the widows and orphans are thrown upon public or private charity for support, and the money which is expended to save them from starvation, to educate them in the public schools, or perchance, to maintain them in the work-house or the prison, if judiciously spent in improving the sanitary arrangements of the city, and instilling into the population knowledge of the means by which their health might be protected, and their lives prolonged and made happy, would have been not only saved, but returned to the treasury in the increased health of the population, a much better state of public morals, and by consequence, a more easily governed and respectably community. . . .

> Sanitary regulations affect the pauper class of the population more directly than any other (. . .) They are more crowded, they live more in cellars, their apartments are less ventilated and more exposed to vapours and other emanations, &c., hence ventilation, sewerage, and all other sanitary regulations, are more necessary for them, and would produce greater comparative change in their condition . . . (cited in Pumphrey and Pumphrey, 1961, pp. 96-98).

Griscom eloquently noted the relationship between poor housing and disease.

Social work's role in public health history

Bracht (1978) reviewed social work's contribution to early public health efforts. Edward Devine established a committee for the prevention of tuberculosis. This committee carried out research on the social and medical aspects of tuberculosis and contributed to the creation of sanitoriums for the care of indigents with tuberculosis. The Charity Organization Society, one of the forerunners of contemporary social work, developed programs to combat infant mortality, rickets, and scurvy. The Association for Improving the Conditions of the Poor, together with the New York City Health Department, established a center for maternal and child health in one of the settlement houses. Bracht cites the following comments by Dr. Rosen, a physician and public health historian, suggesting the early alliance between medicine and social work for improving public health.

> . . . The history of social medicine is also the history of social policy. . . . The roots of social medicine are to be found in organized social work. It was here that medicine and social science found a common ground for action in the prevention of tuberculosis, securing better housing and work conditions (cited in Bracht, 1978, p. 9).

Others also noted the relationship between health, illness, the conditions of life, and social work's role in ameliorating negative social conditions. In discussing the social components of medicine, Dr. Richard Cabot, the physician whose name is associated with starting the first hospital social work department, commented:

> A man is not flat like a card. We cannot get the whole of him spread out upon our retina at once. The bit of him which is recorded in the history of his aches, his jumps, and his weaknesses is built into the rest of his life and character like a stone in an arch. To change any part of him appreciably we must change the whole. The average practitioner is used to seeing his patients flash by him like shooting stars—out of darkness into darkness. He has been trained to focus upon a single, suspected organ till he thinks of his patients almost like disembodied diseases.
>
> 'What is there in the waiting room?'. . . 'There's a couple of good hearts, a big liver with jaundice, a floating kidney. . . .'
>
> Among such flying fragments as these the physician has to pass his days. He couldn't earn a living if he did not attend first and chiefly to the part that is thrust before him.

> He cannot be looking off into space for causes and results. . . .
>
> Disease is not often hard luck, nor 'too bad.' For the most part it is as bad as we—the tax payers—allow it to be and as we . . . recognize it to be. *Preventable disease* stares us in the face. Yet still the rank and file of the medical profession are too busy with cases—to have time for causes. It is only when the social workers stir us into action that the Anti-Tuberculosis Crusade, the Clean Milk Crusade, the Pure Food Law, the Playground Association, and the School Hygiene agitation come into being (Cabot, 1915, pp. 32-37).

The development of medical technology

It is important to note these comments were made well before medical care became established in its present form. According to Flexner's report (1910) American medical education and practice were in disarray, not organized well enough to use the scientific advances being made in Europe. While this report had far-reaching consequences for American health care, the far-flung changes in the technology of health care so much a part of contemporary life were not to be introduced for some years. Specialization in medicine had not yet developed to the extent prevailing now (Palmiere, 1981). Sulfur drugs were first recognized as chemotherapeutic agents in 1937. Penicillin, the first antibiotic, was introduced in 1942 (Goodman and Gilman, 1958). There were not enough dialysis machines available to all those who could benefit from their use until 1972 (Somers and Somers, 1977). Pharmacological means of contraception ("the pill") were not introduced until the 1960s.

Many of the major health problems confronting American society today have a dimension and character that greatly differ from the problems that faced Americans in the nineteenth and early twentieth centuries. Many of these problems are a consequence of progress in medical technology. Nevertheless, as shall become evident from the following discussion, poverty and other inequities continue to take their toll in poor health. What then are the dimensions and scope of the health problems before us?

PREVAILING HEALTH DATA

Synthesizing and organizing the vast amount of information available so that it is useful to health care social workers are complex processes. Like most health care professionals, social workers want and need to know something about those health problems leading to death and whether there are differences by socioeconomic status or ethnic group membership. Social workers also need information about the numbers of people affected by various health problems and how these problems are distributed. In addition, much social work practice focuses on individuals and small groups and how these individuals cope with health problems.

Social workers also need knowledge about how health problems are counted and defined. Knowing how information is typically gathered helps to assess the validity of that information. Acquiring this knowledge is not an easy task. Many analysts have commented on the problems inherent in efforts to answer the question, "What are the health problems before us?" The answers given depend on the various approaches to definitions of disease, illness, and health. The answers also depend on whether the facts presented have been gathered by asking health care providers such as physicians and hospitals about the numbers of people with various kinds of problems who come to them in any given time period, or by asking randomly selected people, both those who do and do not use health services, about how they deal with the various health problems they experience. In assessing information obtained by asking health care providers about the people who come to them, it is important to be aware that not all people with similar problems turn to the health care system. Some manage their problems alone. Others turn to what most people term "nontraditional healers." These issues are sufficiently complex to warrant detailed examination in Chapters 3 and 4.

Notwithstanding these concerns about gathering data, for the present purpose, which is to present an image of the health problems that confront us, it is possible to present information on the major causes of death and on the major discomforts experienced in American society today. The sources drawn on in presenting this information are varied. The bulk of this information is from the massive amount of data made available by the U.S. government.

It is common practice to review prevailing problems in health by beginning with an examination of data on mortality; that is, to review information on the number of deaths occurring in any given period for designated age groups and to ascertain the cause of those deaths. Such data indicate the ultimate failure of the social system in its goal of preserving life. Morbidity statistics are also reviewed to reflect the daily health problems encountered by large segments of the population.

Mortality

Analysis of data providing insight into the causes of death points out that heart disease is the leading cause of death in the United States, followed by cancer and stroke (Pear, 1984).

These as well as other problems to be discussed have replaced the killers of an earlier day. In examining and assessing the available data several factors must be kept in mind.

Although mortality for heart disease, stroke, and cancer is high and represents some of the most challenging health problems, there have been persistent decreases between 1950 and the present. Diverse data can be pieced together to document the overall decline and persistent differences between whites, Blacks, men, and women. Between 1950 and 1982 mortality related to heart disease declined from 307.6 to 190.8 per 100,000. Furthermore, there has been a 25% decrease since 1970 in deaths attributed to heart disease (Pear, 1984; Boffey, 1984).

A more detailed analysis by race and sex shows the following: (1) the age-adjusted death rate for white men declined from 381.1 per 100,000 in 1950 to 288.7 per 100,000 in 1978; (2) comparable figures for white women are 223.6 and 136.4 per 100,000, respectively; (3) rates for Black men declined from 415.5 per 100,000 in 1950 to 321.0 per 100,000 in 1978; and (4) comparable figures for Black women are 349.5 and 201.1 per 100,000, respectively (*Health, United States,* 1981).

Declines in deaths related to stroke and other cerebrovascular diseases are also apparent and dramatic. Between 1970 and 1982 deaths attributed to these health problems declined from 66 to 36 per 100,000. Looking separately at the data for whites and Blacks is instructive. Between 1960 and 1978 the rate for white men declined from 80.3 to 46.8 per 100,000. Comparable figures for white women are 68.7 and 39.3 per 100,000, respectively. Black men and women have considerably higher rates, although decline is apparent. Between 1960 and 1978 the rate for Black men declined from 141.2 to 83.8 per 100,000. Comparable figures for Black women are 139.5 and 68.7 per 100,000 (*Health, United States,* 1981). Clearly, Black men are at greatest risk, followed by Black women. The difference in mortality between Blacks and whites can in part be attributed to the fact that about twice as many Black adults have hypertension as do white adults.

Both whites and Blacks have shown an increased incidence of cancers of the respiratory system. The rate for whites rose from approximately 13 per 100,000 to 35 per 100,000 and from approximately 11 per 100,000 to 45 per 100,000 for Blacks. Explanations for these differentials are only speculative. It has been suggested that Blacks have different smoking patterns and greater exposure to hazardous work environments than whites.

Black/white differences also exist in other health problem areas. While the white suicide rate has increased slightly (from approximately 12 per 100,000 to approximately 13 per 100,000) the Black rate has increased significantly from somewhat over 4 in 1950 to 7.5 in 1977.

These death rates have multiple causes, few of which are clearly understood yet. Sophisticated speculation suggests that the one of the main reasons is the inevitable deterioration of aging; other reasons are life-style factors within individual control such as smoking, dietary habits, and exercise. Blacks and whites both show a declining although different mortality. Gains in living and status levels made by some Blacks are a consequence of the social gain made by the liberation movements occurring between 1960 and 1980. Nevertheless, much can be done to diminish status- and poverty-related differentials.

The discerning reader will have noted that the differences in mortality by ethnicity reported to this point have focused on distinctions between Blacks and whites. The reasons for this relate to the standard manner in which such data have been collected.

Nevertheless, some materials are available that reflect important health problems among other select groups, such as American Indians. American Indians are considered to be among the most disadvantaged groups living in the United States today. However, major efforts to reduce health problems have had a positive effect on mortality. Between 1950 and 1970 the life expectancy of this group rose from 60 to 65 years. This rate is still lower than that for whites. American Indian infant mortality has declined to the point where it is equal to or better than the overall rate for the United States. Death rates for other diseases, for example, tuberculosis, influenza, and early infancy diseases such as gastroenteritis (*Health, United States,* 1979) that were once the great scourge of American Indians and Alaskan natives, have shown remarkable declines since the 1950s. These dramatic improvements are associated with extensive efforts to make health services available through the Indian Health Service. There were also increased efforts to improve the level of sanitation, water supply, and sewage disposal in those areas largely inhabited by American Indians.

Infant mortality. Infant mortality is frequently considered an indication of the degree of commitment a nation has to the health level of its people. According to Anderson (1958) the rate of infant deaths is "a sensitive index of the health level of an area, and one readily responsive to environmental conditions" (p. 11).

The decline in infant mortality has indeed been substantial. Earlier it was noted that in 1850 infant mortality in Massachusetts ran as high as 200 per 1,000 live births. By 1982 the overall American rate was reduced to 11.2 deaths per 1,000 live births. However, mortality for Black infants was twice as high as that for white newborns (Pear, 1984). Other differences by ethnic group membership are of interest. Among American Indians the 1980 rate was 15.6 per 1,000, while the rates for Chinese and Japanese Americans were 5.9 and 6.6, respectively (*Health of the Disadvantaged,* 1980). There are also regional variations. The lowest rates for both whites and Blacks are reported in the Pacific area.

What accounts for the decline and the present differences? To what extent are the conditions of social life and the nature of available health care implicated? The assertion made by Anderson (1958) that "class, occupation and income are very closely related and in turn are associated with given infant mortality rates" (p. 16) still holds true. His data on infant mortality among the ruling families of Europe between 1500 and 1930 provide some vivid documentation of how the level of living affects the capacity of families to nurture and sustain their newborn infants.

By 1930 the infant death rates during the first year of life of infants born to ruling families were only 8 per 1,000. These rates are better than those currently prevailing for the total American population. They also compare favorably with the rates available for a number of countries having consistently lower infant mortality than the United States. For example, in 1979 Sweden, the Netherlands, Switzerland, and Japan had rates between 8 and 10.7 deaths per 1,000 live births (*Health, United States,* 1979). Currently, only Chinese and

Japanese Americans have rates lower than the rate for the whole country.

Although much has happened since Anderson (1958) attempted to ". . . indicate the general social factors which have been associated with the changing infant mortality picture . . ." (p. 11), many aspects of his analysis still help to clarify the connection. He identifies three sets of factors that must be taken into account. First are biological factors that are independent of time and place and those that are responsive to environmental influences. Among the former are certain genetic factors and predispositions to disease. Second are social factors related to income, class, housing, and rural or urban residence. Third are cultural factors that reflect prevailing values, religious beliefs, attitudes toward human life, and hygienic habits.

In reviewing a number of studies done in various areas of the world, a number of factors emerge. From 1890 to 1900 most European countries, as well as the United States, experienced a decline apparently related to hygiene and sanitation improvements. As of 1958 the decline of prematurity and congenital malformations (which usually take their toll in infants aged 1 to 12 months) was associated with hygiene and medical advances. Recent developments have served to save the lives of many critically ill newborns (Watkins and Player, 1981). Neonatal intensive care centers located throughout the country receive children with severe difficulty born in hospitals nearby. All that contemporary medical technology has to offer is brought to bear in the efforts to save these children. These centers are thought to have contributed to the reduced neonatal mortality noted previously.

In assessing the role of culture, Anderson (1958) notes that between 1911 and 1916, the Jewish infant mortality in eight American cities was, in some instances, almost half that of other groups, including native- and foreign-born whites and Blacks. These differences cannot be explained on economic grounds. Jews in that period lived in conditions as crowded as those of other immigrants, had as many children, and had incomes lower than native-born whites. Anderson suggests "a closer examination would probably reveal a pattern of infant care of a high order embedded in the Jewish culture . . ." (p. 23). Jewish people pay particular attention to matters of health and survival, as noted by analysts of Jewish life (for example, Howe, 1975). This characteristic has been related to a lengthy history of dispersion and persecution when tactics for survival become paramount.

A number of factors may explain the patterns of infant mortality. These factors include conditions surrounding childbirth, geographical availability of medical resources, differences in the ages of women giving birth, and the use of prenatal care. Children living in urban centers are more likely to have been born in hospitals having blood banks and special nurseries for premature babies. The relationship between the use of early prenatal care and the birth of healthy infants is well established. But women whose infants are at greatest risk of dying (adolescents, older women, and Black women) are least likely to get early prenatal care. The association between low birth weight and subsequent difficulty is also well established. In 1976 the number of low birth weight infants born to adolescent Black mothers was double that of the rest of the nation.

Despite marked improvements in infant mortality the discrepancies between Blacks and other groups, as well as regional variations, are cause for great concern. These discrepancies reflect what many term a two-class system of health care; they also reflect the effect of poor nutrition and the low esteem in which those at low socioeconomic levels are held.

The importance of medical care. In commenting on these data one observation is particularly important. In the introductory comments I pointed out that the relationship between the availability of health services and health levels is often challenged. There is indeed a clear relationship between infant mortality and living conditions. However, health services also play a crucial part. Prenatal care and prompt attention for low birth weight infants and infants with a variety of handicaps markedly affect infant mortality.

Life related to pregnancy and early child rearing. The human aspirations and turmoil reflected by the data just presented are often neglected in official documents and other writing on health problems. Yet, the importance of this kind of information for social workers lies in the fact that "hard statistics" are just one way of reflecting pain, suffering, and need. Therefore I consider these matters to help social workers gain a better picture of what these data reflect.

History has shown that improvements in the level of living have led to dramatic decreases in infant deaths. Yet it is important to consider the lives of those children and their families still experiencing the agonies of infant death. Young adolescents and members of minority groups sustain the majority of infant deaths (McCormick, Shapiro, and Starfield, 1984). Although the poverty they experience pales by comparison with that of 100 years ago, many are still, by current standards, poorly clothed, housed, fed, and educated. Racism and discrimination are very much with us. So many of the young mothers whose infants die are considered "lesser" persons by the society. Avenues for a positive identity and a sense of self-worth are still not available to many. Medical center personnel, physicians, and social workers often approach people from the perspective of their own experiences and views of life and fail to recognize the extensive fear, insecurity, and lack of resources experienced by many in these groups. Admonitions to see a physician or breast-feed the baby may not take these factors into account. Many women whose infants die are among the most disadvantaged. Neonatal intensive care units are often located at a considerable distance away from home and family. Only now are approaches beginning to evolve by which the parents of such infants may be helped to spend time with them in the hospital. Methods are being developed to help prepare them for the child's arrival at home by educating and rehearsing what to do in case of crisis. Clearly, efforts to save infants must focus on the social and psychological factors that deter people from making use of the facilities available.

Much remains to be done to ensure that mothers of childbearing age and their infants have access to basic health care, economic means above subsistence levels, and supportive services designed to enhance infant care, customs, and practices. In 1958 Anderson suggested that attention be devoted to enhancing the skills of "mothercraft." At this point in history, a more appropriate view is one suggesting the need for help with the complex task of "parenting." This task involves attention to parenting skills, and the economic conditions of life that permit such skills to be used.

Life expectancy. Changes paralleling those in infant mortality can be noted in those related to life expectancy. An American male born in 1900 could expect to live 46 years and a woman 48 years. Life expectancy for all nonwhites was even lower—32.5 years for men and 33.5 for women. By 1982 life expectancy for whites rose to 74.5 years and to 69.3 years for Blacks (Pear, 1984).

The table below, adapted from the 1979 edition of *Health, United States,* illustrates both the dramatic increase in life expectancy between 1900 and 1950 and the persistent but gradual increase between 1950 and the late 1970s. This table also illustrates a number of other factors that hold true for a diverse set of health data. One factor is the different life expectancies of men and women, with women's consistently being higher than men's. The other factor is the persistent disadvantage of most nonwhites or minority group members. Unfortunately, these data obscure class differences.

Violence. The third annual report on the health status of the nation (*Health, United States,* 1978) singles out violence as one of the health problems that are the "consequences of human action and therefore, mostly preventable" (p. 38). The report points out that violence-related death rates were higher in the 1970s than in the preceding two decades. Also stressed is the fact

Life expectancy at birth according to color and sex: United States, selected years 1900-1977*

Specified age and year	Total			White			All other		
	Both sexes	Male	Female	Both sexes	Male	Female	Both sexes	Male	Female
1900	47.3	46.3	48.3	47.6	46.6	48.7	33.0	32.5	33.5
1950	68.2	65.6	71.1	69.1	66.5	72.2	60.8	59.1	62.9
1960	69.7	66.6	73.1	70.6	67.4	74.1	63.6	61.1	66.3
1970	70.9	67.1	74.8	71.7	68.0	75.6	65.3	61.3	69.4
1975	72.5	68.7	76.5	73.2	69.4	77.2	67.9	63.6	72.3
1976	72.8	69.0	76.7	73.5	69.7	77.3	68.3	64.1	72.6
1977	73.2	69.3	77.1	73.8	70.0	77.7	68.8	64.6	73.1

*Modified from Health, United States, 1979, DHEW Publication No. (PHS), 80-1231, Washington, D.C., 1979, U.S. Government Printing Office.

that deaths from violent and accidental causes were higher in the 1930s—a period of economic depression.

Black/white and male/female differences are startling. In 1978 the age-adjusted death rates for homicide per 100,000 population were (1) 9.2 for white men; (2) 2.9 for white women; (3) 65.6 for Black men; and (4) 13.5 for Black women. For all groups, the highest rates are found between the ages of 15 and 44 (*Health, United States,* 1981), an age group that many consider to be the prime of life.

Subsequent studies have investigated socioeconomic conditions as possible contributors to violence-associated mortality. Clues to the prevention of homicide are more likely found in the life circumstances of both victim and murderer rather than in their personal characteristics. The report states:

> Finally, since untimely death for almost all causes and unnecessary disease and disability are higher for the poor and less educated, the overriding factor in their prevention appears to remain in improvement of socioeconomic conditions (*Health, United States,* 1978, p. 41).

Mortality from other causes. There are deaths associated with other diseases. Pneumonia still takes substantial numbers of lives (23 per 100,000 in 1978), as does diabetes, cirrhosis of the liver, and influenza. Each of these is related to living conditions. Low socioeconomic status has a negative effect in all areas.

Impact of mortality data on life. The interest in mortality data reflects concern with deaths that could be prevented or forestalled. Longevity, so clearly on the increase, presents previously unavailable opportunities to experience life in all its dimensions—as child, maturing adult, and senior citizen. Each of these periods has potential for growth, creativity, and widening the scope of the human experience. When the lives of some infants are cut short because the collective "we" does not provide the means to sustain them, the human experience is diminished. Differences in longevity between the sexes and between various groups in the society reflect a complex set of biological and social factors. Nevertheless, as is the case with infant mortality, higher death rates for minorities point to the way in which society views a significant segment of the population. These rates reflect a sense of alienation and a tendency to assign low value to large numbers of people.

Whether focusing on heart disease, cancer, stroke, or violence as the cause of death, some of the data on mortality reflect urban living problems. Some people may question the desirability of living longer as most people do now, as a result of the major diseases of the present as contrasted with those that took so many lives in an earlier day. Most people, I think, prefer the present. Yet, that present is far from ideal. Therefore efforts to reduce mortality need to continue, particularly action to minimize current discrimination against the disadvantaged.

Morbidity

A text on community health defines morbidity as "sickness or the presence of disease" (Smith, 1979, p. 313) and points out that morbidity measures the frequency of illness or disease in a population. A number of analysts (for example, Mechanic, 1978) point out that there can be marked disparities between the way physicians and people affected by varying discomforts view these problems. Physicians think in terms of disease. The general populace tends more to think, feel, and act in terms of symptoms causing discomfort and interfering with daily life.

The increase in the extent of chronic illness has intensified the need to describe experience with illness in terms of its impact on social activity. In keeping with the practice of the National Center for Health Statistics, data are first presented on how people view their health, followed by information on the degree of disruption related to illness or disease reported by various segments of the population. As this information is presented, an effort is made to move beyond the statistics to convey a sense of their meaning in the daily lives of those affected.

Self-assessment of health status. Based on data obtained from the annual Health Interview Survey carried out by the U.S. government, most people report they feel "pretty good." In 1979, 87% of the population (not counting those institutionalized or in the hospital) reported being in good or excellent health.

Age differences are of course pronounced. As age increases, the percent reporting fair and poor health increases. However, less than 9% of people over 65 not institutionalized or hospitalized at the time of the survey reported their health as poor.

Differences by race are readily apparent. Only 36% of Blacks compared to 51% of whites or members of other races consider their health to be excellent. Twice as many Blacks as whites perceive themselves to be in fair or poor health. People who are still victims of discrimination in many spheres of life feel the effects of that discrimination extend to the area of health and illness.

Similar trends are noted when this information is viewed in terms of income. The percent of people reporting their health as excellent doubles as income rises and the reverse is true of those reporting poor health. The relationship provides strong support for the points made earlier. Income, discrimination (or its absence), and the associated ability (or lack thereof) to command resources and respect are related to an individual's assessment of his or her health.

Gender and a subjective sense of well-being are also related. There is a small but persistent difference between women and men, with women tending not to report their health to be as good as do men.

These differences have been the subject of substantial speculation and will be explored at greater length in Chapters 3 and 4 when the components of health and illness behavior are analyzed. For the time being, how can the fact that an overwhelming number of people in all age groups report their health to be excellent or good be interpreted? What, if any, particular use does this information have for health care social workers?

In subsequent sections of this chapter it will become apparent that a large number of people have one or more chronic health problems. This number is quite a bit higher than the number reporting their health to be poor or fair. This disparity indicates how people like to perceive themselves, or at least how they present themselves to government representatives asking how they perceive their health. It also suggests that many people have a reserve of coping strength and capacity. Health workers should not forget this fact as they work to develop programs to identify people having treatable problems. This society values healthiness, strength, and the ability to cope with life's problems. It is essential that these facts be kept in mind when helping people face the inevitable dependency that accompanies some illnesses and the aging process, and when putting forth efforts focused on health and directed in a fashion minimizing the negative effects of being called sick or old.

Activity limitations. Another question raised by the Health Interview Survey data is the degree to which people are limited from carrying on their usual activity because of health problems. In 1977, 7% of the population reported some restriction in activity. As is the case with other morbidity indicators, these data vary by age, gender, ethnicity, and income. The table on p. 20 highlights these variations.

An interesting picture emerges when activity limitations are viewed in relation to income and ethnic group membership. More whites and Blacks than Hispanics experienced limitations in their major activities—7.1% of whites, 7.4% of Blacks, and 4.5% of Hispanics (*Health of the Disadvantaged,* 1980, p. 51). These differences are more impressive when examined according to ethnic group membership and income combined. Income exerted the greatest effect on whether or not people reported activity limitations. In the highest income group only 3.5% to 4.0% of any groups for which information is available reported such limitations; by contrast, 8% of Hispanics, 12.5% of Blacks, and close to 16% of whites at the lowest income level were affected in this manner. The steady decline of the number reporting limitations associated with a rising income level suggests the important effect of income on well-being.

Viewed together, the data suggest that 88% of all people perceive their health to be good or better. Twice as many people over 65 as individuals between 45 and 64 thought their health was fair. Those having lower incomes were more likely to report they were prevented from carrying on their major activity because of chronic limitations; 20% of people over 65 reported such limitations.

Earlier the point was made that 87% of the population claiming good health calls attention to the coping strength and capacity of a large number of people. Lest I conveyed that most people are healthy, I must point out the (1) 12% who reported their health to be fair or poor and (2) 20% who, because of chronic limitations, were not able to carry on some portion of their major activity. There are over 14 million people who do not feel well, and approximately 4 million people who find themselves unable to do all they need or want to do.

Also important is the fact that these data reflect information obtained from a sample of persons not in institutions at the time the studies were carried out. Therefore the data do not reflect information about hospitalized individuals or the 5% of the population over 65 in nursing homes. There are a substantial number of people requiring extensive medical care, as well as a variety of

Limitations in quantity or type of major activity: United States, average annual statistics for 1976-1977 by income and ethnicity*

Annual income and ethnicity	Percent distribution of population with limitation
All incomes	7.0
White	7.1
Black	7.4
Hispanic	4.5
Less than $5000	14.4
White	15.8
Black	12.5
Hispanic	8.3
$5000–9000	8.5
White	9.5
Black	6.5
Hispanic	4.4
$10,000–$14,999	5.9
White	6.1
Black	5.3
Hispanic	3.3
$15,000–$24,999	4.2
White	4.3
Black	4.0
Hispanic	2.2
$25,000 or more	4.1
White	4.2
Black	3.1
Hispanic	3.5

*Modified from Health of the Disadvantaged: Chart Book II, DHHS Publication No. (HRA), 80-633, Washington, D.C., 1980, U.S. Government Printing Office.

social and psychological supports from their families, friends, neighbors, and formal caretaking institutions. These supports include counseling and home health care, Meals on Wheels, and extensive daytime care in day care centers for the elderly or physically handicapped. In short, there are many people afflicted with a variety of extensive health problems. Many of these problems fall under the category of chronic illness.

CHRONIC HEALTH PROBLEMS

In the effort to present an image of current health problems, attention is now focused on the extent and variety of chronic health problems that affect large portions of the American population. There are a number of ways to define and think about chronic illness or chronic conditions. Mayo defined chronic disease as follows:

> All impairments or deviations from normal which have one or more of the following characteristics: are permanent, leave residual disability, are caused by non-reversible pathological alteration, require special training of the patient for rehabilitation, may be expected to require a long period of supervision, observation, or care (cited in Strauss, 1975, p. 1).

The attributes of chronic health problems described by Mayo are those of interest and concern in this book. Their permanence and the fact that they result in some measure of disability requiring long-term attention are conditions of life likely to cause discomfort or fear about possible long-range negative consequences. Such disease affects the way people view themselves, the way others view them, and the way they carry on their lives. Both the individual and society are affected in terms of cost and productivity.

What are these problems? The National Center for Health Services Research (*Health, United States,* 1980) identifies the following:

tuberculosis
benign and malignant neoplasms
diseases of the thyroid gland
diabetes
gout
psychoses and other mental disorders
multiple sclerosis and other diseases of the central nervous system
diseases and conditions of the eye
diseases of the circulatory system, including rheumatic fever, hypertension, stroke, and all heart conditions
emphysema, asthma, hay fever, and bronchiectasis
ulcers and other diseases of the esophagus, stomach, and duodenum
hernia
gastroenteritis and colitis
calculus of the kidney, ureter, and other parts of the urinary system
diseases of the prostate
chronic cystic diseases of the breast
eczema and other forms of dermatitis
cyst of the bone
all congenital anomalies

Alcoholism and accidental injuries also must be added to the list. This list calls the reader's attention to the wide variety of health problems causing the disruption, discomfort, and need for care noted previously.

Not all of these problems can be considered in this book. Discussion is focused on those which, in the view of many analysts, strike many people, are included in every list of major health problems facing western society, and are most likely to be encountered by social workers as they work in hospitals, primary care centers, community facilities, and health planning endeavors.

Before reviewing the nature and impact of the chronic health problems selected for discussion, the scope of chronic disease must be considered. One indication comes from a 1971 analysis made by the National Center for Health Research (Chronic Conditions and Limitations of Activity). That year it was estimated that 94 million Americans, or close to half the population, had one or more chronic diseases. These diseases range from those causing minimal dysfunction (such as mild hayfever without related complications) to those causing total disability (such as quadriplegia following an accident).

This book emphasizes data on selected chronic conditions, people they affect, populations most at risk, their impact on the quality of life, and need for care produced by these conditions. Subsequent chapters (Chapter 5 in particular) consider how epidemiological and public health perspectives can contribute to analysis of and preventive endeavors for chronic health problems.

Hypertension

Hypertension is a major chronic health problem. Essential hypertension (or high blood pressure) is sometimes referred to as the "silent killer." In its early stages it produces no symptoms; therefore detection depends on regular screening. Approximately 60 million Americans have elevated blood pressures. Of these 60 million, 35 million (about 15% of the population) have essential hypertension. Black Americans are more susceptible to hypertension than white Americans; 28% of Black Americans have high blood pressure. Considerable literature exists suggesting that the psychological reality associated with skin color in American society is a probable cause of excess hypertension in Blacks. This suggestion is supported by studies showing no meaningful differences between high blood pressure in Blacks and whites before adulthood. Varying stress states have been suggested as implicated in causing hypertension (for example, Eyer, 1975).

Hypertension is one of the major causes of stroke, heart failure, and kidney failure. Finnerty and Linde (1975) suggest it is a disease that has reached epidemic proportions and perhaps is the leading cause of disability and death in the United States. Approximately 60,000 deaths a year are directly attributed to the disease. However, much high blood pressure can be controlled, primarily by antihypertensive medication. Data from 1960 to 1970 show that the 44% reduction in hypertension-related deaths can most likely be attributed to drug treatment (Caldwell and others, 1970). Other important methods of control are reduced salt intake, other dietary measures, and stopping smoking.

The consequences of hypertension may be critical, but can often be avoided with adequate control. Unfortunately many people are unaware of the disease's possible severity, its control measures, and that they have high blood pressure. In fact, only 50% of those people estimated to have hypertension are aware of it. Also, a substantial number of people who begin treatment drop out. Noncompliance may be related to the problem of patients not understanding the long-term nature of the disease because health care providers fail to communicate effectively its implications. Diverse studies have failed to discover any identifiable patterns related to noncompliance (for example, Finnerty, Matte, and Finnerty, 1973; Ward, 1978).

Efforts to increase screening programs are essential, especially for high risk populations. These populations are all Blacks, men between the ages of 30 and 55, women taking oral contraceptives, and all overweight people. Individuals isolated from the mainstream health care system and those in low income groups also should be targeted for screening (New Jersey State Department of Health, 1980). Social work's involvement with this disease has been too limited. Noncompliance has psychological and social ramifications as well as medical ones. Clearly, the prevalence and risks of hypertension—and the reported Black/white differentials—should alert social workers to the need for preventive activity.

Diabetes

Diabetes mellitus includes a variety of anatomic and biochemical abnormalities sharing a disturbance in the body's ability to metabolize glucose (Cahill, 1975). Like hypertension, diabetes is a life-long condition. Also like hypertension, it is often associated with long-term complications, particularly coronary heart disease, peripheral vascular disease, and diseases of the eyes and kidneys (*Health, United States,* 1981).

The report of the National Commission on Diabetes (1975) estimated that there were 10 million diabetics in the United States, 5 million of them undiagnosed. In 1979, 5.2 million civilian, noninstitutionalized people were known to have diabetes. Diabetic nursing home residents numbered 189,000. The high frequency of association between minority status, low income, and diabetes prevalence affects how help is rendered and the way in which education about the disease is presented.

Essential components of diabetes management include proper diet, exercise, and, for some, insulin administration or oral medication. No known cure exists and "many of the acute and long-term complications of diabetes may be checked in varying degrees by appropriate treatment" (*Health, United States,* 1981, p. 27).

High-risk candidates are women, Blacks, the less educated, and low-income families. Middle-aged Black women have the highest known rate of diabetes. The number of diabetics has increased substantially in the last 20 years. This increase may be related to better methods of detection and to the fact that diabetics now live longer than they have in the past. Diabetes clearly has implications for life-style and self-perception and entails many psychosocial risks.

Psychosocial effect of hypertension and diabetes

Individuals with hypertension or relatively uncomplicated diabetes must be ever-mindful of their diets and extremely careful that they follow the recommended regimen of medication and exercise. The fact that these diseases put them at greater risk for heart disease, stroke, and kidney disease has psychic costs. This increased risk forces these people to take all the precautions a person must take when sick, yet many are symptom free and able, in most respects, to do all they need or would like to do with regard to work, sexual activity, and social relationships.

• • •

The difficulties involved in helping people adhere to a hypertensive and/or diabetic regimen suggest that the tensions evoked by "being sick" while "feeling well" may explain some of the noncompliance. These people may be in the group of those who say their health is excellent or good. Strategies to help people retain positive self-identification as healthy people without incurring the major risks associated with denial of these diseases have yet to be clearly understood and developed.

Cancer

Cancer is a term commonly used for a series of diseases. The causes are thought to be multiple, involving both environmental and genetic factors. Data available for the 1970s suggest its occurrence disrupts the physical and psychological well-being of 25% of all Americans and two out of three families. Stonberg (1981) cites the following quotation from *Cancer Facts and Figures* (1981):

> It kills more children aged 3 to 14 than any other disease, and [it] strikes more frequently with advancing age. . . . In the 1970s, there were an estimated 3.5 million cancer deaths, over 6.5 million new cancer cases, and more than 10 million people under care for cancer (p. 695).

Cancer is a dreaded disease. It involves treatable and reversible conditions as well as those leading to rapid death or periods of extensive discomfort and wasting. People afflicted with cancer may undergo surgery, radiation, or chemotherapy for treatment. The latter can cause hair loss and extensive nausea, as well as other negative side effects. Many affected people feel physically and emotionally debilitated after treatment.

Breast cancer, the leading cause of cancer-related death in women, is inevitably a traumatic experience involving physical and psychological loss that strikes at the core of a woman's sense of self.

The trauma for cancer victims, their families, and the community has been well documented (for example, Stonberg, 1981). Social work's involvement with those who have cancer is extensive and has led to the development of groups of social workers who regularly communicate with each other about particular practice issues confronting them in this area of practice (Stonberg, 1981).

End-stage renal disease

As of 1980 there were 45,565 people receiving dialysis treatments, and 4,697 people had received kidney transplants (Frazier, 1981). People of all ages are affected by the disease.

End-stage renal disease (kidney disease) occurs when the kidneys reduce functioning and fail to remove waste products and maintain fluid homeostasis in the body. Uremia—secondary to kidney failure is a condition in which the kidneys are not capable of removing the end products of metabolism. Reduction of renal functioning to less than 10% of the normal level is fatal unless aided by dialysis or kidney transplant. Dialysis uses a kidney machine to remove wastes and toxins the kidney can no longer remove. Two or three treatments a week, encompassing many hours usually are required. Dialysis commonly involves severe dietary restrictions and side effects. Patients on dialysis are in effect dependent on the machine for survival.

Extensive literature suggests that for many dialysis patients and their families, life revolves around treatment and diet, which generate a variety of psychological and physical discomforts. Fear of death is ever present. Social work's involvement with dialysis patients is extensive because federal legislation involving the funding and organization of this expensive mode of care mandates social work participation (Federal Register, 1976).

Heart disease

The term *heart disease* covers a wide variety of disorders. In 1977, 170,000 people between the ages of 25 and 64 died from heart disease (*Health, United States,* 1980). Approximately 1,300,000 people suffer a heart attack each year. About 4 million people have a history of heart attack and/or angina pectoris (Croog and Levine, 1977). Heart disease is a major cause of permanent disability claims among workers under 65 and is the leading cause of death among men over 40. Diabetics with high blood pressure and high serum cholesterol levels and who smoke have increased risk of heart disease. Premenopausal women are much less likely to get heart disease than men of equivalent age (*Health, United States,* 1980).

Heart attacks are often sudden, dramatic, and painful, calling for immediate emergency measures. Individuals surviving an attack are often hospitalized in coronary care units. An atmosphere of serious and critical illness pervades these units.

Studies that have followed the medical, social, and psychological experiences of a group of men for an extended period following a heart attack (for example, Croog and Levine, 1977; Finlayson and McEwen, 1977) suggest that life may never be quite the same for heart attack victims. Questions about their ability to work, engage in sexual relationships, and view themselves as whole human beings loom large. People who did physically strenuous work before the attack experience more problems than those who were less active. Traditional sex role relationships also require considerable adaptation.

> Clearly, the problems and experiences they have go beyond questions of physical illness and involve such social and psychological dimensions as self image, emotional concerns, work status, relations with family members and level of social participation. Although as many as 96 percent of those who left the hospital survive the first year, approximately one-half the patients in our study had some physical symptoms or difficulties in connection with the illness. This finding suggests the need to mobilize services to provide effective health services to patients. (Croog and Levine, 1977, pp. 371-372)

People with heart disease experience psychological, social, and economic consequences similar to those of individuals who suffer a stroke (discussed next), survive disabling cancers, and live on dialysis.

Stroke

Stroke, also termed cerebrovascular accident (CVA), is the third leading cause of death in the United States. Approximately 75% to 85% of stroke victims survive the first attack. The percentage varies according to age and other factors. One study found that 50% of the people surviving an original attack subsequently die of a heart attack or another type of cardiac failure (McDowell, 1975).

The immediate effects of a stroke can be quite visible, unlike those following a heart attack. They may include weakness, paralysis, and speech and thought disturbances. There is the ever-present threat of recurrence. Rehabilitative processes can be extensive and involve prolonged speech, physical, and occupational therapy (Moos, 1977). Social work often plays a role in coordinating the various therapies offered in rehabilitation centers and works with victims and their families to help them cope with the slow resumption of daily living routines.

Mental illness

Of all of the disorders considered to this point mental health problems are the most elusive and difficult to define. It has been suggested (for example,

Thackeray, Skidmore, and Farley, 1979) that all people have mental health problems and that the difference between persistent and disabling problems and fleeting ones is only a matter of degree. All people at some time experience guilt and fear, engage in irrational behavior, or become childishly dependent. However, for many people, these and related behaviors and emotions persist and sharply diminish their capacity to carry out life's tasks. Whether or not difficulties of this nature are legitimately classified as illness has been a subject of considerable debate (for example, Lemert, 1951; Mechanic, 1978; Scheff, 1966; Szasz, 1960).

Some people take the position that mental disturbances are analogous to physical illness. Others, like Szasz, suggest that

> What the medical model calls mental illnesses are not illnesses at all but rather "problems of living" manifested in deviations from moral, legal, and social norms; . . . To label those deviations "sick" is . . . not only a blatant falsification of the conflict between the individual and the society but also a dangerous sanctification of the society's norms (Thackeray, Skidmore, and Farley, 1979, p. 26).

This debate has generated massive ferment in the mental health field. The debate notwithstanding, there is little question that a substantial number of people suffer acutely and become disabled because of crippling anxiety, depression, and hallucinations, as well as other mood disturbances. These disabilities in turn affect their ability to engage in satisfying emotional relationships, work, and carry out their daily social lives.

Mental health problems are difficult to define. Yet work in this area calls for some definitions that capture the essence of the disturbances involved, imperfect and fraught with potential for disagreement as they may be. In my view the definition offered by Knee and Lamson (1977) serves this purpose.

> Mental illness refers to a range of disorders related to an as yet incompletely elucidated complex of physiological, psychological and sociological factors leading to acute or chronic physical, emotional and/or behavioral disabilities. Many mental disorders are accompanied by a distortion of personality functions associated with greater or lesser distortions of the affected person's social relationships and economic status (p. 879).*

The third annual report on the health status of the nation (*Health, United States,* 1978) refers to these disorders as psychoses, neuroses, personality disorders, behavioral disorders, mental retardation, alcoholism, and drug dependence. Based on this categorization it was estimated that in a given year 15% of the American population has some episode of mental illness, and at any specific point in a year 10% of the population experiences a disorder.

Psychoses and schizophrenias involve hallucinations and delusions that

* Copyright 1977, National Association of Social Workers, Inc. Reprinted with permission, from Encyclopedia of Social Work, 17th Edition, John B. Turner, editor, p. 879, excerpt.

seriously distort perception of reality, produce inappropriate and constricted emotional responses, and may be manifest in withdrawn, regressive, bizarre behavior. A growing amount of literature suggests that schizophrenia is caused by an interaction of inherited and environmental factors. "A genetic disposition is probably necessary if schizophrenia is to occur at all . . . " (The Merck Manual, 1982, p. 1463). However, stressful life experiences do play a part. Mood disorders are characterized by extreme depression or elation; paranoid states are characterized by persecutory or grandiose delusions. The chief feature of the neuroses is anxiety (Margolis and Favazza, 1977).

Children are subject to a variety of mental health problems. A rare but extremely disabling condition is infantile autism. It is characterized "by a lack of human contact." Speech development is abnormal. Children are stiff and unresponsive and often twirl or spin (Mandelbaum, 1977).

Efforts to identify the number of people with mental health problems and the distribution by age, gender, ethnicity, and socioeconomic status are longstanding and plagued with difficulties. Classic investigations (for example, Hollingshead and Redlich, 1958) suggest there may be major differences in the way poor and middle-class people are diagnosed. Recent data suggest more men and minority group members are admitted to specialized mental health facilities than women and nonminority group members. Men are more likely than women to be diagnosed as alcoholic and schizophrenic; women are more likely than men to be diagnosed depressive and schizophrenic. Whites were most frequently categorized depressive, and nonwhites were more likely than whites to be diagnosed schizophrenic (*Health, United States,* 1978).

Considerable literature suggests that the poor and minority group members are more likely to be falsely diagnosed as suffering from the most severe disorders. A recent government study (*Health, United States,* 1978) suggests the discrepancy in diagnoses between whites and nonwhites "may represent bias in the diagnostic process rather than a true difference in the prevalence of this disorder among racial groups" (p. 72).

There is also a substantial amount of work suggesting women are more likely than men to be misdiagnosed as suffering from severe mental illness. These misdiagnoses imply that white middle-class professionals fail to understand culturally specific behaviors. There is, however, an equally impressive body of work suggesting that the diverse conditions of deprivation disproportionately experienced by the disadvantaged generate a high degree of mental health problems (Schlesinger and Schatz, 1977; Vance, 1973).

A major issue involving the care of people with severe mental health problems is deinstitutionalization. In the last 20 years the number of state mental hospital inpatients declined from 559,000 to 191,000 (Linn and Stein, 1981). This decline was triggered by diverse developments, including (1) the advent of psychotropic drugs that made it possible for many severely disabled people to function outside the rigidly controlled institution, (2) the liberation movements of the 1960s that focused on the civil rights of unwillingly committed patients, (3) a developing sense that institutional life did not facilitate subsequent adaptation in the community, and (4) efforts to control care costs.

The movement toward deinstitutionalization was begun enthusiastically; however, the associated problems are numerous. Mechanic's succinct statement (1978) highlights the problems of deinstitutionalizing people requiring extensive care, no matter where they are:

> For the most part, however, community-care technologies are still undeveloped, and in returning impaired patients to the community we do not eliminate illness or the social problems that illness may cause. Rather we shift some of the responsibilities and burdens of care from the hospital to the community (p. 459).

The development of a "technology of care" for the mentally disabled is a task facing many health care professionals. Social work has a long history of involvement with the mentally ill. In this area of work the interaction between individuals, their unique needs, and the development of resources tailored to these complex needs are particularly crucial. Some encouraging experiments (for example, Pasamanick, Scarpitti, and Dinitz, 1967) suggest a large role for social work in meeting this challenge.

Developmental disability

The term *developmental disability* applies to a wide spectrum of people. While in the past, it was more common to speak of the mentally retarded, it has increasingly been recognized that a variety of physical and mental handicaps lead to substantial functional limitations in self-care, receptive and expressive language, learning, mobility, self-direction, capacity for independent living, and economic self-sufficiency. These handicaps include mental retardation, cerebral palsy, deafness, blindness, epilepsy, dyslexia, learning disability, and autism (Andrews and Wikler, 1981). They result in permanent disability and usually involve deficits in cognitive and adaptive functioning. The extent and nature of the deficits involved is such that the handicapped themselves and their families require extensive educational, social, psychological, and economic help.

Evans (1983) points to the difficulty encountered in efforts to identify the number of people affected. He cites data showing that estimates of mental retardation rates vary substantially, depending on the criteria used to identify people who suffer from this type of disability. Despite disagreement, a prevalence rate of 3% is a commonly accepted figure.

As is the case with so many other health problems, the poor are disproportionately affected, especially by less severe impairments. Many factors associated with poverty are implicated as contributory factors, including malnutrition during pregnancy, alcohol and drug use during pregnancy, and lead poisoning. Severe mental handicaps are relatively "class free."

Many developmentally disabled individuals, like those suffering severe mental handicaps, were formerly institutionalized. Now there is more reliance on community-based medical care, day-care centers, education, and interventions designed to improve cognitive capacities, speech, and physical mobility.

PROBLEMS OF THE ELDERLY

The elderly experience many of the same health problems already discussed. Nevertheless, this group is singled out for separate consideration because the need for health care and related social support services is pronounced and increasing. The elderly are "the major consumers of health care and spenders of health care dollars" (Libow, 1981). The group is increasing in proportion to the rest of the population. American society values youth, good looks, vigor, and economic and social independence. Therefore the decline associated with aging is particularly damaging to an elderly person's self-esteem and self-worth. In the preface to *Social Work with the Aging* (Lowy, 1979) cites the following comments made by Maddox:

> In a society which values youthfulness and productivity, older people have the capacity simultaneously to fascinate, to trouble and to embarrass. Older people are a commentary on what it means to be finite. Older people live on a frontier which every man sooner or later must explore (p. xiii).

People over 65 years of age comprise almost 11% of the population; 4% of that 11% is over 75. Individuals over 75 comprise 38% of the total elderly population. Projections are that by the year 2000 these figures will be 12%, 5.5%, and 45%, respectively (Libow, Schechter, and Margolis, 1981). Not only is the percentage of elderly rising, but the percentage of those to whom many refer as the frail elderly also is increasing.

While the elderly comprise 11% of the population, they account for 29% of the monies spent on personal health care. A substantial number of the elderly need extensive medical and social care. Only 5% are in nursing homes. However, 7% of the elderly people living in the community need assistance if they leave their homes, and an additional 5% are homebound.

A substantial number (25%) of the elderly live at or near poverty level. Many people's income is reduced by 50% at retirement. Therefore they cannot afford the care they need.

The difference in life expectancy between men and women greatly affects the lives of the elderly. In 1975 approximately 16% of men over 65 were widowed, compared to approximately 65% of women in the same age group. Therefore elderly women are particularly at risk for the isolation that often accompanies aging and reduced mobility.

Adequate resolution of the elderly's health and social needs constitutes a particular challenge for contemporary society. Meyer (1973) poses the challenge for social work:

> The influence of social workers, using their special knowledge and skill to sustain and at times create pathways between the aged person and his [or her] immediate world, has the potential of becoming a modern-day social convention that will exact intellectual as well as emotional excitement for the practitioner in search of a developing field (pp. 1, 4).

OTHER HEALTH PROBLEMS

Drug and alcohol abuse

Current estimates show that 10 million adult Americans are alcoholics or problem drinkers. The number of minors using alcohol has increased dramatically. The impact of excessive drinking can be found in all spheres of life. It is associated with major family disruption, increased motor vehicle fatalities, and crime. According to estimates made in 1975 by the Alcohol, Drug Abuse, and Mental Health Administration, the types of alcohol-related problems previously referred to cost $43 billion (*Healthy People,* 1979).

Although data on drug use are more difficult to obtain, there is no question that excessive use of drugs such as cocaine and barbiturates affects people negatively. A recent survey suggests that 1 out of 40 residents of New York City is a heroin user (*The New York Times,* June 15, 1982). The dependence increases crime because users need money to "feed their habit." A problem of such proportion is of concern to anyone involved in treating illness and promoting health.

Accidents

Health problems associated with motor vehicle accidents loom large and strike young adults with particular force. "In 1977, motor vehicle accidents were the leading cause of mortality in the 15 to 24 year age group, accounting for 37 percent of all deaths" (*Healthy People,* 1979). A complex of factors lies behind these data. One factor is the attitudes of young adults about risk. Excessive speed contributed to about 40% of the motor vehicle fatalities among the young, as did excessive alcohol consumption. Reduction in speed and alcohol use and increase in safety belt use could reduce these figures markedly. However, more than 80% of Americans, including teenagers and young adults, do not use safety belts.

Sexually transmitted diseases

Venereal diseases have concerned health workers for a long time. According to recent analysis (*Healthy People,* 1979) the term *venereal disease* is no longer adequate to describe the range of diseases now known to be transmitted by sexual contact.

Ten million cases of sexually transmitted diseases were reported in 1977; 86% of the clients were between the ages of 15 and 29. Currently herpes and acquired immune deficiency syndrome (AIDS) are of great concern to many people; AIDS has generated intense governmental activity directed at finding the cause and cure.

Despite growing comfort concerning human sexuality, efforts to control sexually transmitted diseases are still hindered by feelings of guilt and shame. Many health professionals are not trained to deal with this sensitive area. Health care social workers, trained to listen sensitively and be nonjudgmental, can use their skills to help treat this serious health problem.

Environmental hazards and related health problems

Every inhabitant of contemporary, industrialized, urban society is increasingly aware of environmental hazards triggering health problems. Health risks caused by toxic wastes, air pollution, and unsafe work environments are discussed often by the media. *The Surgeon General's Report on Health Promotion and Disease Prevention* (*Healthy People,* 1979) included these hazards in a list of areas requiring major preventive approaches. When dangers posed by toxic agents, occupational hazards, and air pollution are combined with other dangers such as accidents and failure to control against infection, some startling figures emerge.

> Some estimates hold that perhaps 20 percent of all premature deaths—and a vast amount of disease and disability—could be eliminated by protecting our people from environmental hazards. . . . A commitment to safety and elimination of hazards—by everyone from government officials to parents to children—would save millions of Americans from needless pain and disability (*Healthy People,* 1979, pp. 101, 118).

Social work in health care, with its commitment to recognize and work toward elimination of factors that mitigate against positive person-environment interaction, cannot ignore these problems.

The nuclear arms race

Detailed analysis of the nuclear arms race is beyond the scope of this book and my competence. However, it is fitting to comment on this problem and the threat it poses. As social workers assign priorities to various health needs they need to keep in mind Yankauer's comments (1980).

> The rationale for cutting total federal expenditures, as part of an effort to slow the inflationary spiral appears reasonable to most people. The rationale for increasing military expenditures while reducing social sector expenditures is of a different order. To many, this appears to be unreasonable and unnecessary, and to pose a greater menace to the public health than any of the germs, toxins, and degenerative diseases with which public health workers have had to do battle in the past (p. 949).

The nuclear arms race is antithetical to social work values. Social workers committed to promoting individual and collective health cannot ignore this threat.

SUMMARY

This chapter has presented an overview of the diverse health problems predominant in the United States today. Their historical origins were briefly traced, illustrating that major advances in public health measures, standards of living, and medical knowledge and skills have dramatically altered the shape and nature of current health problems. The incidence of the infectious diseases that were the major killers of the nineteenth century has decreased substantially.

Analysis of contemporary mortality and morbidity data showed that chronic illness is the leading current health concern. Heart disease, cancer, stroke, and accidents, especially among the young, are the leading causes of death. Infant mortality, though substantially reduced, is still higher than in other industrialized countries. Infant mortality is often considered an indicator of a nation's commitment to health and to the disadvantaged in the population, and on this measure the nation can be faulted. Rates among the poor and minority groups in the United States are high, exceeding those found among more privileged groups.

Although medical advances have been dramatic, they have been accompanied by a number of disquieting features. New drug therapies, surgical techniques, and medical technology often maintain the lives of many people affected by major diseases. Nevertheless, considerable numbers are not "cured." Many individuals live with varying degrees of disability and have extensive need for supportive services, such as home health care, nursing home care, and counseling, and for opportunities to maintain continued social interaction.

Many current health problems relate to life-style and low standards of living. Therefore considerable attention was paid to the fact that both prevention and management of diverse health problems require changes in public policy.

The implications for health care social work practice were considered throughout. Social workers have and continue to take major responsibility for prevention, efforts to increase the number of supportive services available, and enhancement of the quality of life of those with health problems.

REFERENCES

Anderson, O.W.: Infant mortality and social and cultural factors. In Jaco, E.G., editor: Patients, physicians, and illness: a sourcebook in behavioral science and health. Glencoe, Ill., 1958, The Free Press.

Andrews, S., and Wikler, L.: Developmental disabilities, Health and Social Work (Suppl.) **6**(4):625, 1981.

Blum, H.L.: Planning for health, New York, 1974, Human Sciences Press, Inc.

Boffey, P.M.: U.S. reports gains in nation's health, *The New York Times,* Jan. 18, 1984.

Bracht, N.F.: The scope and historical development of social work, 1900-1975. In Bracht, N.F., editor: Social work in health care: a guide to professional practice, New York, 1978, The Haworth Press.

Cabot, R.C.: Social service and the art of healing, New York, 1915, Moffat, Yard & Co.

Cahill, G.F., Jr.: Diabetes mellitus. In Beeson, P.B., and McDermott, W.: Textbook of medicine, Philadelphia, 1975, W. B. Saunders Co.

Caldwell, J.R., Cobb, S., Dowling, M.D., and deJongh, P.: The dropout problem in antihypertensive treatment, Journal of Chronic Diseases **22**:579, 1970.

Children's Defense Fund of the Washington Research Project, Inc.: Doctors and dollars are not enough, Washington, D.C., 1976, Washington Research Project, Inc.

Conceptual problems in developing an index of health, U.S. Public Health Service Pub. No. 1000 (series 2, no. 17), Washington, D.C., 1966, U.S. Government Printing Office.

Congressional Research Service: The national health insurance debate, 97th Congress Issue Brief 1B81082, Washington, D.C., 1981, U.S. Government Printing Office.

Croog, S.H., and Levine, S.: The heart patient recovers, New York, 1977, Human Sciences Press, Inc.

Evans, D.P.: The lives of the mentally retarded, Boulder, Colo., 1983, Westview Press, Inc.

Eyer, J.: Hypertension as a disease of modern society, International Journal of Health Services **5**:539, 1975.

Federal Register, Vol. 4, No. 8, 1976.

Finlayson, A., and McEwen, J.: Coronary heart disease and patterns of living, New York, 1977, Prodist.

Finnerty, F.A., Jr., and Linde, S.M.: High blood pressure, New York, 1975, David McKay Co., Inc.

Finnerty, F.A., Jr., Matte, E.C., and Finnerty, F.A., III: Hypertension in the inner city: analysis of clinical dropouts, Circulation **47**:73, 1973.

Flexner, A.: Medical education in the United States and Canada, New York, 1910, Carnegie Foundation.

Frank, J.D.: The nuclear arms race—sociopsychological aspects, American Journal of Public Health **70**(9):950, 1980.

Frazier, C.L.: Renal disease, Health and Social Work (Suppl.) **6**(4):755, 1981.

Fuchs, V.R.: Who shall live? health, economics and social choice, New York, 1974, Basic Books, Inc., Publishers.

Goodman, L.S., and Gilman, A.: The pharmacological basis of therapeutics, New York, 1958, Macmillan Publishing, Inc.

Griscom, J.H.: The sanitary condition of the laboring population of New York, New York, 1845, Harper. In Pumphrey, R.E., and Pumphrey, M.W., editors: The heritage of American social work, New York, 1961, Columbia University Press.

Gruenberg, E.M.: The failures of success, Milbank Memorial Fund Quarterly; Health and Society, **55**(1):3, 1977.

Guidelines: chronic disease services, Trenton, N.J., 1980, New Jersey State Department of Health.

Hanlon, J.J., and Pickett, G.R.: Public health: administration and practice, ed. 8, St. Louis, 1984, The C.V. Mosby Co.

Health of the disadvantaged: chart book II, DHHS Pub. No. (HRA) 80-633, Washington, D.C., 1980, U.S. Government Printing Office.

Health status of minorities and low-income groups, DHEW Pub. No. (HRA) 79-627, Washington D.C., U.S. Government Printing Office.

Health, United States, DHEW Pub. No. (PHS) 78-1232, Washington, D.C., 1978, U.S. Government Printing Office.

Health, United States, DHEW Pub. No. (PHS) 80-1232, Washington, D.C., 1979, U.S. Government Printing Office.

Health, United States, DHEW Pub. No. (HRA) 79-633, Washington, D.C., 1980, U.S. Government Printing Office.

Health, United States, DHHS Pub. No. (PHS) 82-1232, Washington, D.C., 1981, U.S. Government Printing Office.

Health, United States, DHHS Pub. No. (PHS) 83-1232, Washington, D.C., 1982, U.S. Government Printing Office.

Healthy people, The Surgeon General's report on health promotion and disease prevention, DHEW Pub. No. (PHS) 79-55071, Washington, D.C., 1979, U.S. Government Printing Office.

Holden, M.O.: Dialysis or death: the ethical alternatives, Health and Social Work **5**(2):18, 1980.

Hollingshead, A.B., and Redlich, F.C.: Social class and mental illness, New York, 1958, John Wiley & Sons, Inc.

Howe, I.: Immigrant Jewish families in New York: the end of the world of our fathers, New York **8**(41):51, 1975.

Interim report of the graduate medical education national advisory committee to the secretary, department of Health, Education, and Welfare, DHEW Pub. No. (HRA) 79-633, Washington, D.C., 1979, U.S. Government Printing Office.

Knee, R.I., and Lamson. W.C.: Mental health services. In Turner, J.B., editor: Encyclopedia of social work, Washington, D.C., 1977, National Association of Social Workers, vol. 11, p. 879.

Lemert, E.M.: Social pathology, New York, 1951, McGraw-Hill Book Co.

Libow, L.S.: General concepts of geriatric medicine. In Libow, L.S., and Sherman, F.J.: The core of geriatric medicine, St. Louis, 1981, The C.V. Mosby Co.

Libow, L.S., Schechter, Z., and Margolis, E.: Demographic and economic aspects, including Medicare and Medicaid. In Libow, L.S., and Sherman, F.J.: The core of geriatric medicine, St. Louis, 1981, The C.V. Mosby Co.

Linn, M.W., and Stein, S.: Chronic adult mental illness, Health and Social Work (Suppl.) **6**(4):545, 1981.

Lowy, L.: Social work with the aging, New York, 1979, Harper & Row, Publishers, Inc.

Mandelbaum, A.: Mental health and retardation. In Turner, J.B., editor: Encyclopedia of social work, Washington, D.C., 1977, National Association of Social Workers, vol. 11, p. 869.

Margolis, P.M., and Favazza, A.R.: Mental health and illness. In Turner, J.B., editor: Encyclopedia of social work, Washington, D.C., 1977, National Association of Social Workers, vol. 11, p. 849.

McCormick, M.C., Shapiro, S., and Starfield, B.: High-risk young mothers: infant mortality and morbidity in four areas in the United States—1973-1978, American Journal of Public Health **74**(1):18, 1984.

McDowell, F.N.: Cerebrovascular diseases. In Beeson, P.B., and McDermott, W.: Textbook of medicine, Philadelphia, 1975, W. B. Saunders Co.

Mechanic, D.: Medical sociology, ed. 2, New York, 1978, The Free Press.

The Merck Manual, ed. 14, Rahway, N.J., 1982.

Meyer, C., editor: Social work with the aging, New York, 1973, Columbia University Press.

Moos, R.H., editor: Coping with physical illness, New York, 1977, Plenum Medical Book Co.

National Center for Health Statistics: Chronic conditions and limitations of activity and mobility, Series 10, No. 61, Washington, D.C., 1971, U.S. Department of Health, Education, and Welfare.

New Jersey State Department of Health: Guidelines, chronic disease services, Trenton, N.J., 1980, The Department.

Newsholme, A., Sir: The ministry of health, London, 1925, G.P. Putnam's Sons, Ltd.

The New York Times, June 15, 1982.

Palmiere, D.: Specialization in medicine and nursing: implications for social work, Health and Social Work (Suppl.) **6** (4):135, 1981.

Pasamanick, B., Scarpitti, F.R., and Dinitz, S.: Schizophrenics in the community: an experimental study in the prevention of hospitalization, New York, 1967, Appleton-Century-Crofts.

Pear, R.: Interpreting the results of the yearly U.S. physical, *The New York Times,* The week of news in review, Jan. 20, 1984.

President's Commission on Mental Health: Task Panel Report 3, Appendix, Washington, D.C., 1978, The Commission.

Pumphrey, R.E., and Pumphrey, M.W., editors: The heritage of American social work, New York, 1961, Columbia University Press.

The National Commission on Diabetes: The long range plan to combat diabetes, 1975, vol. 1, The Commission.

Sackett, D.L., Haynes, R.B., Gibson, E.S., Taylor, D.W., Roberts, R.S., and Johnson, A.L.: Hypertension control, compliance and science, American Heart Journal **94**:666, 1977.

Scheff, T.J.: Being mentally ill: a sociological theory, Chicago, 1966, Aldine Publishing Co.
Schlesinger, E.G., and Schatz, J.L.: Competence and social disability: a conceptual framework for HBSE content, Journal of Education for Social Work **13**(3):84, 1977.
Smith, B.C.: Community health, New York, 1979, Macmillan Publishing Co., Inc.
Somers, A.P., and Somers, H.M.: Health and health care: policies in perspective, Rockville, Md., 1977, Aspen Systems Corp.
Stonberg, M.F.: Oncology, Health and Social Work (Suppl.) **6**(4):695, 1981.
Strauss, A.L.: Chronic illness and the quality of life, St. Louis, 1975, The C.V. Mosby Co.
Szasz, T.S.: The myth of mental illness, American Psychologist **15**:113, 1960.
Thackeray, M.G., Skidmore, R.A., and Farley, W.O.: Introduction to mental health field and practice, Englewood Cliffs, N.J., 1979, Prentice-Hall, Inc.
Vance, E.T.: Social disability, American Psychologist **28**:498, June 1973.
Ward, G.W.: Changing trends in control of hypertension, Public Health Reports **93**:31, 1978.
Watkins, E.L., and Player, E.C.: Maternal and child health care, Health and Social Work (Suppl.) **6**(4):465, 1981.
Yankauer, A.: The pseudo-environment of national defense, American Journal of Public Health **70**(9):949, 1980.

Newark
Beth Israel
Medical
Center
OUTPATIENT SERVICES
ADULT MEDICINE
•Eye
•Ear, Nose, Throat
•Heart
• Allergy
•General Medical
•Other Specialties
PEDIATRIC HEALTH CENTER
WOMEN'S HEALTH CENTER
•Family Planning
•Prenatal
•GYN
DENTAL HEALTH CENTER

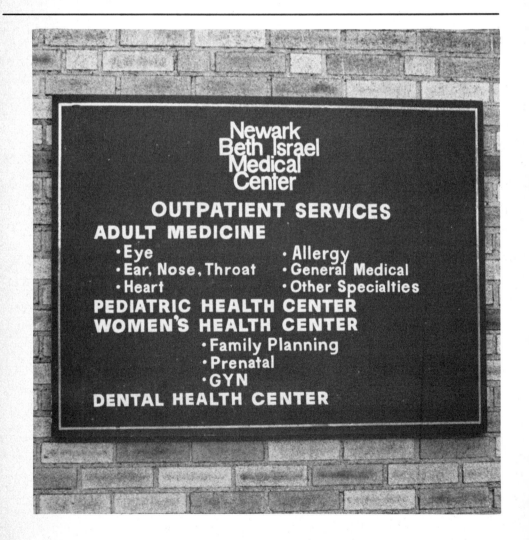

Chapter 2

Health policy, costs and financing, delivery systems, and providers

The Jones family

Mr. Arthur Jones is a 75-year-old man who has been confined to a wheelchair since an accident left his legs paralyzed 10 years ago. Additional chronic health problems have since appeared. He has limited control of his bladder function and needs a catheter. He needs to be lifted when he has to move his bowels and has to have skilled nurses who can supervise the care of his catheter. He also needs help with bathing.

He is married and lives with his 72-year-old wife Mary, who herself has a number of chronic health problems. Arthritis results in stiffening of her joints and her movements are slow. She has mild diabetes, which she controls with diet.

A married son, John, and his wife, Joan, live nearby with their own two grown children Frank and Susan. They are all employed. Although John and Joan are not able to help Mr. and Mrs. Jones with all of their daily needs, they take care of much of the shopping and are able to provide transportation for visits to their physician. A married daughter, Anne Brown, lives about 1 hour's drive away and visits regularly.

Mr. and Mrs. Jones have no savings. They live on Social Security payments supplemented by SSI. Their son and daughter-in-law are both postal employees whose income allows them to live in reasonable comfort but does not afford them many extras for themselves or their parents.

The family lives in a state that has made relatively generous provisions for home health services for the elderly via the Medicaid program. Because of this, arrangements have been made for a homemaker to spend 8 hours a day in the home. A visiting nurse visits regularly to check the catheter, to make sure that medication is being used properly, and to monitor the work of the homemaker. In addition to helping with Arthur's physical care, the homemaker tries to help Mary with light household tasks.

A social worker visits once monthly to determine whether the arrangements that have been made are working smoothly. Her visits give Mr. and Mrs. Jones Senior an opportunity to express some of their concerns about their health and their isolation. She has told them about a service established by some local churches to visit the elderly and to care for some routine chores. This is of great relief to them, since they worry that their son and daughter-in-law devote so much time to them that they have little energy left to enjoy life.

Because of the help provided by the homemaker, the nurse, the home health aide, the social worker, and the volunteer services of the church, Mr. Jones is able to live at home. Without these services he would probably have to go to a nursing home.

The Bernstein family

Saul and Sadie Bernstein find themselves in circumstances quite similar to those of Mr. and Mrs. Jones. Because both had worked, they both receive Social Security payments and small pensions from employer-employee negotiated pension plans. Refugees from Hitler's Germany, they also have received a few thousand dollars in reparations payments.*

Beyond this they have a few thousand dollars in savings. Between their income from Social Security, pensions, and interest earnings on their small savings account, their annual income just exceeds the upper limits for eligibility for SSI and the Medicaid program. Current regulations make Mr. Bernstein eligible for some home health services under the Medicare program following a hospital stay.† But Mr. Bernstein really does not need hospital care. Periodically, his physician hospitalizes him just so that he can "order" home health services for a few weeks.

At other times, they draw on their meager savings to pay a young man to come in 1 hour daily to care for Mr. Bernstein's basic needs. Their son David looks in daily and finds he has little time to rest or relax between working at his job, looking in on his father, and worrying about his elderly parents. When Sadies' arthritis grew worse, it became increasingly difficult for her to do the housework and tend to Mr. Bernstein.

The family has had a conference, and with much sadness they decide to put Saul on the waiting list for one of the better nursing homes. Sadie will go to live with her son. Once their limited savings are depleted, in paying for the nursing home, the Medicaid program will pick up the cost.

All will feel an additional strain. Mr. Bernstein knows the nursing home is "the last stop." He will die there. Mrs. Bernstein will feel like an intruder in her son's home. She knows her son, daughter-in-law, and grandchildren care for her, but "after all, they have their own lives." Most importantly, she has lived with this man for over 50 years. They really wanted to live out their days together, as they laugh about the past, enjoy what they still have, and commiserate about their failing health.

Unfortunately, nursing home care for Mr. Bernstein will probably cost the public treasury more than would the provision of home health care.

The Bernsteins and the Jones are elderly people with modest incomes who have worked hard. Both couples have families who care for them—but who lead their own busy lives. The fact that Mr. Jones can remain at home while Mr. Bernstein must resort to nursing home care in large measure reflects the pluralistic and uneven provisions for health care financing and the varia-

* Payment for lost earnings and compensation for other indignities and harm caused by the Nazi regime.

† Detailed information concerning the number of hours/days of eligbility are omitted, since these are continually changing with shifting federal regulations.

tions in policies and philosophy found in health care today. A philosophical stance that views home care as desirable, when at all feasible, is often not supported by financing mechanisms that make it possible to provide humane, sound care at home. These mechanisms vary by state and by income levels. Many people "fall between the cracks" in the prevailing pluralistic system.

Ms. Mary Tavatti

Ms. Tavatti is a young single woman in her thirties who has periodic bouts of depression. For many years she was sufficiently depressed to be considered disabled and entitled to SSI. During these years she took advantage of the mental health services at the local community mental health center. With a combination of counseling and use of psychotropic drugs the chronic depression subsided, and she got much better and began to work regularly as a clerk, commuting to a state adjacent to her home state. The company for which she works provides a health benefits package. She continues psychotherapy with a psychiatrist in private practice.

Not yet quite ready to live totally on her own, she lives with an older brother and his family. Other relatives are nearby. Not long ago she again began to suffer from a severe depression. The psychiatrist recommended a short (perhaps 3-week) stay in a small, psychiatric facility with a reputation for being able to help people mobilize themselves and quickly regain lost levels of functioning. This facility was conveniently located where family and friends could visit and provide evidence of concern and love. Most of the psychiatrist's patients for whom he had made similar recommendations had had the cost of short-term care in this institution covered by their employment-related health insurance plans.

The family took Ms. Tavatti to the hospital. In the process of making the necessary arrangements in the admitting office, they found that her "out of state policy"—unlike those usually available through employment in the state where she lives—did not cover the cost of private, inpatient psychiatric care. At this point the family decided they would have to bear the cost (somewhere between $3,000 and $5,000) themselves. Though they are professional and business people, this sum will strain their finances considerably. They are trying, for the period of the crisis, to keep knowledge of this fact from Ms. Tavatti, for she was already feeling that she was a burden to her family.

Examples of these kinds of gaps between health care needs and resources to meet them are legion. Every health care social worker, physician, and other health care personnel can tell similar tales.

I believe it is fitting, in a book on health care social work practice, to introduce the discussion of health care policy, costs and financing, personnel, and services by presenting such examples. They begin to illustrate the kind of obstacles that confront health care consumers and providers in the effort to address health problems in a humane, meaningful manner.

No one effort to understand prevailing and emerging patterns of health care structure and financing can possibly encompass the range, complexity, and diversity that comprise the health care system. Thus no claim is made that this chapter provides an in-depth or complete overview of the current situation. Decisions concerning material to be included and assessment of policies and programs are based on a professional judgment concerning the kind of information health care social workers need to carry out their daily work—whether that is primarily focused on the provision of day-to-day services to individuals and small groups or on administrative and planning concerns.

The other, and perhaps more important, criterion derives from the assumption that the provision for basic human needs is an intrinsic responsibility of modern industrial society and must be built into the basic institutional structure (Reichert, 1983; Wilensky and Lebeaux, 1965). This translates into support for policy positions that endorse equal and unlimited access to health care, independent of ability to pay or status in the social structure. This position is reflected in the official professional endorsements of a national health service that would provide for such access (National Health Policy, 1979). Of equal importance are the values concerning how people are to be treated. In health care these naturally generate questions about the relationship between the way health services are organized, available financing, and attention paid by health care providers to dignity, privacy, and culturally derived dispositions to care.

MAJOR THRUSTS IN HEALTH CARE POLICY

During the 1960s and early 1970s it was fashionable to speak and write about the "health care crisis." The popular and professional literature devoted special issues of magazines and journals to this "crisis" and projected numerous solutions. Among the frequently cited concerns were fragmented and depersonalized care, the high cost of care, and health care personnel shortages, particularly in the inner cities and rural areas. The view was widespread that Congress would shortly enact national health insurance legislation to provide universal coverage and diminish problems of access to health care. In an incisive analysis Dana (1977) suggests that "what was termed the 'health care crisis' in the rhetoric of the Great Society is now considered a chronic problem that will require a multifaceted approach to both the definition of the problem and corrective intervention" (p. 544).

To support this view she identifies several basic weaknesses in the structure and support of health services: (1) the problems inherent in current funding mechanisms and resources as they attempt to keep pace with the rising costs of care; (2) inadequate provisions for primary, preventive, and long-term care; (3) unequal access to health care for large segments of the population; (4) failure to reconcile the needs for holistic, comprehensive care with the advances related to specialized care; and (5) depersonalized health care.

The health care system has frequently been described as a "nonsystem" characterized by a patchwork of services lacking any coherent or unified policy direction. A number of major thrusts can nevertheless be identified.

Dana (1977) suggests that prevailing laws, regulation efforts, and practices represent responses to persistent policy questions faced by generations of policy makers. Among these are questions about (1) who should be entitled to publicly financed health care and under what conditions, (2) what services should be covered, (3) what institutional mechanisms and auspices would be developed, and (4) how the designated rights would be protected. It is her contention that the policies that have evolved in response to these questions are a reflection of scientific knowledge and related social, economic, and political developments.

The social elite that determined health care policy in the eighteenth and nineteenth centuries was replaced during the twentieth century by a scientific and professional elite. That elite promoted "the purposes, priorities, and style of biomedical science and its attendant technology" (Dana, 1977, p. 546). The consequences of this thrust have resulted in some of the prevailing issues confronting health care today, as noted in Chapter 1.

Dana (1977) has identified some of these issues as follows: (1) the disease orientation of health care practice, research, and education; (2) the displacement of the generalist by the specialist who focuses attention on specific organs or diseases; (3) the centrality of the hospital in scientific medicine's approach to disease; (4) the separation of preventive and long-term services from the mainstream of scientific medical concerns; (5) the separation between medicine as taught in the schools and that in community-based practice; (6) the dominance of the physician and the "medical model" in the education of health care professionals; and (7) the continuation of a fee-for-service system as the dominant mode of payment for health services.

The deficits of this basic thrust have become increasingly evident. Distrust in the health care establishment coupled with the focus on human rights so characteristic of the 1960s began to change the perceptions and definitions of health. Social definitions of health problems emerged as it became clear that prevailing approaches had failed in many respects. These include the discrepancies in health status between the poor, minorities, and others that have already been detailed in Chapter 1. The concerns for equity and justice focused attention on the fact that health care was beyond the financial reach of many. Environmental health hazards were increasingly identified. These and other developments triggered increasing governmental involvement in financing health services and increasing efforts to protect the public from health hazards. A number of legislative initiatives can be identified. These relate to methods of financing health care and, increasingly, to controlling health care costs. In this section I will first focus on various ways in which health care is currently financed. Next I will review various proposals, long advanced, for altering the present system.

PAYING FOR HEALTH CARE

The methods by which the costs of health and medical care are met are complex and multifaceted. It is not possible in this book to make a thorough analysis of the political and social forces that have contributed to the present and ever-changing picture. However, some brief comments concerning the political philosophies and economic tenets that shape the current situation are indicated to serve as a backdrop for understanding the present system. These philosophies and tenets include reference to diverse views concerning government's role in ensuring access to health and social services and the role played by health care consumers in making judgments about how, where, and why they use those resources available to them.

Government's role in health care provision and financing

As I pointed out earlier, a number of developments have converged to generate increasing governmental involvement in financing and organizing health services. Nevertheless, to date no legislation has emerged that provides a universal system of health care financing unrelated to such factors as age, employment, or other indicators of socioeconomic status. Those whose philosophical and political views have been predominant in the legislative arena view government's role to be supplementary. Stevens (1983) suggests this view may be characterized as "residual and regulatory" (p. 282).

The view that health care is a right, although espoused by many, has not been translated into programs and financing mechanisms backed by legislation. This contrasts sharply with the developments in other western industrialized countries. The National Health Service in Britain is an example of these developments. In that country health care is universally available. Commenting on the philosophy that generated the British system, Stevens (1983) suggests that government was seen as "a necessary vehicle for achieving a reasonable social distribution of health care" (p. 282). She further indicates that the national health service was developed on the assumption that "health services are a national resource which should be shared across the population so that services are, as far as possible, apportioned on the basis of medical need rather than the ability to pay" (p. 282).

The "marketplace model" of health care

Closely related to the philosophical and political stance that seeks to keep government's role to a minimum is a perspective suggesting that in health care, as in other sectors of the economy, the consumer is in a position to determine how resources will be used. This perspective has been termed the *marketplace model* (Mechanic, 1978). In his critique of this model Mechanic points out its failure to distribute health care in a fair or cost-effective manner. He suggests that the health care consumer is often not in a position to make judgments about the complex care decisions that need to be made. In addition, there is a high degree of uncertainty and unpredictability about when and what kinds of services will be needed.

Other factors limit the consumer's capacity to affect the cost and quality of care by wise purchasing decisions. Entry to the health profession is highly restricted. Competition among health care providers has been limited, and needs for care are often triggered by life-threatening conditions. In the latter situation the consumer's capacity to choose between various providers is limited further.

Although many adhere to the view that the government's role in health care should be limited and others see an increasing role for the consumer in determining the shape of health care, there is no question that the government's role in health care financing has increased substantially. A variety of legislative decisions illustrate that the marketplace model is not successful in bringing health care within the reach of various populations.

Currently health care is financed in myriad ways. Federally based programs such as Medicare and Medicaid defray some of the costs of health care for those over the age of 65 and for those who are poor. Private health insurance plans available to people through their employers cover various portions of health care costs for a substantial number of people. However, few people do not incur some out-of-pocket expenses for medical care. Total health care, without cost, is available only to the members of Congress, other federal officials, and members of the armed forces. Virtually no other plan pays for all the health care costs incurred.

As I present the major aspects of these various schemes I also offer a word of caution. This chapter is being written at a time when the Reagan administration is making extensive efforts to reduce the federal involvement in paying for health care. Legislative changes are rapid. Therefore emphasis is on major thrusts, both those that have been in place for some time and those that are currently being proposed.

Medicare.* Medicare, or Title XVIII of the Social Security Act, was first enacted in 1965. Originally designed as a nationwide health insurance program for those over 65, it was subsequently amended to include a group of younger disabled individuals.

This federal program, available to insured people without regard to their income or assets, consists of two parts: (1) Part A—the Hospital Insurance Program and (2) Part B—the Supplementary Medical Insurance Program. The vast majority of people are eligible for Part A on reaching age 65. Also eligible are disabled widows and disabled dependent widowers between 50 and 65, those over age 18 who receive benefits because of disability before reaching age 22, and disabled railroad workers. Those workers insured and their depen-

* Much of this discussion and the one on Medicaid that follows is based on a summary of material contained in O'Sullivan, J.: Medicare and Medicaid: issue brief No. 1B76028, Congressional Research Service, Major Issues System, updated Nov. 19, 1981.

dents who have chronic renal disease are considered disabled for life.

Part A is financed through a special hospital insurance tax levied on employees, employers, and the self-employed. Part A pays for hospital care. This care is not unlimited. Regulations concerning covered costs, those for which a patient must contribute part of the cost, and the "deductible costs" are in constant flux. At present, cuts are being proposed. Also covered under Part A are a designated number of days of posthospital care in a skilled nursing facility, for which recipients must make a contribution to the daily cost. A limited number of hours of home health visits following hospitalization are also included.*

The kinds of services to which Medicare recipients are automatically entitled in Part A are limited to a designated number of hospital days, a limited amount of nursing home care, and a limited number of home health visits. With few exceptions, eligibility for these services is linked to evidence provided by physicians concerning the presence of specified disease that generates short-term care needs. For the most part they do not encompass the range of care needs that persist following the acute episode of an illness. Earlier reference was made to Dana's comments on the inadequacy of funding mechanisms needed to cover long-term care needs. The first two case examples presented at the beginning of this chapter highlight these inadequacies. The services available to Arthur Jones were *not* via his Medicare entitlements, but rather through special supplementary programs. Saul Bernstein, who has just *slightly more* money *and* who lives in a different state, is not covered for these services. Mr. Bernstein's physician periodically hospitalized Mr. Bernstein to make him eligible for short-term home health care.

Care required because of more broadly defined social or emotional needs is not available. For example, the elderly who may need help with shopping are not covered unless they have had a recent, medically diagnosed illness. Yet Chapter 1 pointed to the cumulative effects of aging that often result in the presence of persistent, chronic conditions not readily classifiable as acute, time-limited episodes of illness.

Unlike Part A, Part B is a voluntary program. It is financed jointly by monthly premium charges paid by enrollees and by the federal government. It pays 80% of "reasonable" charges, after certain deductibles have been met.

Covered items include the services of independent practitioners (usually physicians/related services), outpatient hospital care, and laboratory work. Currently *not* covered is most long-term care, medication prescribed on an outpatient basis, eyeglasses, dental care, hearing aids, and routine physical examinations. It is estimated that approximately 44% of the health care costs incurred by those over 65 are covered by Medicare.

Among the costs incurred for many are the bills levied by physicians who

* The number of days of care available is subject to continuing regulatory change.

do not consider the "reasonable charges" allowed by Medicare as sufficient payment for their services. The reader may have noted signs in physicians' waiting rooms that state: "We do not accept Medicare assignments."

At present a number of proposals are being considered to repeal certain benefits and to further control costs.

Assessment. A cursory review of the intent and effect of the Medicare program highlights the advantages and disadvantages from a value perspective. Medicare represents the first major federal effort to make health care available through a universal tax system without the requirements of a means test. That is, recipients are not required to provide evidence or information concerning their financial resources to be eligible for service. All who have contributed to the Social Security system are eligible for Medicare on reaching age 65. In a limited sense, Medicare represents a policy and program in accordance with the view that modern industrial societies are responsible for meeting basic human needs through arrangements built into the institutional structure. However, coverage is limited and does not extend to many long-term health care needs. Based on the perspective developed in Chapter 1, which will be elaborated on in subsequent chapters, a number of glaring gaps are noted. Nowhere does the program truly tend to the long-term needs for services to support or supplement medical services. Failure to cover care in extended-care facilities or for supplementary services required by the elderly is a serious deficit. Reference was made (Chapter 1) to the fact that approximately 12% of those elderly who live at home need some assistance with their daily care needs. Except for those who are eligible for such services under Medicaid (to be described shortly) or those with adequate resources of their own, there is virtually no guarantee that these needs will be met.

Since physicians are allowed to bill for what they consider "reasonable charges," many people over 65 continue to be subject to certain indignities in their use of the program. Confronted with the sign "We do not accept Medicare assignments," many people sit in the waiting room, fretting and worrying about whether they can afford those extra charges. Perhaps they should "forget it" or go elsewhere. When they need eyeglasses, dental work, or hearing aids—as many elderly do—these indignities are compounded by having to meet the cost for these out of pocket. Since 25% of those over 65 are at or below poverty level, medical care is in fact not accessible independent of economic status. Those who must apply for Medicaid to supplement the care available under Medicare suffer all the degradation that relates to having to "prove" that one is worthy of assistance. In sum, the program falls far short of making the range of health services needed by the elderly accessible and comfortably available.

Medicaid. The Medicaid program, Title XIX of the Social Security Act, is a medical assistance program for those who demonstrate financial need. It is designed to provide care for low-income persons who are aged, blind, disabled, or members of families with dependent children. It is based on a federal-state matching formula, and states have the option not to participate. Some states have taken that option.* The federal portion of program costs ranges from 50% to 83%, with certain reductions being planned. Since states administer and operate their own programs, subject to federal guidelines, variability from state to state is extensive.

Eligibility for Medicaid assistance is tied to the levels pertaining for eligibility for Aid to Families with Dependent Children (AFDC) and the Federal Supplemental Security Income Program (SSI) for the aged, blind, and disabled. While all states cover those eligible for these categorical programs, they have the option to apply more restrictive criteria to SSI recipients.†

All states *must* offer the following services for those eligible: inpatient and outpatient hospital services; laboratory and x-ray services; skilled nursing care; home health services; health screening for those under 21 (early and periodic screening, diagnosis and treatment [EPSDT]); and family planning services, including needed supplies and physicians' services. They *may* pay for drugs, intermediate care facilities,‡ eyeglasses, and inpatient psychiatric care for people between 21 and 65. There are certain options, such as limiting the number of physicians' services or the number of days of hospital care for which payment will be made. States have leeway in the amount they reimburse providers.

Health care providers who agree to participate in the program are required to accept the amount of reimbursement provided by the state for federal services. The levels of reimbursement to physicians for services rendered to Medicaid patients are, in most instances, substantially below those they charge routinely, whether by fees paid directly by consumers or by other forms of third-party reimbursement. For these reasons many physicians take advantage of the option not to accept Medicaid patients. In fact, then, many low-income people do not have access to private health care providers.

A number of other types of problems are associated with the program. The low reimbursement rates, when compared to the fees customarily charged for similar services, invite abuse and there are frequent exposés of abuse. O'Sullivan (1981) points out that such abuse is much *more* extensive among those who *provide* than among those who *use* services. The "Medicaid mills" are a case in point. Centers set up to provide health services in communities largely inhabited by the poor, they process large numbers of people in a perfunctory manner. Since fees are charged on a "per visit" basis, many questionable repeat visits are scheduled. A number of examples can be cited. For example, an individual complaining of fever, sore throat, cough, and headaches usually has all necessary examinations performed in one visit. Medicaid patients may be

---

* As of November 1981, Arizona did not participate.

† Readers who are interested in knowing the requirements that pertain in their states should contact their state welfare offices and state legislators.

‡ Those facilities in which skilled nursing care is not essential.

asked to return "the next day" to have their throat checked. Former employees of methadone clinics attended by Medicaid recipients have told of being discouraged in their attempt to help people "get off the drug." The "cured addict" no longer needs regular visits.*

The varied and difficult eligibility requirements also make the program difficult to administer. Since eligibility is tied to actual receipt of public assistance (or financial eligibility for such assistance), many low-income people are not eligible. "Further, a person with a specified income could be eligible automatically for benefits in one state, forced to incur substantial medical expenses before gaining eligibility in a second state, and not be eligible at all in a third state" (O'Sullivan, 1981, p. CRS-11). For example, had Mr. Bernstein (whose situation was described at the beginning of this chapter) resided in another state, he might have been eligible for certain programs available under the Medicaid but not the Medicare program.

Further, primary emphasis has been on institutional rather than home care. Yet despite the high proportion of Medicaid monies allocated for institutional care, many in need of such care are not receiving it. Every hospital social worker can readily report on the substantial numbers of elderly waiting for a nursing home bed available to Medicaid-eligible people. Because levels of reimbursement for Medicaid-funded beds are low, many nursing home owners keep only a limited number of beds available for this population group. In Chapter 1 it was pointed out that close to 42% of payments are used for care in long-term institutions, compared with 1% for home health services. Only 5% of those over 65 are in institutions; however, 12% of those at home require some help to get about or get out of the house. How much more reasonable it would be to bring policy in line with prevailing need.

Assessment. The Medicaid program was, in part, intended to make fee-for-service, private medical care available to economically disadvantaged people who in the past had to rely on free services available in dreary clinics. Though this option is used, the stigma of poverty often haunts those who use private services. The process of establishing eligibility and identifying oneself as a "Medicaid patient" is not without its psychic costs. Clerks, receptionists, physicians, nurses, and other health care personnel are quick to recognize who "those people" are and can generate a rejecting and demeaning ambience.

• • •

The fact that the major portions of both Medicare and Medicaid are tied to "diseases" is indicative of some of the problems identified by Dana and others. The lack of fit between this approach and prevailing health problems has been touched on in Chapter 1 and is a major focus of discussion in Chapter 5. Surely

* Information based on papers written and reports made by students in my classes on health services.

a social work value perspective compels social work action designed to remedy the deficiencies of these programs.

Private health insurance. Private health insurance is a mechanism designed to cover the cost of inpatient and outpatient health services. Although they can be purchased privately, most plans are part of an employee benefits package negotiated between employers and employees. These plans mushroomed following World War II; union-management health and welfare funds have played a large part in their growth. By 1977, 88% of employees worked in firms that offered a health insurance plan. Those working in firms employing fewer than 26 people were least likely to have coverage. Of this group, 45%, or 9 million people, worked for employers who provided no coverage (*Health, United States,* 1981). Although an overwhelming number of workers and their dependents have some kind of coverage, such coverage can be tenuous. Job loss, death of an employed family member, divorce, and disability can leave people without coverage.

The rise in unemployment during the early 1980s showed how rapidly coverage can be lost. At this writing, legislation is pending to provide continuation of health coverage for those who lose their jobs.

The amount of coverage offered by private health insurance varies extensively. Some plans, such as "major medical coverage," pay up to 80% of all costs, including those incurred because of catastrophic illness; some plans barely cover a limited number of hospital days. Domestic workers and many people who by choice or necessity change jobs frequently are unlikely to be covered. It has been estimated that 25 million people, or approximately 12% of the population, have no health insurance protection through either private programs or the public programs that have been discussed (for example, Davis, 1983). Those with higher incomes are more likely to be covered.

• • •

Although each of the major financing provisions involves distinct patterns of coverage and guidelines, they clearly define some of the major parameters governing the delivery and use of health services. For the most part they are firmly based on a fee-for-service system in which time equals money. Further, money is more available for some services than for others. How this is played out in daily decisions about practice is illustrated later.

At present, there are increasing efforts to incorporate training on the social and emotional components of care into the education of physicians, especially those in the primary care specialties. Substantial numbers of such programs have social workers on the faculty so that they may contribute expertise in this area (Bracht, 1978). In studies focused on those involved in such programs, questions about how this training will be used in practice are often raised. Social workers and physicians alike frequently respond with cynicism or skepticism, saying, "It's all well and good; but nobody's paying us to listen, to make referrals to community resources, or to spend time with families explaining what's wrong. We get paid the same whether we spend ten minutes or even an hour. And we get paid for x-rays, and laboratory tests, and other procedures. And if we include social workers in our practice, they're going to have to generate fees to make their presence financially worthwhile" (Schlesinger, 1982).

These comments reflect in part on the fact that third-party reimbursement mechanisms (whether via Medicare, Medicaid, or private health insurance) are essentially limited in coverage to clearly designated "medical problems." They also point out that health care providers, especially physicians, benefit financially from these plans, which in turn give some direction to emphasis in the care rendered.

Clearly the present system has many flaws. Recognizing this, alternatives have long been proposed.

Proposals for comprehensive coverage for health services. There has been extensive debate in this country on the need for comprehensive national health insurance or a nationally based health service. At this writing it appears most unlikely that any proposal of major scope and substance will be enacted within the near future. A brief review of the major types of legislation introduced with some regularity is nevertheless indicated. Several major approaches are reflected in the proposals put forth.

1. Build on the present system, based on a mix of government programs and private insurance. For those who work, private insurance schemes would be retained, but employers would be required to offer insurance plans. Simultaneously, a uniform government program for the unemployed and the poor would be established, jointly financed and administered by federal and state governments. The Medicare program would be integrated into the government plan. Proposals of this type have been endorsed by the hospital industry, the commercial insurance companies, and some business groups.

2. Base the system on social insurance principles to cover the entire population, without differentiating between categories of people. These plans have been favored by the labor movement and would be financed by taxes on employers and employees and by contributions from general federal revenues; they would be federally administered.

3. Base the system on the principle that only illness of catastrophic dimensions, in which unusually high expenses are incurred, would be covered through government responsibility (Rice, 1977).

4. Create an independent federal agency to deliver health care. This approach is encompassed by the concept of a United States Health Service. Financed from a special health service tax or other revenues, this system would cover the spectrum of medical, preventive, occupational, and home health services. Community health boards, elected locally, would be responsible for the planning and operation of local systems (Klebe, 1982). The basic principles

involved in such a scheme have been endorsed by the National Association of Social Workers and the American Public Health Association. This endorsement is based on the assumption that inadequate financing is but one of many factors that contribute to the inequitable distribution of health care. A national health service, as envisioned in the proposed legislation, would link preventive and treatment services, involve lay persons and consumers in planning, and be organized around the particular needs encompassed by community and population groups.

Although a proposal such as the last one mentioned is even less likely to be enacted in the near future than the others, the basic conceptions involved bear close scrutiny by social workers. It is of some interest to note that Congressman Dellums, who has introduced legislation embodying the principles outlined, is a social worker. Also, though not a replica of the British National Health Service, the proposals draw heavily on the basic conceptions encompassed by that program. This fact—that such a program exists (albeit not without flaws) in a major western, industrialized nation—suggests that the conceptions do not represent the fantasies of some "wild-eyed liberals." Rather, as suggested earlier, this proposal involves a country's basic commitment—and choices—concerning how to respond to a universal human need.

Most American social workers who study the British program are immediately struck by the total access to care available to all and the fact that fee-for-service medical care plays a negligible role in British health care.*

HEALTH CARE COSTS

It is hardly possible to pick up a newspaper or a piece of scholarly or journalistic writing on health care that does not contain reference to the alarming increase in health care expenditures. A number of factors are said to be responsible for the increases: (1) the growth of private health insurance programs, (2) third-party payment mechanisms such as Medicaid and Medicare, (3) the growth in use and cost of hospital care, (4) the advances in medical technology that generate costly procedures, and (5) the increase in the proportion of the population over age 65. Important also is the fact that the availability of the previously mentioned public and private insurance mechanisms has increased the use of both hospital and ambulatory care services by the lowest income groups, who experience more illness than those with higher incomes.

A cursory review of the available data on the nature of cost increases

*This is notwithstanding the fact that recently there has been a small growth of private-sector medicine. Readers interested in a more detailed yet brief analysis of health care financing mechanisms and comparisons between the American and other systems may find the following of interest: Terris, M.: "The Three World Systems of Medical Care: Trends and Prospects," American Journal of Public Health **68**(11):1125, 1978; Stevens, R.: "Comparisons in Health Care: Britain As Contrasted to the United States." In Mechanic, D., editor: Handbook of Health, Health Care and the Health Professions, New York, 1983, The Free Press, pp. 281-304.

suggests why many view these with alarm. One way of examining these is to look at actual cost figures; a second is to compare the rate of increase in health care costs with those of other sectors of the economy. A third method of reviewing these data involves examining the proportion of the gross national product (GNP) accounted for by health care costs.* In 1982, $322 billion was spent on health care in the United States (Davis, 1983). Data presented in 1981 and 1982 showed $286 billion annual expenditures (*Health, United States,* 1982), $104 billion of which was taken from public funds (*Health, United States,* 1981). The average per person expenditure was $1,225.

Health care costs have increased at a faster rate than costs in other sectors. They have been rising at an average annual rate of over 11% during the past 20 years, thus claiming an increasing share of the gross national product. This phenomenon is also observed in other western industrialized countries (*Health, United States,* 1981). Between 1979 and 1982 "health spending increased by 50 percent—considerably faster than either inflation in the economy or growth in family incomes," (Davis, 1983, p. D2).

Expenditure for Medicare and Medicaid increased from $51 billion in 1979 to $83 billion in 1982. "One in 10 families representing 18 million people, spent more than 10% of its income on health care. More than 3 million families, or 7.6 million people, had truly catastrophic out-of-pocket expenses exceeding 20 percent of family income" (Davis, 1983, p. D2). These trends have accelerated efforts to curb the rising costs of health care.

Cost control efforts

Efforts to reduce the cost of health care, especially that portion financed by the varying levels of government, are commanding considerable attention. They are diverse and variously targeted at finding ways by which (1) the consumer's share of costs is increased; (2) the consumer's propensity to use services is reduced; (3) the provider's incentive to provide excessive care—especially hospital care—is reduced; and (4) care can be reorganized to provide quality service in a more efficient, cost-effective manner. In this brief discussion, emphasis is on a few of those proposals and mechanisms that clearly have an impact on those groups of consumers of special concern to social workers—the poor, the elderly, and the chronically disabled.

Increasing the consumer's share of costs. Review of material issued by the Congressional Research Service (Markus and O'Sullivan, 1983; O'Sullivan, 1983) points to a series of already enacted or proposed changes in Medicare and Medicaid provisions that increase the cost to the consumers of care or impose charges for services previously covered without costs. For example, proposals by the federal government call for new cost-sharing requirements for

* The following data are those available as of November, 1983. Given the rapidly changing picture, some of these figures will be outdated by the time of publication. They are, nevertheless, presented to give the reader a sense of the nature and pace of cost increases.

the first 60 days of inpatient care by Medicare recipients. Other proposals would mandate states to impose some charges on Medicaid recipients for physician and hospital services. Such charges were initially prohibited.

While extensive analysis is not possible here, the materials prepared by the Congressional Research Service clearly outline efforts to increase the share of costs paid by those consumers who can least afford to pay. Although few would question the need to control escalating health care costs, developments of the type reviewed here are of major concern to health care social workers. The brunt of these efforts should not be borne by the poor elderly, Medicaid recipients, and others most in need. In their role as policy analysts and systems change agents, health care social workers need to take an active role in assessing and making efforts to reverse these thrusts.

Reducing the propensity to use and provide services. Reference was made to the view that all third-party payment mechanisms are thought to increase costs because neither consumers nor providers have direct incentives to reduce or keep costs down. Hospital expenditures are thought to be particularly high. For these reasons, alternate mechanisms for reimbursing hospitals for patient stays were instituted in October, 1983.

A major departure from past practice that relates to the cost of hospital care for Medicare recipients is the development of a prospective payment system for hospital reimbursement implemented in October, 1983. Hospitals are reimbursed on the basis of length of stay expected for specific diagnoses using a diagnosis-related group (DRG) system rather than one based on the actual length of stay. A variant of this system has been operative for some years in New Jersey hospitals for all patients. These reimbursement formulas are intended to provide incentives to reduce length of stay and thereby hospital costs. Under the new system the reimbursement rate is essentially the same if the length of stay for a designated diagnosis is exceeded or reduced, thus creating the incentive for shortening hospital stays.

It is too early to assess the social impact of this new hospital reimbursement mechanism. As a New Jersey resident and social work educator, I have obtained informal reactions of some New Jersey hospital social work directors. A number find that the pressure for early discharge—without adequate consideration of psychosocial issues—has been accelerated. Others agree with this but find that the new system poses a challenge for social work and facilitates creative discharge planning initiated early in the patient's hospital stay. Obviously reduction in the number of hospital days, without a commensurate increase in posthospital services (whether community or institutionally based), can only intensify the problems of those elderly needing long-term care. Socially oriented early planing for hospital care after discharge is thought to aid in the hospital's effort to reduce length of stay. Social work, through its involvement in discharge planning, can play a key role in this component of cost control efforts. Social work must develop knowledge and strategies to respond to this development.

Reorganization of care: the case of HMOs. In the prevailing fee-for-service care system, physicians and other providers benefit financially when the number of patient visits is high. One potential solution to this cost-escalating structure of care is the health maintenance organization (HMO). Luft (1983) summarizes the essential features of this concept of prepaid care. The HMO (1) assumes contractual responsibility for providing care to enrollees on a prepaid basis; (2) serves defined populations who are enrolled voluntarily; (3) requires fixed periodic payment independent of use of services; and (4) assumes some financial risk in the provision of services. The services may be provided by group medical practices (that may include social workers); by individual practitioners who contract to provide services for enrollees, as in individual practice associations (IPAs); or by unions, universities, and other organizations. The prepayment mechanism alters the usual economic incentives and gives providers a stake in keeping costs down. "A review of all substantive research on health-care expenditures leads to the general conclusion that HMO enrollees have lower total expenditures for medical care . . . than comparable people with conventional insurance coverage" (Luft, 1983, p. 322). By July 1980, 9 million Americans were enrolled in these programs. Whether they will grow, maintain the lower costs, and provide care of equal quality relative to other modes of care are matters of continuing inquiry. As is the case with the prospective reimbursement rates for hospitals, social workers will want to ascertain whether the psychosocial components of care receive sufficient attention and whether those population groups in special need of care benefit from this form of delivery (Chapter 11).

Perspectives on health care costs

In considering the impact of the various cost-control proposals and whether alarm about the rising costs of health care is justified, social workers need to consider a number of questions:

1. How do rising health expenditures compare with costs for other sectors of the economy that benefit the standard of living—those for education, housing, welfare, and reduction of environmental wastes?

2. Who will bear the brunt of the various cost control measures already initiated or now being proposed—relatively high paid providers, such as physicians, or the most needy segments of the population?

3. How do total health expenditures compare with expenditures for a burgeoning defense industry?

4. Of the total health care package cost, what is the relative benefit for each sector of the population? For example, how much of the increase in prices in a 15-year period is accounted for by high profits for suppliers (for example, of hospital equipment or pharmaceuticals) and how much by wage increases for semi-skilled hospital employees? The latter have traditionally represented one of the more underpaid employee groups. Successful unionizing drives in

some sections of the country have resulted in wage increases, thus adding to the cost of care.

5. Within the health sector, what is the distribution of costs between such areas as preventive care, "disease-oriented technology intensive care" (the benefits of which are not thoroughly understood), and long-term, humane, supportive care, such as home health care or community supportive services for the deinstitutionalized population, the elderly, and others.

I have already considered many of these questions. Prevailing financing mechanisms funnel disproportionate amounts of money into hospital-based care, nursing home care, and care that is "technology intensive." Proportionately less money is spent on home care and community services for varying segments of the disabled and elderly populations.

There is no clear-cut answer as to whether the services currently underfunded "deserve" higher priority than those more generously funded, assuming the same availability of funding. Specifically, should there be more cautious use of respirators for people who clearly are going to die? Or should funds be cut back for hospital-based kidney dialysis treatment in favor of less costly home-based treatment, as has been proposed (*The New York Times,* July 31, 1983)? Should the funds saved in these areas be diverted to long-term care and other areas currently being underfunded? Are current health needs in the areas of prevention, treatment, and long-term care sufficiently great to warrant increases in expenditures relative to expenditures for other sectors of the economy? Fuchs (1974) suggests that the answer to each of these and related questions entails a choice; choosing one, we must accord lower priority to another, given a finite set of resources.

No textbook can presume to provide answers to each set of questions. Rather, these questions are presented to alert health care social workers to the kind of issues they will confront when making decisions. Further, these questions point to the areas of resource deficits that social workers face daily in their work, such as the shortage of nursing home beds, few home health aides, lack of community services for the disabled, inadequate transportation for costly treatment, inadequate funds for screening for hypertension and diabetes, and underfunded, understaffed social work departments. Much of the discussion of rising health expenditures masks these and related issues. To make the choices they must make, social workers need to know about sources of costs and be committed to specific values that will guide decisions about financial allocations. Such allocations always involve setting implicit or explicit priorities.

HEALTH CARE DELIVERY SETTINGS

The review of health financing mechanisms and health care costs has pointed to the mix between public and private responsibility that characterizes financing of health care. This mix also exists in relation to the sponsorship and nature of health service settings.

Fuchs (1974) has commented on this, suggesting that these patterns:

> Reflect the diversity and pluralism characteristic of American life in general. Unlike the small homogeneous democracies of Western Europe or the large centrally controlled nations such as the USSR and China, the United States has refrained from establishing a national medical care system (pp. 128-129).

Because of the pluralistic nature of health service systems, they are not easy to classify.

Inpatient and ambulatory care settings

One distinction that can be made is between care provided on an inpatient basis and that delivered on an ambulatory basis. Inpatient care is provided in hospitals, nursing homes, personal care homes that do not involve extensive nursing care, group homes for the mentally retarded, and large state institutions. To this list must be added the growing number of institutionally based hospice programs that provide inpatient care for the terminally ill, adhering to a particular philosophical stance about how to make the terminal phase of illness most comfortable for the dying and their families.

Ambulatory services are extremely varied. Physicians practicing alone or in groups on a fee-for-service basis represent the most common pattern. Most hospitals have ambulatory care centers or outpatient clinics. Health maintenance organizations, which are designed to provide comprehensive care to subscribers who pay a fixed fee in advance are recent developments, on the increase, that are intended to deal with the problems of cost and fragmented care. These, like other special programs, usually involve many disciplines, including social workers. Important among the ambulatory facilities that have developed in the last 15 years or so are neighborhood or community health centers and community mental health centers. Much of the care rendered in these types of facilities is characterized as primary care.

It is almost impossible to provide an exhaustive or logically organized listing of the variety of settings outside the hospital where ambulatory health care is provided. Major among these are (1) the physician's office and (2) ambulatory care centers such as community health centers and health maintenance organizations. Family planning clinics, well baby clinics, abortion centers, free clinics, and mental health centers are also among the better known health service centers.

Many, but not all, of these focus on efforts to provide front-line, first-contact care. With few exceptions they are staffed by multidisciplinary health workers, including social workers.

Personal health services

Personal health services include (1) hospital services; (2) physicians' services; (3) the services of such personnel as physical therapists and social workers; (4) nursing services; and (5) services connected with provision of appliances and medication. To the list developed by Anderson and Anderson (1979) should be added those that complement, supplement, and sometimes precede, in time or importance, those focused on medical care: home health services, health education, outreach to populations at risk for particular health problems, and prevention focused on the hazards related to the workplace. Although some of these are difficult to locate by "delivery site," they have been frequently identified as crucial health care activities.

Not to be neglected are the services provided by self-help groups, ranging from Alcoholics Anonymous to those developed by cancer patients or people with various physical disabilities. Informal networks, based on membership in communities of residence or church or based on ethnic group membership, often play a vital role in health promotion and care.

A public health perspective and major public health services

A public health or population perspective derives "from the wide range of continuing concerns for morbidity and disability and the means for prolonging and improving life. The preoccupation over the past few decades has been with the vulnerable sectors of the national population—the people at risk—and with means of identifying, treating and educating them" (Wittman, 1978, p. 203). This approach is of increasing conceptual and strategic importance in health care social work. The view that health care social work is responsible for, and accountable to, diverse population groups is a fundamental theme of this book; the basic rationale and conceptualization encompassed by this view are elaborated in Chapter 5, which is devoted to conceptual approaches to health care social work practice. In this chapter, focused on prevailing health policy, organization, and financing, the discussion is limited to a few major public health services.

Public health services are extensive and multifaceted. According to Anderson and Anderson (1979), they traditionally include services provided for populations as a group without special regard for individual needs or differences. Some are carried out under the auspices of the United States Public Health Service, whereas many are administered by state departments of public health. Among these services are the better known programs to assure a sanitary environment with pure air, water, and food and the well-known efforts to control communicable disease through mass immunizations. In addition, a range of public health programs are targeted to special population groups, for example, programs to identify and refer people with hypertension and diabetes for treatment, programs focused on prevention of alcoholism that provide genetic screening, and programs in the area of maternal and child health, which are outlined here in more detail to show a major involvement of social work.

Insley (1977) traces the history of public health programs in maternal and child health and points to social work's extensive involvement. A long-standing focus of these programs has been on health promotion and prevention, with less emphasis on medical care. Of particular concern have been programs to educate the public on the importance of prenatal care, child development, accident prevention, and nutrition. The Children's Bureau, created in 1912 "to investigate and report on all matters pertaining to the welfare of children and child life among all classes of our people," is still active. It has been involved in research and in the development of training programs to provide coordinated health, educational, and social services for young mothers and their children. Special nutrition projects, for example, Women's and Infant Care, (WIC) designed to assure adequate nutrition for women and infants, are efforts to promote public health.

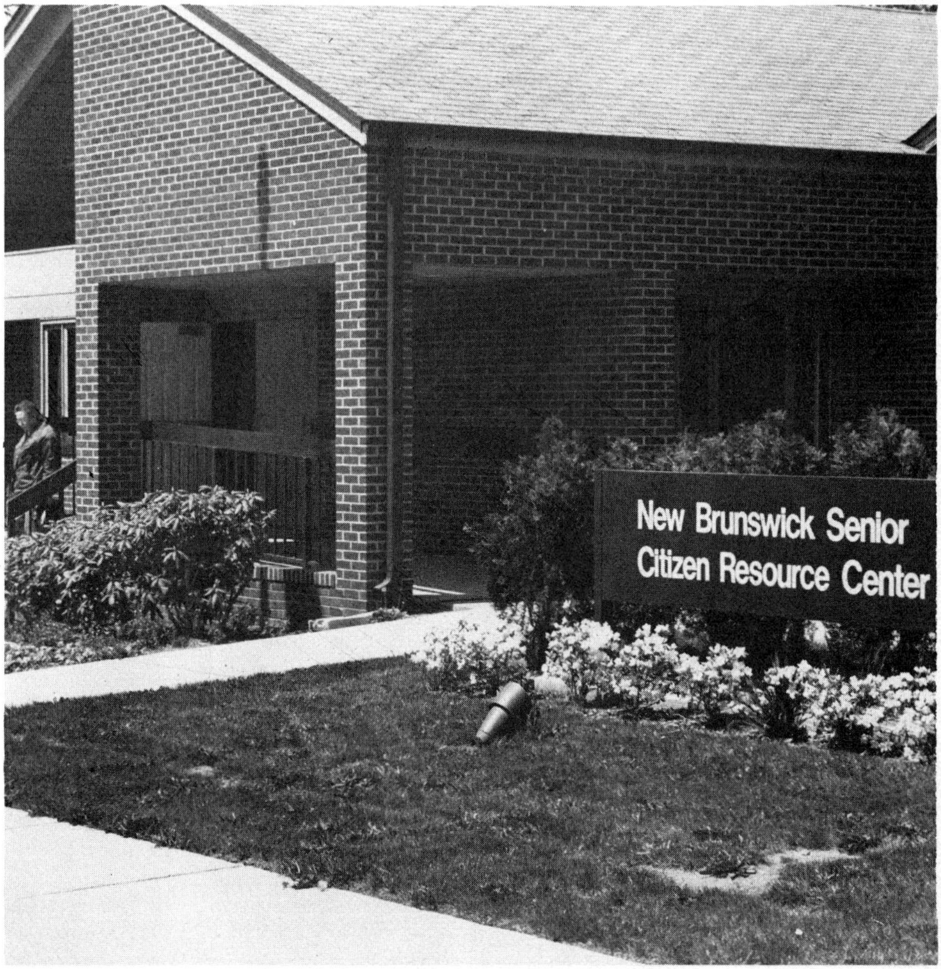

Watkins and Player (1981) point to the role of maternal and child health care in reducing infant mortality and developing guidelines for family planning. A comprehensive, integrated approach to service is emphasized.

Maternal and child health services are provided in various health settings, including the private and public ambulatory facilities discussed earlier, where direct services are provided. State health departments and centralized regional offices carry out planning. Watkins and Player (1981) point to the integration of direct services and program planning that characterizes efforts in this field.

> The use of direct-service interventions in combination with program planning or administrative services is a common occurrence in maternal and child health. Social workers in this field of practice frequently use the public health approach and focus on the improvement of the health status of the community. Social workers involved in direct services to individuals, families, and groups often use their knowledge of the etiology and impact of the health condition to plan changes in the health and welfare systems of the community (p. 465).*

Thus efforts directed at enhancing knowledge, health services, and changing dysfunctional behaviors have joined earlier public health efforts focused on sanitation, sewage, and water supplies.

As social workers explore the contribution to health of these and other settings, they will find enormous potential for dealing with the various health problems identified in Chapter 1. Family planning clinics, for example, work with those who want to limit their families; they pay special attention to young people, who are at particular risk for having premature newborns or children with whom they are not equipped to cope. "Free clinics" sprang up during the sixties in response to what many young people perceived as depersonalized, mechanized care. Home health services, to which reference has been repeatedly made, are crucial. To qualify for reimbursement under the Medicare and Medicaid legislation, home services must offer skilled nursing care plus one other therapeutic service, such as physical therapy, speech therapy, occupational therapy, or social work.

Other settings and modalities have already been mentioned. They all bear on social work's concern with health care.

HEALTH CARE PERSONNEL

The list of those who provide health care is extensive and includes not only those professionals of whom we customarily think when talking about health care personnel. People who sit at reception desks, who bring food to patients confined to hospital beds, and who service emergency medical transport units all comprise the vast health care work force that includes over 4 million individuals.

Limitations of space and time as well as a parsimonious approach to analysis of the issues of major concern to health care social workers necessitate a limited focus. In this section, I will discuss physicians, nurses, and social workers, commenting on how many there are, how they are distributed in the health care system, and what education and training are involved. It is almost impossible to consider the distribution of health care personnel without mentioning the hierarchical relationships between them. The work of other health professionals and social work's relationship with them will surface throughout the remainder of the book.

Physicians

"Medical dominance" and concerns about the negative impact of such dominance on health, as contrasted with medical care, are central in much social work literature on health care. Considerable literature implicitly or explicitly characterizes physicians as the central villains in the faulty drama of health care as we know it. Yet much of the preceding discussion has suggested that considerably more is at stake. If physicians can be faulted—and in many respects they can—the root causes are many. First, the system grants physicians control over matters about which they claim limited competence; second, an educational system focuses their energies into narrow channels; and third, payment mechanisms reward a narrow range of functions.

However, at present physicians generally function as "captains of the health care team." Social workers cannot understand, function in, or hope to change the prevailing health care delivery system without information concerning physicians' social role.

Many aspects of this role and its origin are analyzed in detail in Chapter 5, which distinguishes between cure and care and discusses the dysfunctional aspects of the medical model. Some data on basic physician characteristics and dimensions are presented after a look at specifics of the physician population.

In 1980 there were 426,350 practicing physicians in the United States. This represents a 34% increase over the period 1970 to 1980. Past and projected increases suggest that by 1990 there will be about as many physicians for every 10,000 people as are needed. Thus there is no anticipated shortage of physicians, a sharp contrast with the past when major physician shortages were identified. Despite these optimistic estimates about availability, there is concern, especially involving distribution both by specialty and by urban-rural location. Also problematic is the fact that a relatively small number of physicians are drawn from the ranks of women and minorities (*Health, United States,* 1980).

Problems in distribution

Primary care and specialized physicians. Understanding the distinctions between primary care and specialized physicians and the implications for social workers relies on identifying specific terms and roles. The concept of *primary care* has been evolving and shifting in health care services organization and delivery, complicated by the difficulty of defining primary care physicians as distinct from primary care services and primary care problems (*Interim Report,* 1979, p. 27). The Health Professions Educational Assistance Act of 1976 defined those physicians engaged in the practice of family medicine, general internal medicine, and general pediatrics as primary care specialists.

Over a period of years, a number of developments converged to reduce the number of physicians engaged in primary or first-contact comprehensive care. By 1969 close to 40% of physicians were engaged in primary care practice, and approximately 60% were classified as specialists. Although this figure has not changed perceptibly to date, several federal initiatives have led to increased numbers of medical school graduates preparing for primary care practice. A 75% increase in primary care physicians is expected by 1990, which is more in line with projected need (*Interim Report,* 1979).

The types of specialized physicians and the various kinds of specialty practice in which they engage are extensive and varied. Approximately 5% are engaged in branches of internal medicine not considered a part of primary care, 27.7% are in various surgical specialties, and 27% practice other specialties. Among these latter specialties 7% are psychiatrists, less than 1% are engaged in occupational medicine, and 1% are public health physicians.

What, then, are the areas of concern involving these two groups of physicians? At a fundamental level, primary care physicians are more likely oriented to comprehensive, preventive care. As suggested in the discussion of prevailing health problems, many specialists, despite their skill, are unable to "cure" many of the major health problems. There is therefore a discrepancy between the knowledge of specialized physicians and the approach required to manage contemporary health problems.

At another level, the optimistic projections for availability of primary care physicians mask some underlying difficulties. Though internists are classified as primary care physicians, many subspecialize and perforce focus on what Dana terms "organ-oriented care." Still other developments suggest a move toward comprehensive care. For example, by 1973, 75% of medical schools had divisions of family medicine. A specialty board in family medicine has also been established. There were 5,400 family practice residents in training and 11,000 physicians certified by the American Board of Family Practice. This group of physicians is committed to a holistic concept of health care. Eduction in the behavioral sciences, in identification of psychosocial problems, and in the skills of managing these areas is required graduate medical education in family practice (Schlesinger, 1982).

Incomes between primary care physicians and those engaged in specialties differ substantially. Data for 1975 show that radiologists had the highest median incomes, followed by surgeons. The lowest median incomes were earned by general practitioners, pediatricians, and psychiatrists (*Interim Report,* 1979). The fact that radiologists are least involved with care and rely on extensive new technology suggests the relatively low value placed on diagnostic and direct patient care skills and the high value assigned to skills in mastering emerging technology.

Finally specialists in physical medicine and rehabilitation can contribute much to the rehabilitation of stroke victims, yet they constitute less than 1% of practicing physicians. The formation of the Graduate Medical Education National Advisory Committee to the Secretary of the Department of Health, Education and Welfare in 1975 was one response to this "alleged physician specialty maldistribution" (p. v).

Geographical distribution. It has frequently been noted that physicians tend to cluster in urban areas. In the 1970s, 87% of all physicians were located in the 300 major metropolitan counties where 75% of the population resides. There were 145 counties, mostly sparsely populated, that had no physicians. Although primary care physicians represent a higher proportion of physicians in the sparsely populated states, the proportion is still low. People in rural areas are relatively underserved both in primary and in specialized care.

Representation of women and minorities among physicians. Although the numbers of women and minority member physicians have increased, their numbers still fall well below what might be expected, given their representation in the population. By 1977 only 7% of all practicing physicians were women. Despite a sharp increase in female enrollment in medical schools, it is expected that by 1990 women will constitute only 16% of the physician labor force. From 1980 to 1981, 5.7% of students enrolled in American medical schools were Black, and 4.2% were Hispanic (*Health of Minorities and Women,* 1982). Although these figures represent increases over past trends, they hardly point to a situation in which women and minority members will be represented in proportion to their numbers in this prestigious profession.

The nature of medical practice: physicians' autonomy and social workers. The context, organization, and nature of medical practice have been studied extensively (Freidson, 1979; Fuchs, 1974; Mechanic, 1979). Freidson (1979) points out that physicians place a high premium on professional autonomy and independent decision making. Studies of medical education show that learning to assume ultimate responsibility for personal decisions is a basic norm stressed in medical training (Becker and others, 1961).

Many factors increasingly mitigate against physicians' ability to exercise total authority over their work. The growing role of the hospital, the prevalence of group practice, the increased role of nonphysician providers (including social workers), and a technology that compels dependence on others converge to diminish that control. Yet social workers who work with physicians feel physicians' actions are consonant with a perspective suggesting the physician is in charge. Such a sense is perhaps best illustrated when aspects of physician control are removed by legal or organizational mandate. In England social workers have been granted considerable authority involving involuntary commitment of mental patients. In exercising that authority they sometimes clash with physicians. Interviews with British social workers and physicians suggest physicians are less than benign about this state of affairs; as stated by one British general practitioner, "You know how we doctors are. We don't like the idea that anybody can tell us what to do" (Schlesinger, 1982). Physician authority and dominance are crucial in contemporary health care delivery.

Authority is evident, not in numbers but in the prestige and impact physicians have on other segments of the health care delivery system. Fuchs (1974) identifies physicians' influence on the cost of care as reflected in volume of surgery performed, number of hospital admissions, number of prescriptions written, and types of procedures carried out. To illustrate, only about 8% of the 4.5 million Americans employed in health services delivery are physicians, and only 20% of health care costs reimbursed physicians for their services. Hospital care and drugs account for approximately half of health care expenditures, and these expenses are incurred almost directly as a result of decisions made by physicians (Fuchs, 1974).

Mechanic (1979) points to influences in yet other respects:

> They have vast control over the organization and provision of all medical services and the work settings of most other health professionals. Also disproportionate is their influence on health and social policies because of their high social status and their network of interest groups which serve political as well as professional purposes (p. 177).

Physician autonomy and prestige have impact on the work of other health professionals as well as on consumers of health care. Old approaches to work, some of them myths, "die hard":

> The stereotypical mode of medical practice in the United States is "solo practice"—a person working by himself in an office that he equips with his own capital, treating patients who have chosen him as their personal physician and for whom he assumes responsibility. He usually has no formal connection with colleagues (Freidson, 1979, p. 299).

The solo, fee-for-service practitioner, though by no means extinct, is no longer the only mode of medical practice. Increasingly physicians practice in groups and function as salaried employees of hospitals. By the mid-1970s close to 24% of physicians were in group practice (*Health, United States,* 1979), a dramatic increase.

There have been many incursions on physician autonomy. One stems from efforts to reduce health care costs. Health maintenance organizations reduce physician-induced costs (*Health, United States,* 1981) and minimize autonomy. Professional standards review organizations (PSROs), mandated by federal law in 1972 to review services provided under Medicare, Medicaid, and maternal and child health programs, were to determine whether services financed by these programs were medically necessary, provided in accordance with professional standards, and rendered in appropriate settings (O'Sullivan, 1981), also providing a check on the autonomous practitioner. Various schemes for setting reimbursement rates in hospitals and for review of utilization procedures have similarly affected autonomy. When physicians work together in groups, formal or informal mechanisms are set into play whereby they review each other's work. Other team members are also in a position to reflect on their work. When third parties pay substantial portions of the fees incurred by patients (as in the case of Medicare, Medicaid, and private insurance), they are in a position to exercise some control over quantity and perhaps quality of care.

Medical practice is, then, a changing phenomenon, and the physician who truly works in isolation is increasingly rare.

> As the images of medicine change, younger physicians may see organized practice as more rewarding and less frustrating. And medical organizations will develop new ways of coping with the frustrations of bureaucracy and with new types of patient relationships. Transitions are usually slow and difficult due to the resistance of the old guard. Yet, medical science and technology have gone too far to easily accommodate the physician as an entrepreneur. Like an old soldier, he is unlikely to die soon but will slowly fade away (Mechanic, 1979, p. 190).

It is important that social workers understand and recognize the prevailing sources of physician autonomy and control so as to distinguish between those areas where such control is legitimate and those where it derives from political and economic forces that bear limited relationship to quality patient care.

Understanding can also help to avoid petulance and the sense of being unloved or misunderstood that health care social workers often experience when working with physicians. It can also facilitate social workers' efforts to assert their own professional autonomy and expertise in areas where legitimate claim can be made. For example, claim can be made about social work's ability to make judgments about the geographical distribution of physicians, the need for greater representation of women and minorities, the need for mechanisms to monitor the cost and quality of care, and the need for care not part of the physician's expertise. As the discussion focuses on the issues involved in health and illness behavior (Chapters 3 and 4) and on the increased need for a caring stance by health professionals, the legitimacy of social work's claim for autonomy in other areas will become clear.

Nurses

Few people think about health care delivery without an image of the nurse—clad in white, efficient, attentive, always ministering to the needs of those in hospitals, physicians' offices, and, not infrequently, the home. The word *nurse* is derived from the Latin *nutriere,* meaning to nourish or suckle. By the eighteenth century, the term had "crystalized to mean a person, generally a woman, who attended or waited upon the sick." Hence this link to female role images has persisted throughout history, even though men have been involved in nursing tasks since the Crusades (Reeder and Mauksch, 1979, p. 210).

The history of nursing is closely tied to Florence Nightingale and her activities in the Crimean War. The efforts emanating from her work brought the role of the nurse into association with that of the physician. Closely related is the history of physician control and jurisdiction over nursing activities.

The "employed nursing labor force" in the United States can be characterized in numerous ways. One focuses on distinctions between levels of education and training. Thus from one perspective only those nurses who have undergone professional training are included in the term. Others researchers include nursing aides, orderlies, attendants, and home health aides among the nursing labor force. They estimate the nursing labor force to be 48% of the total health care labor force (Cannings and Lazonick, 1975). Assigning numbers to these percentages, in the United States there are over 1 million registered nurses and 400,000 practical nurses (*Health, United States,* 1979). Clearly, nurses and the more inclusively conceived nursing labor force constitute a major segment of the health care labor force.

Reeder and Mauksch (1979) identify three educational routes by which people can become registered nurses: (1) a 4-year baccalaureate program; (2) a 2-year associate degree program; or (3) a 2- or 3-year diploma-granting hospital program. During past years, nurse practitioner training programs have proliferated. This training, available to those who are already registered nurses, involves work for either a master's degree or a certificate.

Recent developments in nursing education have intensified efforts to increase the numbers of nurse practitioners. With these developments it is estimated that by 1990 there will be over 38,000 trained nurse practitioners (*Health, United States,* 1979). These efforts in part derive from the primary care shortages that still exist. Nurse practitioners, along with other nonphysician health care providers (particularly physicians' assistants), are "individuals who have been trained to perform tasks that have traditionally been performed only by physicians, such as taking a complete medical history or performing a routine physical examination" (*Health, United States,* 1979). When functioning as nonphysician health care providers, nurse practitioners operate in expanded nursing roles. They may, in addition to certain medical functions, provide counseling, guidance, and emotional support and coordinate health and social service resources.

Despite the expansion of some nursing roles and a thrust for autonomy, a number of studies suggest that the physician remains the leader of the team or the "superconsultant" (Brody, 1976; Zola and Miller, 1973). In the introduction to this section, reference was made to the fact that nursing is identified as a woman's profession that has traditionally functioned in a subservient role in relation to physicians. Reeder and Mauksch (1979), Lurie (1981), and others have commented on the persistent struggle for autonomy and the greater collegial relations with physicians in which the nursing profession has been engaged. Though traditional work relations are bureaucratic (both within nursing and in nurses' relationship to other professionals, mainly physicians), a number of developments have expanded diagnostic, treatment, and patient care education functions carried out by nurses. One study of a nurse practitioner training program (Lurie, 1981) found that the program emphasized the importance of patient education, counseling, and psychosocial care functions.

Like the other health professionals nurses confront issues of specialization and efforts to carve out work roles consonant with levels of training and patient care needs. Promotion, or further education, is often equated with carrying out fewer "bedside" nursing tasks. The increase in the number of nurse practitioners suggests that some nurses are moving into counseling roles that social work has long considered as falling in its domain.

This movement entails some strain, turf battles, and blurring of functions between nurses and social workers. As schools of nursing increase the portion of their curriculum devoted to psychosocial issues and skills, some nurses view themselves as capable of carrying on traditional social work roles. As nurses' training expands to include attention to the social components of care, some role blurring is inevitable. Public health nurses are familiar with community resources. Psychiatric nurses have considerable skill in managing patients with severe emotional disturbance. Inevitably, some strains surface. Too often, efforts to carve out complementary areas of function—and to live comfortably with the overlap where such exists—are diminished, and attention instead is focused on irritants that increase the strain. Banta and Fox (1972) report that nurses on a team found social workers unwilling to communicate readily about clients.

Some nurses resent what they perceive to be the relatively leisurely pace at which social workers function. This is understandable when, as is the case in one home health agency, social workers are expected to make five home visits per week; nurses, by contrast, make six per day. In turn, some social workers have a view of nurses as authoritarian and bureaucratic, more concerned with patient care routines than with feelings. On several occasions, when I have engaged my students in role play, they have portrayed the nurse as an unfeeling partner on the health team.

The work of nurses and social workers is an essential component of the health care system. Therefore social work educators and practitioners need to take the lead in finding the means to develop greater clarity and knowledge of the respective roles. The development of harmonious working relationships that promote effective patient care is crucial.

Social workers

Medical social services have been an integral part of health services since 1905 when Dr. Richard Cabot "recognized the need to add another dimension to patient care through a deeper understanding of a patient's social situation as it affected his total medical problems" (Phillips, 1977), p. 615). Since then social work has been an integral part of health services in hospitals, departments of health, maternal and child health services, primary care centers, and nursing homes. Increasing numbers of social workers function as faculty members in medical schools and in other centers for the education of health professionals. Their roles are diverse, including the provision of direct service, consultation, planning, and administration.

Bracht (1978), drawing on a variety of data, points out the following:

1. As of 1974, 40,000 social workers were estimated to be employed in various facets of health care. Approximately one third of all members of the National Association of Social Workers identify themselves as being employed in the health and mental health field.
2. As of 1976, one half of the nation's hospitals provided social services. In this connection it should be noted that the Joint Commission on Accreditation of Hospitals now mandates social work services in accredited hospitals. Hospitals are the largest employers of social workers (Phillips, 1977).
3. The Veterans Administration has a long tradition of employing social workers in its hospitals and other health service centers.
4. A 1976 study showed that social workers represented the largest employed group of professional staff in federally funded health planning agencies. To this should be added that as of 1980* one half of the directors of health systems agencies (HSAs), which are federally mandated health planning bodies, were social workers.
5. Social workers account for 42% of the staff of all mental health facilities. Psychiatrists, psychologists, and psychiatric nurses constitute much smaller percentages of the staffs of such facilities.
6. The number of social workers who hold appointments as faculty members in schools of medicine, dentistry, nursing, public health, and other health professions schools has increased substantially.

* Data based on presentation by Stanley Matek, Council on Social Work Education Annual Program Meeting, Los Angeles, Calif., Spring 1980.

7. Social work participation in centers providing renal dialysis is federally mandated.
8. Social workers work in the armed forces and hold administrative and planning positions in the Department of Health and Human Services.

Their past and present participation in public health activities has already been noted.

As Bracht (1978) suggests, today it is far easier to point to areas where social workers are not involved in health care delivery than to areas where they participate actively.

Presently the educational levels of social workers involved in health care vary from those with no professional education to a few who have doctoral degrees. Three basic levels of professional social work education are identified: (1) the bachelor's (BSW) level, (2) the master's (MSW) level, and (3) the doctoral (DSW or Ph.D.) level. Bachelor's level education is by definition education for generalist practice involving training for provision of services to individuals, families, and groups. Training at the master's level is organized by focus on the needs of population groups, on social problems, or on social work methods (Council on Social Work Education, 1982). Those who hold doctoral degrees function as social work educators, researchers, and often administrators of social work departments in prestigious teaching hospitals and other health care settings. Many of the groundbreaking contributions to social work in health care cited throughout this book have been made by doctoral-level social workers.

At all levels of education, but especially at the advanced levels, social work function increasingly includes involvement in research. The need for more research on health care social work is pressing. Some of the knowledge gaps and fruitful areas for inquiry are identified in Chapter 12.

A note on coverage for social work services. Before concluding these remarks, some comments on financing of social work services in health care are in order. The discussion on Medicare, Medicaid, and private health insurance has reviewed, in broad outline, those health services that tend to be reimbursed by the various programs. The reader will have noted that nowhere was reference made to reimbursement for social work services. For the most part, such services, when rendered by varying health care institutions, are paid for out of a general budget and not directly reimbursed, although there are some exceptions.

Third-party reimbursement for social work services is viewed by many as a desirable goal. Many believe that there would be several potential advantages if social work services in hospitals and other health care institutions were directly reimbursed. The financial benefits that acrue to health care organizations from social work services would be readily demonstrable. Social workers engaged in private practices would have the costs of their services reimbursed.

But some view such possibilities with skepticism. Reichert (1983) points out that the National Association of Social Workers (NASW) public policy statements oppose fee-for-service medical practice, while promoting fee-for-service practice in social work. He suggests that this intrusion of market mechanisms into social work delivery may be antithetical to basic social work tenets.

Given the uneven, patchwork nature of present financing mechanisms, social work's efforts to have its services recognized by financial remuneration analogous to those available to other providers are not surprising. Particular efforts have been made supporting inclusion of social workers as third-party venders of psychotherapeutic services. Without such inclusion, social workers in private practice must often refer clients to other professionals whose services are reimbursed. Currently reimbursement is available for psychiatrists and psychologists, yet these social workers, ineligible for reimbursement, provide the bulk of mental health services in transitional facilities for the mentally ill. Although the picture is changing, Blue Cross, Medicaid, and private insurance carriers have been opposed to reimbursement for social work services. The stated reasons are that there are not sufficient standards governing the title and practice of social work.

Health care social work specialization. Health care social workers, like physicians and other health care professionals, are confronted with decisions about specialized as contrasted with generalized practice. A recent issue of *Health and Social Work* (Specialization, 1981) was devoted to "specialization and specialty interests." In the introduction to that issue the editor points out that "social workers have engaged in more than a half century of dialogue about what makes them the same and different from each other" (Kane, 1981, p. 25). This book is written because I share the view that "at this juncture, health is recognized as an educational and practice specialization within social work" (Kane, 1981, p. 25). But specialization within health care raises questions whose answers are not clear-cut. Should health care social workers specialize by health problem area, or by the different practice settings within which they are involved? Should there be oncology workers, nephrology workers, and those with expertise in mental health, or should health care social workers have command of the range of knowledge and skill required for the broad range of practice in the health field?

Brengarth (1981) points out that health care social workers must understand biomedical issues and the impact they have on human development. Further, they need to be familiar with the variations in effect of disease processes, drugs, and illness behaviors.

Basic social work mandates and values identify the common core of social work practice directions in health and in subspecialized areas. How to avoid the negative effects of extensive specialization in patient care described for medicine is a question with which we must continually grapple.

There are no easy answers. However, there is a constellation of basic social work knowledge and skill, specialized knowledge about illness and disease and its social and psychological antecedents and consequences, as well as insight into health care organization and financing that characterize the well-educated health care social worker.

Given the basic physician autonomy and authority reviewed earlier, it is not surprising that social workers often experience frustration. Yet, as the definitions of health care expand to include social components, social workers can be optimistic about increased participation and autonomy. Mechanisms whereby social workers identify populations at risk for illness and for the psychosocial crises associated with illness are being developed and increasingly used. Social workers are uniquely equipped to develop, use, and coordinate the diverse resources for the chronically ill and others with special health problems. The knowledge and skill base clearly has been found useful in health planning efforts and in work designed to minimize the insult to body and psyche associated with major health problems. The rest of this book focuses on efforts to further conceptualize, clarify, and refine the knowledge social workers need to carry on these tasks.

SUMMARY

This chapter focused on selected issues in health care policy, financing mechanisms, the key organizational structures within which health care is rendered, and some of the characteristics of three groups of health care providers—physicians, nurses, and social workers.

Several case examples, presented at the beginning of the chapter, illustrated the point made by many health care analysts that the present system of financing is pluralistic and uneven, varies in some respects from state to state, and presents many obstacles in the effort to address health problems in a humane and meaningful manner. The United States is the only industrialized nation lacking a system whereby universal access to health care independent of ability to pay is available. Several legislative proposals have been made to remedy this situation.

I reviewed key components of three major financing mechanisms: Medicare, Medicaid, and employer-supported private health insurance schemes. These go a long way toward providing needed health service, although there are gaps between services provided and those needed. For example, Medicare covers less than 40% of the health care costs incurred by those over 65 and does not cover the costs of many supportive services related to the long-term, chronic problems experienced by the elderly. Medicaid requires a means test and is usually tied to state standards of eligibility for public assistance.

The federal-state matching component of the program makes for uneven coverage of services between states. In a period of high unemployment, many people, formerly covered by private health insurance, lose their coverage. Coverage is uneven, ranging from payment only for hospital care to financing of a broad range of inpatient and outpatient services. Social workers are making efforts to be defined as health care providers whose services are reimbursable under these various financing schemes.

The pluralistic nature of financing was shown to have its counterpart in the multiple and pluralistic pattern of health care organization—hospitals, ambulatory care centers, the private practice of medicine, and various special programs such as maternal and child health services rendered by various providers in many locations. Review of the major characteristics of physicians, nurses, and social workers pointed to the unique educational patterns for each, highlighted the source of physician dominance, and identified possible sources of role conflict as well as areas for productive collaborative effort.

REFERENCES

Anderson, R., and Anderson, O.W.: Trends in the use of health services. In Freedman, H.E., Levine, S., and Reeder, L.G., editors: Handbook of medical sociology, ed. 3, Englewood Cliffs, N.J., 1979, Prentice-Hall, Inc.

Banta, D.H., and Fox, R.C.: Role strains of a health care team in a poverty community, Social Science and Medicine **6**:697, 1972.

Becker, H.S., Geer, B., Hughes, E.C., and Strauss, A.: Boys in white: student culture in medical school, Chicago, 1961, University of Chicago Press.

Boaz, R.F.: Health care system. In Turner, J.B., editor: Encyclopedia of social work, Washington, D.C., 1977, National Association of Social Workers.

Bracht, N.: The scope and historical development of social work. In Bracht, N., editor: Social work in health care, New York, 1978, The Haworth Press.

Brengarth, J.A.: What is "special" about specialization? Health and Social Work (suppl.) **6**(4):135, 1981.

Brody, E.M.: A social work guide for long-term care facilities, DHEW Pub. No. (ADM) 76-177, Washington, D.C., 1976, U.S. Government Printing Office.

Budetti, P.P., Butler, J., and McManus, R.: Federal health program reforms: implications for child health care, Milbank Memorial Fund Quarterly **60**(1):155, 1982.

Cannings, K., and Lazonick, W.: The development of the nursing labor force in the United States: a basic analysis, International Journal of Health Services **5**(2):185, 1975.

Dana, B.: Health care: social components. In Turner, J.B., editor: Encyclopedia of social work, vol. 1, Washington D.C., 1977, National Association of Social Workers.

Davis, K.: Economic scene: health care's soaring costs, The New York Times, Aug. 26, 1983, p. D2.

Devore, W., and Schlesinger, E.: Ethnic-sensitive social work practice, St. Louis, 1981, The C. V. Mosby Co.

Freidson, E.: The organization of medical practice. In Freeman, H.E., Levine, S., and Reeder, L.G., editors: Handbook of medical sociology, ed 3, Englewood Cliffs, N.J., 1979, Prentice-Hall, Inc.

Fuchs, V.R.: Who shall live? health economics and social choice, New York, 1974, Basic Books, Inc., Publishers.

Health, United States, DHEW Pub. No. (PHS) 80-1232, Washington, D.C., 1979, U.S. Government Printing Office.

Health, United States, DHEW Pub. No. (HRA) 79-633, Washington, D.C., 1980, U.S. Government Printing Office.

Health, United States, DHHS Pub. No. (PHS) 82-1232, Washington, D.C., 1981.

Health, United States, DHHS Pub. No. (PHS) 83-1232, Washington, D.C., 1982, U.S. Government Printing Office.

Insley, V.: Health services: maternal and child health. In Turner, J.B., editor:

Encyclopedia of social work, vol. 1, Washington, D.C., 1977, National Association of Social Workers.

Interim Report of the graduate medical educational national advisory committee to the secretary, Department of Health, Education and Welfare, DHEW Pub. No. (HRA) 79-633, Washington, D.C., April, 1979, U.S. Government Printing Office.

Kane, R.A.: Social workers in health: commonalities and differences, Health and Social Work (suppl.) **6**(4):25, 1981.

Levy, C.: The value base of social work, Journal of Education for Social Work **9**:34, Winter 1973.

Luft, H.S.: Health maintenance organization. In Mechanic, D., editor: Handbook of health, health care and the health professions, New York, 1983, The Free Press.

Lurie, E.E.: Nurse practitioners: issues in professional socialization, Journal of Health and Social Behavior **22**(1):31, 1981.

Markus, G., and O'Sullivan, J.: Medicare, issue brief no. IB82044, Congressional Research Service, updated June 8, 1983.

Mechanic, D.: Physicians. In Freeman, H.E., Levine, S., and Reeder, L.G., editors: Handbook of medical sociology, ed. 3, Englewood Cliffs, N.J., 1979, Prentice-Hall, Inc.

National Health Policy, 1979: Compilation of public social policy statements, Washington, D.C., 1979, National Association of Social Workers.

The New York Times, July 31, 1983.

O'Sullivan, J.: Medicaid, issue brief no. IB82041, Congressional Research Service, updated June 17, 1983.

O'Sullivan, J.: Medicare and Medicaid, issue brief no. IB76028, Congressional Research Service, Major Issues System, updated Nov. 19, 1981.

Pernice, J., and Markus, G.: Health insurance: the procompetition proposals, issue brief no. IB81046, Congressional Research Service, Major Issues System, updated April 6, 1982.

Phillips, B.: Health services: social workers in. In Turner, J.B., editor: Encyclopedia of social work, vol. 1, Washington, D.C., 1977, National Association of Social Workers.

Reeder, J., and Mauksch, H.: Nursing: continuing change. In Freeman, H.E., Levine, S., and Reeder, L.G., editors: Handbook of medical sociology, ed. 3, Englewood Cliffs, N.J., 1979, Prentice-Hall, Inc.

Reichert, K.: Social work in the health field: the years ahead. In Dinerman, M., editor: Social work futures, New Brunswick, N.J., 1983, School of Social Work, Rutgers University.

Rice, D.P.: Financing social welfare: health care. In Turner, J.B., editor: Encyclopedia of social work, vol. 1, Washington, D.C., 1977, National Association of Social Workers.

Rubin, A.: Statistics on social work education in the United States: 1981, New York, 1982, Council on Social Work Education.

Schlesinger, E.: Unpublished data, 1982.

Specialization and speciality interests, Health and Social Work (suppl.) **6**(4):entire issue, 1981.

Stevens, R.: Comparisons in health care: Britain as contrast to the United States. In Mechanic, D., editor: Handbook of health, health care and the health professions, New York, 1983, The Free Press.

Terris, M.: The three world systems of medical care, American Journal of Public Health **68**(11):1125, 1978.

Watkins, E.L., and Player, E.C.: Maternal and child health care, Health and Social Work (suppl.) **6**(4):465, 1981.

Wilensky, H.L., and Lebeaux, C.N.: Industrial society and social welfare, New York, 1965, The Free Press.

Wittman, M.: Application of knowledge about prevention to health and mental health practice. In Bracht, N.F., editor: Social work in health care: a guide to professional practice, New York, 1978, The Haworth Press.

Zola, J., and Miller, S.: The erosion of medicine from within. In Freidson, E., editor: The professions and their prospects, Beverly Hills, Calif., 1973, Sage Publications, Inc.

WE COLLECT USED EYE GLASSES
WE COLLECT USED HEARING AIDS
OVER 1,000,000 LION'S DEDICATED TO MANKIND
FREE AUDIO·VISUAL SCREENING

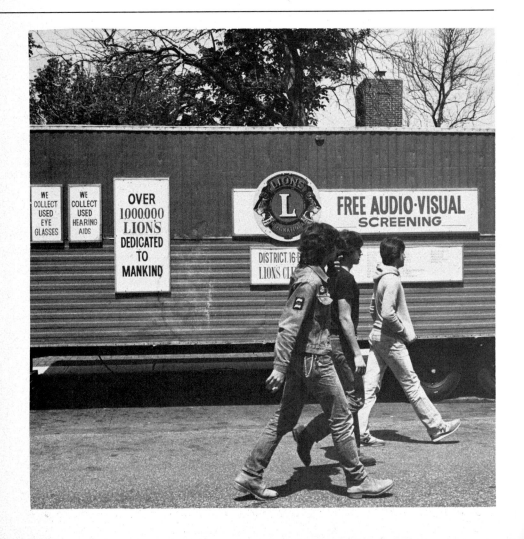

Chapter 3

Health, disease, and illness: social work, sociological, and medical perspectives

Injury, pain, and death are universal human experiences. The same is true for the intense sensations of fear or the periodic feelings of melancholy or despair that often seem unrelated to any apparent external threat. Illness is viewed negatively by all social groups. Without exception it disrupts human lives and activities and causes discomfort.

Although these experiences with physical and emotional distress are universal, how such afflictions are defined and how a society develops consistent, organized responses vary substantially. The differences relate to available knowledge about effective remedies and treatment, the way a society defines various signs of pain and disability, how a society views people who are incapacitated by physical or psychological distress, and the social structures developed to deal with such distress.

This chapter will examine some of the perspectives and conceptual approaches that have been brought to bear on these issues. In this chapter a number of these are examined and analyzed. This assessment is guided by one major objective: to determine to what extent these formulations can aid in sharpening the practice principles that guide social work practice in health care.

I will first discuss the distinctions among *health, disease,* and *illness.* These distinctions have an impact on the thought and behavior of those who use and those who provide health services.

Second, I will examine the variations in human response to the physical and emotional states termed disease and illness. These responses are called *health and illness behavior.* The discussion will focus on the sources of uniformity and variation in response to the nature of symptoms, how the response and symptoms are interpreted, and how these affect the decisions people make about whether or not to seek health services.

I will also review concepts developed to explain the factors that trigger decisions to engage in health behavior—that is, actions designed to prevent illness. Much of the work on health and illness behavior indicates that several factors are important in an individual's decision to seek care: social class, ethnic group membership, availability of services, and the financial means to pay for services. Earlier findings on these relationships have recently been questioned. An impressive body of work has found the extent of morbidity to be the major determinant of care-seeking behavior. I will review the basis of the discrepancy and assess the implications that both viewpoints have for social work practice.

I have made an effort to relate these various perspectives to the prevailing health needs identified in Chapter 1 and to certain policy and delivery issues reviewed in Chapter 2.

WHAT ARE HEALTH, DISEASE, AND ILLNESS?

At first thought, the definitions of health, disease, and illness seem evident. Isn't a healthy person one who is not sick? Aren't "disease" and "illness" just different words meaning the same thing?

My experience, and much that has been written on the subject, suggest that the answers are not that simple or clear-cut.

There are many reasons for this lack of clarity. Differences exist between the way lay people and health professionals, especially physicians, think about these phenomena. For example, in Chapter 1 it was noted that over 80% of all Americans state that they are in good health. Yet close to half of the population has at least one chronic health problem. Clearly many people do not equate the fact that they have some pathological condition with the subjective sense of being ill.

Some confusion also rests with the definition of health. Is health equated with the ability to work, and play, and love? Or are people "healthy" only if they clearly have no pathological condition demonstrated by "objective" physical and psychological examination? To find the answers to these questions, it is useful to review some of the formal definitions that have been advanced and the implications that these may have for work in the health field.

Health

As early as the second century the Greek physician-writer Galen described health as "a condition in which we neither suffer pain, nor are hindered in the functions of daily life [and are able] to take part in government, bathe, drink and eat, and do other things we want" (cited in Kosa and Robertson, 1975, p. 41).

This somewhat "utopian" perspective (Kosa and Robertson, 1975) is incorporated in current definitions. Consider the one offered by the World Health Organization: "Health is a state of complete physical, mental and social well being, and not merely the absence of disease or infirmity" (World Health Organization, 1948, p. 100). These definitions, though lofty, provide limited insight into etiological factors, therapeutic approaches, or health and illness behavior.

The idea that the absence of disease and symptoms is equated with the capacity to carry out a series of life tasks is too simplistic. Many people work and enjoy life despite the presence of disease or symptoms. Indeed, many of the activities of health care professionals, especially those of social workers, are intended to promote healthy functioning despite the presence of disease, symptoms, or ailments.

A more appropriate perspective on health focuses on efforts to minimize disease and to maximize dynamic involvement in life, even when discomfort or disease is present. An alternative definition of health—one that appears consonant with social workers' perspective on social functioning—is offered here. The definition focuses on people's capacity to function, whether or not discernible symptoms are present.

- Health involves not the absence of disease but the capacity to cope in physical or psychological terms.
- Health is related to the quality of social relationships and the ability to carry out a variety of activities consonant with age, interests, and physical and mental capacities.

This definition pertains to both physical and mental health and permits a focus on the promotion of strength and coping capacity, regardless of one's physical or psychological state. The relationship between this definition and the coping-adaptation models presented in Chapter 5 will become quite apparent. Those models focus on approaches for enhancing the skills needed for coping with health problems.

Disease and illness

If health involves not only the absence of disease, but also the capacity to cope and enjoy even when problems are evident, what is disease and how does it differ—if at all—from illness?

In making distinctions between *disease* and *illness,* some analysts focus on the difference between disease as a "biomedical condition or entity" (Fabrega, 1974) and illness as a subjective reaction to a physical state. "It is the subjective reaction and not the physical state which is the measure of the person's illness" (McKinlay and Dutton, 1974, p. 252). Mechanic (1978) suggests that disease is a deviation from the norm that can be explained by biomedical and neurophysiological processes.

Biomedical and biopsychosocial models. The principles and approaches intrinsic to this model are either applauded for their contribution to much that medicine offers or held responsible for many of the problems that beset contemporary health care. Engel (1977) succinctly identified the components of the model:

1. The dominant model of disease is biomedical, and molecular biology is its basic scientific discipline.
2. Disease is accounted for by deviations from the norm of biological variables.

3. Implicit in the model is the expectation that disease be dealt with as an entity that is independent of social behavior.
4. Behavioral "aberrations" can be explained on the basis of disordered biochemical processes.
5. Mental and somatic phenomena are distinct; in other words, a mind/body dualism is involved.

Engel also suggested that this model, though scientific, shares a characteristic with all other models: it involves a shared set of assumptions based on the scientific method. It was developed as an approach for categorizing and understanding the puzzling phenomena of physical discomfort. The model assumes that "the language of chemistry and physics will ultimately suffice to explain biological phenomena" (Engel, 1977, p. 130). In Engel's view certain aspects of the model have acquired the status of "dogma" and require that all disease, including "mental disease," be conceptualized in terms of "derangement of underlying physical mechanisms."

The distinctions between the model as a useful research tool and its application to issues of adaptation are not usually clarified. The biomedical view of disease is intrinsic to our culture and readily reinforced during medical education.

The dominant conceptions of the biomedical model make it difficult to incorporate psychosocial factors and other experiences into efforts to explain and treat disease and illness. An alternative or expanded version proposed is the "biopsychosocial model." This model focuses on the clusters of symptoms experienced by people in discomfort and takes into account the social, psychological, and biological factors that influence the onset of disease and variations in the course of the disease.

When disease or illness processes are not necessarily "reduced" to "the smallest isolatable component having causal implications, for example, the biochemical" (Engel, 1977, p. 131), the practitioner's attention is perforce focused on a wider range of phenomena. This enlarged conception, in Engel's view, encompasses a wider range of action. He proposes that the biomedical model leaves no room for consideration of the social, psychological, and behavioral dimensions of illness. The biopsychosocial model, by contrast, "provides a blueprint for research, a framework for teaching, and a design for action in the real world of health care" (Engel, 1977, p. 135).

This perspective makes it more likely that the problems for which people seek care and what they define as "illness" will be incorporated in the biopsychosocial model. Vague headaches, stomachaches, depression, and other symptoms are not readily reduced to clinical entities. Nevertheless, when people seek help for these kinds of problems, they do view themselves as ill. Also important is the assertion that the subjective reaction is the measure of the person's illness. Many rehabilitation efforts are directed toward helping people to alter a subjective sense of despair, helplessness, and dependence so that they may make progress within the limitations imposed by a physical state.

Mechanic's view of illness is relevant to this discussion. He suggested that the term refers to "any conditions that cause or might usefully cause an individual to concern himself with his symptoms and to seek help" (Mechanic, 1978, p. 249). Illness then would thus involve deviation from a comfortable physical or psychological state. Whether people are more concerned with the discomfort associated with their symptoms or with whether their symptoms indicate that they have an underlying disease varies with their level of medical knowledge and is affected by ethnic, cultural, and personality variables.

Practice implications of disease or illness distinction. Clearly the distinctions between disease and illness, especially as these terms are commonly used, affect the work of health professionals, especially social workers. The following case examples serve as a starting point for considering the importance of these distinctions.

Mrs. Goldie Solomon

Mrs. Solomon is a 55-year-old Jewish woman who has been told by her physician that she has a mild form of diabetes. This was determined during a routine physical examination. Although she had experienced some minor dizzy spells, she hadn't paid too much attention to them.

The physician tells her that since she is somewhat overweight, she should lose about 20 pounds. If she loses weight and generally pays attention to her diet, he feels that they will be able to keep the diabetes under control without medication.

Mrs. Solomon is quite worried about this diagnosis. She has heard that some people with diabetes need insulin and that sometimes they have complications leading to eye problems, kidney disease, or the loss of a foot.

Although she is worried, she will go on with life as usual, even though she has to take certain precautions. She likes sweets, but she expects to be able to follow the prescribed diet. It should be fairly easy, since she has no one to cook for but herself. Her husband is dead, and her grown children are on their own.

Mr. Chou Won-Lee

Mr. Won-Lee, a Chinese man who recently arrived in the United States from Hong Kong, has seen a physician about vague stomach pains, headaches, and chronic fatigue. Examination reveals no discernible organic basis for these complaints. Since Mr. Won-Lee arrived alone from Hong Kong, leaving his wife and family behind, the physician wonders if the symptoms might be masking some underlying distress—perhaps even depression. Mr. Won-Lee responds to the physician's attempt to discuss these aspects of his life by assuring her that everything is all right. His demeanor makes it very clear that he prefers not to discuss these matters.

John Wolensky

The parents of John Wolensky, a 20-year-old Polish schizophrenic man, have been referred to the social worker for help in making plans for his care at home. The young man spent a brief period in a psychiatric hospital following the acute onset of hallucinations, bizarre ideation, and withdrawal from everyday social relationships. The psychotropic drugs prescribed seem to have reduced the hallucinations and bizarre behavior. Now, at home, he is still withdrawn and does little to care for his own needs.

Mr. and Mrs. Wolensky would like to help in "drawing him out" and finding a place where he might go to socialize. They present a rather stoic appearance—expressing little overt distress about their son's problem.

How do the definitions of health, disease, and illness considered to this point help in understanding the situations of Mrs. Solomon, Mr. Won-Lee, and John Wolensky?

None of them is healthy by classic definition—that is, free from disease or ailment—yet only Mrs. Solomon has a disease in the sense that a clear-cut known biological basis is present. Her response to the disease is not unlike that of many other Jewish people: she worries about the long-range meaning of the illness—and carefully follows physician's orders (for example, Zborowski, 1952).

The organic basis of some of the schizophrenias has not been clearly established, although many do classify schizophrenia as a disease. The Wolenskys do not readily show their sadness over the turn of events. A certain stoicism in the face of troubles is not atypical of Poles (for example, Lopata, 1976). No underlying pathology can be detected as a cause of Mr. Won-Lee's vague symptoms. Rejection of the idea that somatic complaints may mask psychological concerns is not uncommon among some Chinese people.

The three situations presented shed some light on the distinction between illness and disease as defined here. Each illustrates the view of health I proposed earlier—that is, involvement in life's activities and efforts to minimize the effect that the disease or illness has on these. The consequence of illness as defined by patients and their families and the promotion of reasonably healthy functioning is health care social work's main focus. Mrs. Solomon seems relatively resilient in response to diagnosis of a lifelong condition. However, it will be difficult to help Mr. Won-Lee recognize an association between his cultural and personal isolation and his symptoms. Perhaps he would be responsive to subtle suggestions that he become more socially involved with other recent Chinese immigrants. An approach focused on social functioning, geared to his ethnic disposition, may be appropriate. The Wolenskys surely need help in dealing with their son's social needs.

It is important to understand disease and its consequences, because disease has a number of clear-cut physical and psychological manifestations. Appendix A presents an approach to helping social workers gain the kind of knowledge of disease they need in their daily work. Together with the view of health, disease, and illness reviewed here, such understanding can contribute much to effective intervention.

ILLNESS BEHAVIOR AND HEALTH BEHAVIOR

The terms *illness behavior* and *health behavior* are used to describe the kinds of actions people take when their physical and emotional well-being is threatened. The processes involved have been studied extensively, and much of the investigation has focused on the factors that lead individuals to seek the care of a physician.

Review of this literature points to two major and, to some extent, contradictory sets of findings. One, derived from studies in medical sociology, economics, and health services research, explores a variety of sociocultural, organizational, and psychosocial factors that affect decisions about (1) when and under what circumstances people pay attention to symptoms and (2) to whom they turn when they believe such attention is warranted. Much of this literature suggests that how illness and symptoms are defined is largely a function of a variety of social and psychological characteristics.

Factors that have been identified as affecting an individual's decision to seek care include ethnicity, household structure, informal influences, stress, access to medical care, and values and attitudes that relate to inclinations to use services. The availability of health insurance coverage and medical care has also been shown to be related to decisions to use care (Mechanic, 1979). For example, hospital use increases with the increase in health insurance coverage, as discussed in Chapter 2. When health services are expanded in a previously underserved area, use of these services increases.

Increasingly health professionals are using data derived from such studies in their efforts to tailor services that are congruent with the needs for care as identified by various segments of the population.

> Indeed, our entire understanding of the functioning of health services systems is premised on the common observation that increased insurance coverage and increased access to providers of care result in greater demand and use of services (Mechanic, 1979, pp. 357-358).

More recently a group of studies has questioned the importance of social, psychological, economic, and other determinants of health and illness behavior. Unlike findings derived from the first body of work mentioned, morbidity seemed to emerge as *the* critical factor affecting use of care.

Because these studies are important and their findings, interpretations, and major themes conflict, I will briefly review both bodies of work and attempt to explain and reconcile the discrepancies between the two types of investigations and their conclusions. Following this discussion, I will analyze those elements of health and illness behavior related to age, gender, and social class and ethnicity. Each of these areas of thought have major implications for practice. They affect our thinking about the relative importance of making health care financially accessible, of how services are organized, and about how to interact with people of various backgrounds when they are in pain or are fearing the life disruptions caused by illness.

I will first examine the concepts and findings from studies focused on a number of social, psychological, and organizational factors that have been found to be related to illness behavior.

Three types of behavior related to health and illness have been identified—*illness behavior, health behavior,* and *sick role behavior* (Rosenstock, 1975). In this chapter, I will discuss the first two.

Illness behavior

Mechanic (1977) proposed a useful definition of illness behavior. It refers to:

> The varying perceptions, thoughts, feelings and acts affecting the personal and social meaning of symptoms, illness, disabilities and their consequences (p. 79).

How individuals respond to symptoms is affected by their prior experience with illness, knowledge about the meaning of symptoms, and differences in their coping skills and sensitivity to symptoms. This view of illness behavior has generated substantial work on (1) how various people define symptoms (Mechanic, 1972) and (2) the factors that trigger the decision to seek medical care (Suchman, 1965; Zola, 1964). A large, important area of investigation attempted to identify how members of different social classes and ethnic groups define illness and the use they make of various delivery systems.

Symptom definition. Much of this work has sought to clarify what people do when symptoms are fuzzy, vague, and not clearly indicative of major pathological conditions. There is little room for doubt when someone has a badly broken leg, is bleeding uncontrollably, or has suffered a stroke that dramatically affects speech and mobility.

Mechanic (1972) presented data on "factors afffecting the presentation of bodily complaints." In any given month, three out of four people experience symptoms of sufficient consequence to warrant their taking some action. This ranges from self-medication or restriction of activities to consulting a physician.

There is extensive overlap in symptoms between people who ignore them and people who seek medical and other attention. For example, at any given time, some people will be found sitting anxiously in a physician's office, worrying about a headache of particular intensity. At other times, experiencing an "objectively similar headache," these same people may not even take an aspirin. Most of us can recall times when we ignored symptoms; at other times the same symptoms may have been frightening and worrisome.

The way in which an individual appraises symptoms seems related to how unusual the symptoms are, what is currently happening in the individual's life, and knowledge of or prior experience with those symptoms.

Mechanic (1978) used an interesting analogy—"medical student's disease"—as a way of clarifying the process by which people may assign meaning to symptoms and make decisions about action. The experiences of medical students and those of lay persons are comparable in some respects. Medical students are usually under stress; the same can be said for many other people some of the time. The students are accumulating information about disease, although their knowledge is not yet complete. Lay persons also have various degrees of incomplete knowledge about disease. Stress resulting from frequent examinations and new clinical experiences is high among medical students. Like others they have a great many symptoms, most of which are transient. While these may have been viewed as normal in the past and ignored, their new knowledge leads some to try to explain these symptoms and attribute them to disease. As they acquire additional medical information they alter their "diagnoses," recognizing their error. For example, heart palpitations may be recognized as a manifestation of anxiety about a forthcoming exam rather than as heart disease.

Explanations for the relationship between availability of information and emotional response to symptoms are offered by Schachter and Singer (1962): Review of their work suggests that most people tend to blame ordinary symptoms on factors they can explain. If they have exercised, they are likely to attribute their muscle aches to unusual exertion. If they ate more than usual, indigestion is blamed on this. However,

> When such ordinary symptoms occur concomitantly with emotional arousal and when they are not easily explained within conventional and commonly available understanding, external cues become important in defining their character and importance. Such cues may be fortuitous or they may be the consequence of prior experience, cultural learning, or personal need for secondary gain (Mechanic, 1978, p. 259).

For example, with the advent of health education through schools and the media, many people are more aware that prolonged "indigestion" may be indicative of a heart attack. Or it is possible, for a limited period, to ascribe an adolescent's withdrawal from friends and school to adolescent turmoil. However, when the behavior is prolonged, the definition may change to "perhaps he's really emotionally ill."

Similarly, when repeated visits to the physician for "heart palpitations" indicate that there is nothing wrong with the heart, concern may subside. In turn, how prolonged "indigestion," adolescent withdrawal, or palpitations are originally perceived may derive from many factors. Stress is often thought to determine whether symptoms are perceived as serious or not; so is the availability of accurate information. Frequently a person's perception of seriousness may stem from the way particular symptoms and illness experiences are usually interpreted by those with whom people are in close contact and in whose judgments they have confidence.

Individual personality differences are of course a major factor. Some people are likely to "dismiss all," while others become terribly fearful about the slightest symptom.

These insights can prove useful in work with people who feel vaguely uncomfortable or repeatedly seek help for symptoms for which no clear-cut disease processes can be established. For example, family physicians and social workers in family practice residency programs have commented on this phenomenon (Schlesinger, 1982). Frequently such vague symptoms result from personal problems that heighten tension. Investigating the underlying problems often yields useful information. A woman's headaches may be more pronounced when her alcoholic husband returns from a drinking spree or when she finds herself unable to cope with the growing independence of her adolescent children. Helping people to cope with these kinds of "symptom-generating" life conditions is essential; assurance that there is no remediable organic base is very important.

It is equally important to help people to recognize serious symptoms. Increased knowledge about certain symptoms indicative of a heart attack has already been mentioned. People should also know that symptoms such as bloody stools or unusual and frequent thirst should not be ignored. There have been massive educational efforts to inform women about the significance of lumps in the breasts.

Factors affecting the decision to seek care. Substantial evidence suggests that the relationship between the appearance of symptoms and care seeking is not direct or clear.

Varying models have been developed that focus on the particular factors that trigger use of health services. Many of these are derived from studies of people who go to health care facilities. Other studies have sampled large groups of the population—including both people who did and did not seek health services.

Mention was made earlier of the extensive overlap between those symptoms brought to the attention of health professionals and those for which no care is sought. This diversity has caused some to propose that a review of the literature on health service use "undermines the notion of 'objective illness'" (McKinlay and Dutton, 1974, p. 252). According to this view, emotional stress, cultural definitions, and membership in various social classes and ethnic groups determine what is or is not defined as a problem of sufficient severity to warrant medical intervention. These definitions may or may not coincide with what physicians would classify as disease.

Turning then to the various models that have focused on the decisions to seek care, Dingwall's classification (1976) is useful. He suggests that the approaches to categorizing care-seeking behavior can be characterized by the degree to which they are "individualistic" or "collectivity oriented." Individualistic models explain illness behavior in terms of people's individual characteristics or those of a sociodemographic nature of those based on psychological assessment. Collectivity-oriented models seek to explain illness behavior through social factors that affect action taken in relation to illness.

Individually oriented models. A classic study of individualistic models was that of Mechanic and Volkart (1961), involving 600 students at one university. A major concern was the assessment of the relationship between stress and illness behavior, as conceptualized in the study, and their joint effect on the use of medical facilities.

Stress was measured by getting indications of how "lonely" and "nervous" the students were. Illness behavior was measured by presenting the students during an interview with a series of vignettes about different conditions that might determine whether or not they were inclined to use the university health service. Their actual use of the university health service was also measured. Those who were under a great deal of stress and had a high inclination to use health services used medical services frequently (73%). Of those scoring low on "stress" and "inclination to use," only 30% used medical services frequently.

Another classic individualistic model is the one developed by Kosa (1966). It is based on examination of episodes of illness compiled from absentee records in the workplace and on symptoms reported in family health diaries. The following represents a summary of suggested response to "illness episodes" derived from this study:

1. People perceive some symptoms that they assess as threatening to their physiological and psychological functioning (Figure 1).
2. This perception arouses anxiety.
3. Medical knowledge is used to interpret the disturbance.
4. Some actions designed to remove the anxiety and the disturbance are taken.

In the Kosa study, as in the Mechanic and Volkart study, individual emotional reactions in response to symptoms were seen as the major factors that lead to use of health care services. Dingwall (1976) was critical of these studies because they do not take into account those factors in the social situation that lead to one or another kind of action. It might be asked, "What were the conditions in the workplace?" and "Would absenteeism lead to loss of pay, or were there sick leave plans that made it 'all right' or even advantageous to take time off?" People might be fearful of recording these kinds of motivations, believing they could be used against them.

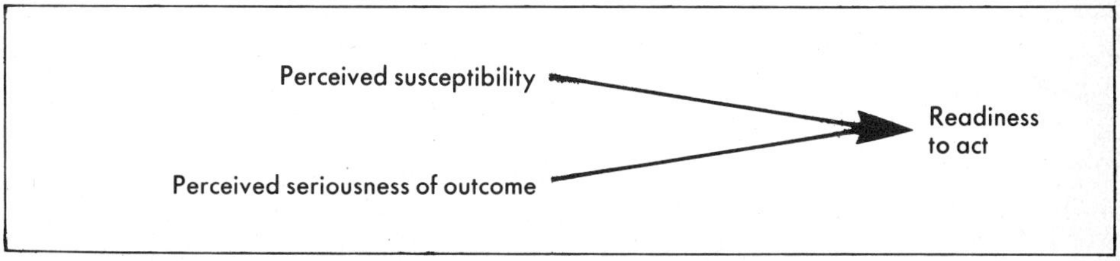

Figure 1. Perceived susceptibility. (Adapted from Dingwall, R.: Aspects of illness, New York, 1976, St. Martin's Press, p. 3.)

Collectivity-oriented models. Through an analysis of data from a study of illness behavior of some ethnic groups in the Boston area, Zola examined why medical aid is sought at a particular time. His findings suggest that the decision to act on symptoms was not systematically related to their severity. Rather, the action seemed to be precipitated by "five triggers":

1. The presence of an interpersonal crisis
2. The perception that the symptoms would interfere with personal relationships
3. How ready others in the person's network are to acknowledge that the symptoms are of sufficient magnitude to seek help
4. Perceived interference with work or physical activity
5. A sudden change in symptoms

Ethnic group membership and educational level were strongly related to the action taken. Both these variables contributed to how symptoms were defined and understood.

Another major body of work within the collectivity orientation is that by Suchman (1964, 1965) and Rosenblatt and Suchman (1965). Suchman tried to relate orientations to medical care and related behavior to the types of social relationships and groups in which people were involved. The work was based on information obtained from a random sample of people living in an ethnically heterogeneous neighborhood in New York City. The original thesis was that social status (position in the class structure) and group structure (the nature of social networks in which people participate) shape people's orientation to medical care. That orientation was thought to affect decisions about whether to use care. The reasoning went like this: In some kinds of groups people interact largely "with their own kind" in the family and in the neighborhood. This usually involves people of the same ethnic group. These close and "exclusive" types of relationships were characterized by Rosenblatt and Suchman as "parochial." He further assumed that these parochial relationships led to limited knowledge of disease as defined by the medical care system and generated skepticism of medical care. This in turn was thought to be related to the use of medical services. In fact, the original analysis did not bear out Suchman's hypothesis. Individual attitudes about the usefulness of the medical care system were more related to socioeconomic status than to the kind of parochial relationships he postulated. Based on these findings he revised the model, now conceptualized as follows: Demographic characteristics (for example, age, gender, ethnicity) and involvement in cohesive groups generate a tendency to be unfavorably inclined to the medical care system and shape response to symptoms. These all affect people's perceptions of their health and what they do about episodes of illness. Out of this new conception he identified the following model to account for the decision to seek medical help: (1) the symptom experience, (2) deciding that one is sick, leads to (3) medical care contact.

The findings of Geertson and others (1975) shed some interesting light on Suchman's thesis. Repeating many features of Suchman's original work, they found that if people:

> Come from a sociocultural milieu that supports modern medicine, then close and exclusive group ties will increase the likelihood that a health problem will be recognized and subsequent action will result in the seeking of medical care. If they do not, then close ties will have an opposite effect. In addition, the more scientific knowledge individuals have of disease, the more likely they are to recognize a health problem and seek medical care (pp. 234-235).

This work does suggest that the nature of symptoms per se does not explain many of the actions people take when they are ill.

Another important work that relates the symptom experience and immersion in family and other groups to the seeking of medical care is Freidson's conception of the "lay referral system" (Freidson, 1961). Basing his premise on his studies in New York City, Freidson suggested that people go through a definite set of steps in handling illness. The concept "is predicated not in a set of attributes that an individual may possess, but on a career, a patterned sequence of events through which individuals pass" (p. 146). He suggested that on initially experiencing a symptom, people tend to diagnose themselves (for example, "Is this headache worth taking an aspirin?"). If after self-diagnosis and perhaps self-treatment (taking the aspirin) the symptom persists, the advice of friends and relatives is sought. This step usually precedes and often leads to seeking of medical advice. The process of "lay consultation" does not stop after the visit to the physician. Family members, neighbors, and friends may then be consulted about the physician's advice. In this process people draw on their own experience with similar problems. "When I had a cold the doctor gave me penicillin," or "When I had that lump on my breast my doctor didn't say anything about operating." This kind of reflection and advice in turn may generate further advice seeking. People may return to the same physician, or based on advice from the lay referral system, they may seek another physician.

Freidson identified some basic differences between working-class and middle-class people in the way the lay referral system was used. Working-class people were more fearful of physicians and passive in their response. They feared rebuff and were more reluctant to ask questions. They were more likely to consult the lay system before going to the physician. Upper-middle-class people were more likely to make decisions on their own and much more likely to go directly to the physician without stopping to consult family, friends, and neighbors.

Abstract as these considerations may be, review of our personal experiences with illness episodes suggests the validity of these observations.

Many of us may muse as follows:

> I've had that cold for a week now, and I'm still coughing. Maybe I'll make an appointment to see Dr. Jones. No, first I'll ask my mother. Besides, I have an important date Friday night. No, she'll worry too much. What if I have lung cancer? I must ask her what Mary's symptoms were when she had lung cancer. Oh, I'll go right to the doctor.

And after the visit:

> I wonder why he didn't take an x-ray? Maybe I should go to somebody else. I'm still coughing.

And, of course, analogous kinds of thinking and consulting go on in relation to emotional problems and stresses related to illness:

> Jane said that the social worker really helped her when she was so upset because she had to put her mother in a nursing home. But social workers are for poor people. I'll go ask Jane again. But if I go to the social worker, is she going to ask me about the fights I used to have with my mother? They always want to know about your past life. I'm not sure what difference that makes now that Mom's so sick. Of course, it would be nice if I could tell her now how sorry I am for being so nasty. But will the social worker really understand?

Clearly, seeking medical care or the services of a social worker or other trained helpers can produce tension and fear that must be understood by all those involved in the helping process.

Both the individually oriented and collectivity-oriented models often fail to deal with the kinds of experiences that some people have with the medical care system once they seek care. Reflecting on their review of behavior related to use of health services, McKinlay and Dutton (1974) suggested the following:

> We believe it fairly accurately reflects the predominant emphasis of past work—concern with important factors in the process of seeking care. In other words, attention has been principally directed at variables that exert some influence up to the point of utilizing some service, and not at what goes on between all those involved when a service organization is actually being utilized. In the light of recent developments in organizational theory, it is clear that what goes on between clients and agencies may be as highly related to utilization behavior as the personal characteristics that so many have highlighted (p. 275).

How organizations are structured, how they often select those to whom they render care, and how they deal with those who come for care will be considered throughout this book.

Clearly criticism can be leveled at some of the work on illness behavior. One may wonder, as did Dingwall, whether paper and pencil tests or diaries really give an accurate picture of people's subjective experiences. Do they trust the interviewer or the person who is going to read their responses? Have we gotten a true image of what is really going on in their minds as they try to decide what to do about a symptom that may appear life threatening? How important does the symptom seem in comparison to other things that have to be done in life such as working or caring for children or other family members? Freidson's work on the lay referral system, based on extensive interviews, begins to provide some of these insights.

These efforts nevertheless represent a remarkable body of work intended to present an image of how people feel and what they worry about when they experience discomfort. Understanding that people do not automatically turn to physicians even when they experience severe distress is most important. That the response to illness is affected by age, gender, and life circumstances generates much room for action by consumers and health care providers. If it is true that membership in cohesive groups can trigger efforts to get care or can deter such efforts (Geertson and others, 1975), such knowledge can be used to guide health care planning. Social networks have been identified as a potential locus for preventive health action by social workers (for example, Schlesinger and Devore, 1982). For example, as noted in Chapter 1 American Blacks are at particular risk for hypertension. Community groups such as churches can serve as screening and educational sites. Centers where the elderly gather to socialize and eat nutritional lunches are paying increasing attention to the amounts of salt and sugar they use in foods. The models highlight the role of nonmedical factors in illness behavior and point to the persistent relationship among individuals, their social characteristics, and the environments in which they function. These factors are important to social workers, whether they are trying to change the structure of health delivery or working with an individual coping with disability.

The work reviewed begins to clarify the relationship between symptom experience and the way this experience is interpreted in light of group membership, perception of disease, feelings about caretakers, and action.

Health behavior

The discussion just completed has focused on how people are thought to deal with discomforts once they are experienced. Another important group of work has tried to assess how people make decisions on whether to take action designed to preserve their health. For example, the work by Rosenstock (1966), called the "health belief model," focused on this. Citing research on whether people will seek preventive dental care, chest x-ray examinations, and similar actions designed to prevent problems or identify them early, Rosenstock proposed a model based on the assumption that people need motivation to act. Thus any preventive health action involves a feeling of vulnerability or fear that illness may occur and have serious consequences. This sense of vulnerability (susceptibility) and the relationship to action have been diagrammed in Figure 1.

Closely related is the knowledge or feeling that action is available and that the action may have beneficial consequences (Figure 2).

For example, some people may know that there is a strong history of hypertension in their family and understand that this may put them at greater risk for a heart attack or stroke. They then view themselves as susceptible to serious trouble. Perceiving this, they may be more likely to have their blood pressure checked regularly than individuals who sense no such threat.

This model, although simple in its conception, facilitates the analysis and planning of much action. To be useful the model must of course take into account cultural and other variations associated with illness behavior. For example, those members of a cohesive group who reject prevailing medical conceptions of illness may insulate themselves from information about the risks of hypertension. Others, knowing such risks, may nevertheless fail to take action. They may not like the way the care is rendered, lack resources for care, or take a fatalistic attitude toward their own ability to affect fate. Faced with such ingrained beliefs, health care professionals have a big job to do in trying to understand and to help people modify behaviors known to be antithetical to their health.

Health status and the use of services.

Reference was made on p. 83 to the findings of a number of studies that cast serious doubt on the importance and implications of the type of work reviewed.

Studies by Aday and Eichhorn (1972), Anderson, Kravits, and Anderson (1975), Kohn and White (1976), and Wolinsky (1978) found the effects of the psychosocial and organizational factors that were reviewed previously to be trivial (Mechanic, 1979). Instead, most physician visits could be explained (Anderson, Kravits, and Anderson, 1975) by actual health concerns, disability days, and symptoms.

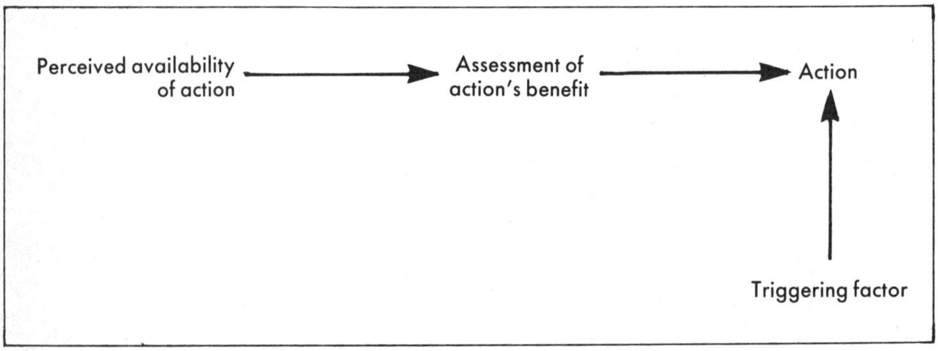

Figure 2. Perceived availability. (Adapted from Dingwall, R.: Aspects of illness, New York, 1976, St. Martin's Press, p. 3.)

To understand how these studies differ from those considered earlier, a brief review of how they were carried out is essential.

One major difference relates to focus. Mechanic (1979) pointed out that the "illness behavior" studies tended to involve small samples in which intensive interviews were carried out. The group of studies now under consideration, known as "large multivariate studies," involve large surveys and less detailed measures to specify the concepts under consideration.

The study by Anderson, Kravits, and Anderson, (1975) deserves particular examination. According to this study, use of physicians results from three sets of factors: *predisposing variables, enabling variables,* and *need variables.* Predisposing variables include those prevailing before the onset of illness such as demographic characteristics, ethnicity, occupation, age, and gender. Enabling variables include income, health levels, health insurance coverage, and the regular availability of care. Illness need variables include perceived and evaluated need. The latter includes those kinds of factors used as indicators of morbidity in the large-scale studies done by the federal government referred to in Chapter 1: (1) reported bed days and restricted-activity days and (2) number of symptoms (for example, feeling weak) checked off from a list of such symptoms.

Using these and other variables, findings were remarkably consistent throughout these types of studies. Although predisposing variables exert some influence, the need variables are the most pronounced in accounting for the use of services. Self-reliance and fatalistic attitudes toward care showed very little relationship to actual use. Most surprisingly, availability of resources was not as important as previous studies had suggested.

> One of the puzzling aspects of the findings from large-scale physician utilization studies is the lack of support for the importance of enabling family and community variables such as family income, insurance, residence, region and M.D.-to-population ratio (Mechanic, 1979, p. 392).

It is beyond the purview of this book to make a detailed assessment of the strength and weakness of the research methodology used in these two bodies of work. Nevertheless, some comments can be made. We have seen that symptoms are variously perceived. In Chapter 1 considerable attention was paid to the fact that morbidity or illness episodes are hard to measure. How these are reported may be a function of the social-psychological factors examined by many. Further, the discrepancy between self-perceived health status and the amount of chronic illness that afflicts large numbers of people was noted. Together, all of the studies have not yet captured the complex interplay of these factors; yet the discrepancy is of concern.

Clearly, those workers whose research was designed to clarify the factors that determine health and illness behavior have a great deal of unfinished business. Their findings and interpretations are nevertheless of major importance to those who plan and provide health services. To date, their interpretations are inconclusive. Intervention must and does take place on the basis of incomplete and changing information. Further, values and political realities shape the interpretation and use to which scientific data are put.

How can social workers use and respond to the competing and somewhat conflicting data on health and illness behavior? Adherence to a social work value perspective can guide use and interpretation of the rich though conflicting literature on health and illness behavior.

There is an impressive body of work that indicates that not all people interpret similar discomforts in the same way. The differences in interpretation are thought to relate to what is happening in their lives and to how these events tend to be viewed by the social groups to which they belong. These responses translate into feelings about the kind of care that makes people comfortable. Surely social work's view that people are self-directing and entitled to self-determination mandates that the kind of understanding derived from these studies be translated into planning efforts and delivery mechanisms. Understanding of attitudes toward care is a case in point. For example, Geertson and others (1975) found that members of cohesive groups that value health care will use such care more than members of groups that are apprehensive about the delivery system. When the distrust of groups of the latter type results in underuse of care and is detrimental to the health of the group, health workers have a responsibility to tailor their services to minimize that distrust, which may mean changing customary ways of delivering care.

People who are reluctant to go to a physician or clinic to have blood pressure readings taken may consent to do so if this is offered as part of a church's educational program. The formal office as a site for marital counseling may be threatening to those who view any admission of such difficulty as a cause for shame. Approached informally on their own "turf"—at the church, the social club, or the workplace—many people may be more comfortable. In such settings discussions of intimate matters may be more commonplace. These and similar approaches, based on understanding of health and illness behavior, are in keeping with a view that people have a right to determine the direction of their own lives.

The data that show how stress, poverty, and availability of care are related to use of services are most important, despite the fact that the extent to which these affect health care use has been questioned. Social work's commitment to the view that health and welfare services should be an intrinsic component of modern industrial life is deeply embedded in the profession's value system. Data that suggest that people will use care when they are ill, regardless of the nature of services and financing available, are important in implementing this component of the value system. These data must be thoroughly examined, understood, and used in planning.

One other issue is important to interpretation and use of the work on health and illness behavior. In commenting on the conflicting findings of the two types of studies, Mechanic states: "Examining the role of cultural and social-psychological processes within the constraining influences of economic and organizational factors will result in better theory" (Mechanic, 1979, p. 395). The constraining influences of economic factors are in great evidence at the time this chapter is being written (summer 1982). The United States is currently experiencing the highest rates of unemployment since the economic depression of the 1930s. Although unemployment insurance and health insurance offset the negative effects of this recession to some extent, effects on health behavior are immediately apparent. Information released by the American Medical Association and other organizations points out that visits to physicians have dropped by 10% to 15%. This is especially true for visits to primary care settings. Two factors account for this. Prevailing insurance plans are less likely to cover the costs of such care. Furthermore, primary care facilities are often used for those "fuzzy" symptoms where danger is not clearly imminent as well as for preventive care. This includes visits for hypertension screening, review of progress in maintaining blood pressure control, and blood sugar checks for diabetes. In the terms used by Anderson, Krevits, and Anderson (1975), "evaluated need" does seem related to ability to pay.

The relationship between perceived need and economic wherewithal is thus subject to economic fluctuations. The following case examples, drawn from current practice, illustrate this interplay.

Mrs. Mary White

A physician who sends reminders about the need for regular visits to her patients with hypertension received a call from one of her patients, Mrs. White, asking if her prescription could be renewed over the telephone. Since she was now unemployed, she could not afford the cost of the visit.

Mrs. Joan Young

A social worker at a family health center had been seeing Mrs. Young, a young mother, on a regular basis to help her plan the care needed by her young child with Down's syndrome. They were looking into the availability of schools, discussed the child's progress, and explored Mrs. Young's feelings that somehow she had done something bad and was responsible for the child's defect. The mother had said often that she found these discussions to be quite helpful.

One day she called to say that the recent increase in bus fares made it difficult for her to continue to come to the center weekly. Perhaps the social worker could visit her at home.

The social worker had wanted to make home visits from the beginning. However, shrinking agency funds had limited the social workers' budget for home visits to those involving major emergencies such as child abuse or neglect.

Mr. John Marvin

Mr. Marvin suffered a heart attack a year ago. A former construction worker, he had been able to get a desk job in his company and was making good progress. Because of the decline in the construction industry he was laid off. His physician advised him to apply for disability benefits, but this made him feel like "less than a man." When the opportunity came along for part-time work loading heavy materials onto trucks, he took the work. Fearing the physician would disapprove, he stopped going for regular checkups.

Each of these examples illustrates how health behavior is immediately constrained by shifting economic circumstances. Mrs. White, Mrs. Young, and Mr. Marvin all have a perceived need to use health services for their problems. The importance these assume alongside other problems varies.

The literature on health and illness behavior related to use of health services provides some guidelines, albeit incomplete, for understanding what people do when they feel ill or believe that certain actions might prevent them from becoming ill. These actions are guided by a sense of vulnerability and of threat to their ability to carry on. They are also influenced by an individual's ability to pay for services. Within these broad dimensions there is great variability. Attention to the unique needs of individuals and groups is a hallmark of social work activity. This rich literature can guide efforts to ascertain unique needs and their social source.

SUMMARY

This chapter has presented a number of definitions of health, disease, and illness. A social work view of health, focused on social functioning rather than on the absence of disease or illness, was proposed.

The distinctions between disease and illness were illustrated, and a number of formulations on "illness behavior" and "health behavior" were discussed. The social and individual sources of variation in response to pain and discomfort were reviewed. A large body of work attributes many of these and the related decisions on whether or not to seek care to social class membership, ethnic group membership, and availability of health services. Another series of studies has cast doubt on these long-standing views, suggesting instead that the degree of morbidity is the major determinant of the decision to use health services. The implications of these two somewhat conflicting perspectives were analyzed in terms of how these affect social work's obligation to assure that health services, consonant with people's needs and dispositions, are available. The reduction in use of health services noted in the currently declining economy suggests that social work values compel attention to any factors that limit the availability of care. A series of case examples highlighted the relationship between economic factors and care decisions.

REFERENCES

Aday, L.A., and Eichhorn, R.: The utilization of health services: indices and correlates: a research bibliography, National Center for Health Services Research and Development, DHEW Pub. No. (HSM) 73-3003, 1972.

Anderson, R., Kravits, J., and Anderson, D.W., editors: Equity in health services: empirical analyses in social policy, Cambridge, 1975, Ballinger Publishing Co.

Dingwall, R.: Aspects of illness, New York, 1976, St. Martin's Press, Inc.

Engel, G.L.: The need for a new medical model: a challenge for biomedicine, Science **196**(4286):129, 1977.

Fabrega, H., Jr.: Disease and social behavior: an interdisciplinary perspective, Cambridge, 1974, M.I.T. Press.

Freidson, E.H.: Patients' views of medical practice, New York, 1961, Russell Sage Foundation.

Geertson, E., Klauber, M.R., Rindflesh, M., Kane, R.L., and Gray, R.: A reexamination of Suchman's views on social factors in health care utilization, Journal of Health and Social Behavior **16**(2):226, 1975.

Kohn, R., and White, K.L., editors: Health care—an international study: report of the World Health Organization/international collaborative study of medical care utilization, London, 1976, Oxford University Press.

Kosa, J., et al.: The place of morbid episodes in the social interaction pattern, Paper presented to Sixth Congress of the International Sociological Association, 1966, Evian, France.

Kosa, J., and Robertson, L.S.: The social aspects of health and illness. In Kosa, J., and Zola, I.K., editors: Poverty and health: a sociological analysis, Cambridge, Mass., 1975, Harvard University Press.

Lopata, H.Z.: Polish Americans: status competition in an ethnic community, Englewood Cliffs, N.J., 1976, Prentice-Hall, Inc.

McKinlay, J.B., and Dutton, D.B.: Social-psychological factors affecting health service utilization. In Mushkin, S.J., editor: Consumer incentives for health care, New York, 1974, Prodist.

Mechanic, D.: Social psychologic factors affecting the presentation of bodily complaints, The New England Journal of Medicine **286:**1132, 1972.

Mechanic, D.: Illness behavior, social adaptation and the management of illness, The Journal of Nervous and Mental Disease **165**(2):79, 1977.

Mechanic, D.: Medical sociology, ed. 2, New York, 1978, The Free Press.

Mechanic. D.: Correlates of physician utilization, Journal of Health and Social Behavior **20**(4):387, 1979.

Mechanic, D., and Volkart, E.H.: Stress, illness behavior and the sick role, American Sociological Review **26:**51, February 1961.

Rosenblatt, D., and Suchman, E.A.: Blue-collar attitudes and information toward health and illness. In Shostak, A.B., and Gomberg, W., editors: Blue-collar worlds, Englewood Cliffs, N.J., 1965, Prentice Hall, Inc.

Rosenstock, I.M.: Why people use health services, Milbank Memorial Fund Quarterly; Health and Society, **64:**94, 1966.

Schachter, S., and Singer, J.: Cognitive, social and physiological determinants of emotional state, Psychological Review **69:**379, 1962.

Schlesinger, E.: Unpublished data, 1982.

Schlesinger, E., and Devore, W.: Ethnic networks: conceptual formulations and interventive strategies, Paper presented at the annual meeting of the American Public Health Association, Los Angeles, November 1982.

Suchman, E.A.: Sociomedical variations among ethnic groups, American Journal of Sociology, **70:**319, 1964.

Suchman, E.A.: Stages of illness and medical care, Journal of Health and Social Behavior **6:**114, 1965.

World Health Organization: Official records, No. 2, June 1948.

Zola, I.: Illness behavior of the working class. In Shostak, A.B., and Gomberg, W., editors: Blue-collar worlds, Englewood Cliffs, N.J., 1964, Prentice-Hall, Inc.

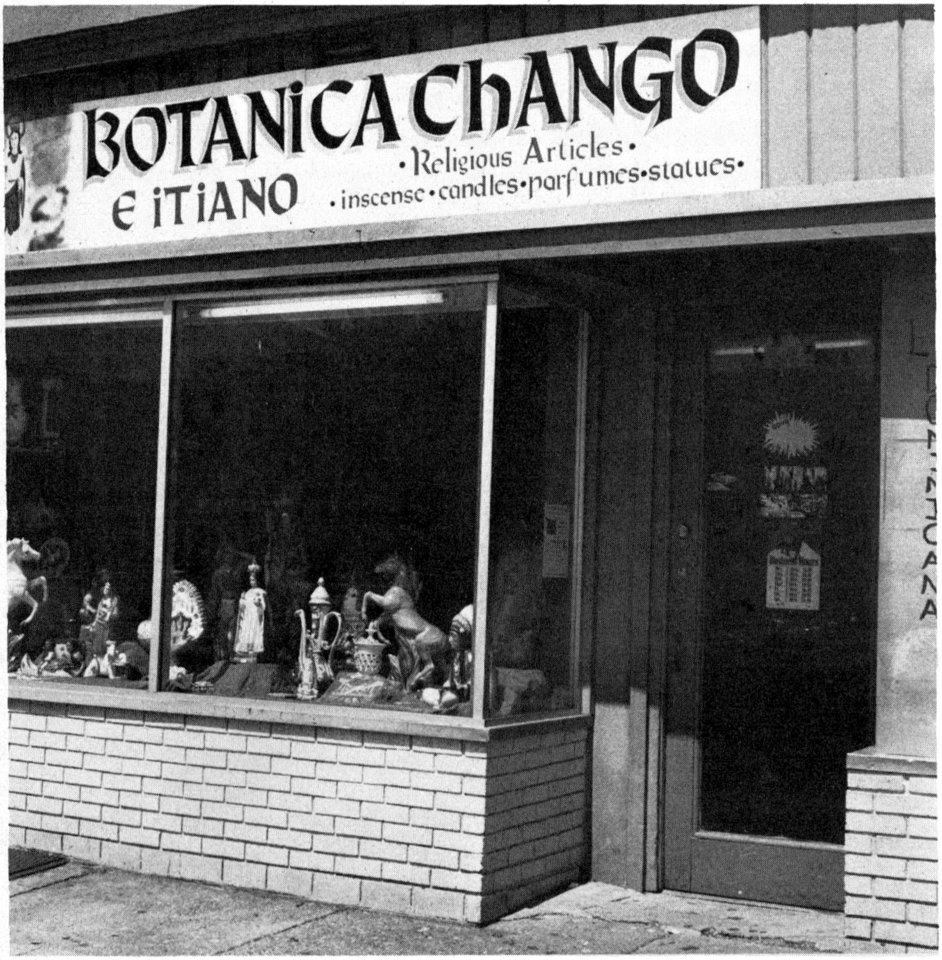
BOTANICA CHANGO
E ITIANO
• Religious Articles •
• inscense • candles • parfumes • statues •

Chapter 4

Variations in response to health and illness

Chapter 3 presented a number of basic concepts on health and illness behavior. This chapter builds on those themes by examining the relationship among age, gender, ethnicity, and health and illness behavior, with considerable attention to differences in how men, women, and members of various social classes and ethnic groups perceive and react to physical and emotional symptoms. The importance of this knowledge for social work practice has already been suggested. To the extent that variations in use of health services are related to these factors, such understanding can enhance the profession's efforts to improve the "fit" between the way services are financed and delivered and the needs and perceptions of those most in need of care.

How individuals and societies respond to illness relates to deeply ingrained beliefs about nature and the supernatural. Characteristic views about whether people can control their lives or whether they believe themselves to be hapless victims of forces beyond their control are expressed in societally approved norms about response to illness and explanations for its cause.

Because of the disruptive effects of illness, all societies and social groups define rights and obligations associated with being ill and develop mechanisms to control illness and its consequences. This fact has generated a number of concepts to explain how societies develop rules and norms about how people are supposed to behave when they believe themselves to be ill. One major formulation is the view of "the sick role" (Parsons, 1958). Another involves an extensive set of deliberations about whether the rules governing the behavior of and attitudes toward "the sick" bear similarity to those pertaining to deviants (Freidson, 1970; Gove, 1975; Mechanic, 1978; Parsons, 1958). A great deal has been written analyzing various illness-related responses in terms similar to those used to study forms of deviance. The extent to which these affect the way social workers approach their clients is of considerable importance in health care practice.

Another formulation involves the concept of illness behavior as a way of coping with diverse stresses (Mechanic, 1978). Closely related are various conceptions of stress and its impact on health and illness.

Study of the biological and physiological causes of disease are clearly within the purview of medicine and related physical sciences. However, the way in which life conditions contribute to disease is of concern to various health professionals. Social work, with its particular focus on the "person-environment interaction," has a special obligation to try to understand these connections.

THE ELDERLY AND ILLNESS BEHAVIOR

Chapter 1 presented data on life expectancy, the numbers of elderly people who are institutionalized, and those who, although they live in their own homes, require a substantial amount of help with the routine activities of living. Substantial numbers of people over 65 years of age report they are in reasonably good health. Nevertheless, as age increases, the number reporting their health as fair or poor increases (*Health, United States,* 1982).

This finding is not surprising. The older people get, the greater the likelihood that they will suffer from one or more chronic *diseases.* The fact, nevertheless, that so many state that they are "ok" supports the definition of health proposed earlier—the capacity to function in a variety of important ways despite the presence of disease or illness.

The elderly do use health services extensively. Their perspectives on how they are received by care givers, what they feel they need, and how they respond to health services deserve detailed examination. Although Chapter 10 will probe more deeply into some of the issues of long-term care as they are encountered in daily practice, some general comments are in order here.

Ours is a youth-oriented society. Virility, youth, vigor, and good looks are equated by many people with all the goods things of this world. When the elderly seek health care, they are confronted not only with their own declining vigor, but also with a mixture of stereotypes and negative feelings harbored by caretakers. Thus it is not surprising that many elderly people do not perceive the health system as "caring."

Considerable research on health care of the elderly shows that significant numbers of those over 65 are skeptical of physicians: many view physicians as detached and lacking interest in their concerns. The elderly visit physicians with greater frequency than any other age group, yet when asked by a group of researchers about their use of health services, many elderly people reported going less often than they thought indicated.

Of particular interest is the finding that people who were most impressed with physicians' technical knowledge were least likely to ask for help with mild discomfort. Many didn't think that their symptoms were in line with those the doctors were interested in treating.

This finding has enormous implications for health care delivery. It points to the lack of fit between the emphasis of much contemporary health education and service and the needs of many people. For some of the elderly, technology intensive care means lack of concern. For highly trained specialists, the care of many of the problems of the elderly provides limited opportunity to use their expertise. This costly care is not meeting needs as defined by both providers and consumers. Alternative approaches to monitoring failing hearts and swollen feet and above all minimizing the isolation of the elderly are clearly needed. Such approaches are being developed; the research findings reported should spur those efforts.

GENDER AND ILLNESS BEHAVIOR

The relationship between gender and illness behavior has long been of interest, especially as it reflects on differences in longevity, morbidity, and the use of health services. Recent interest has been triggered by concerns raised by the women's movement. These areas of thought and inquiry are related to core social work concerns—the quality of life in the family as it relates to the respective roles of women and men, the work they do, and real or perceived inequity.

Health status

The relationship among gender, health status, and illness behavior reflects an interesting paradox: Women report far more illness than men do—but they live longer. This has been true throughout the centuries (Marcus and Seeman, 1981). Many factors are thought to explain this difference, including presumed biological differences and differences in the way women and men are socialized. This in turn is thought to affect how men and women view health and illness and the extent to which they are ready to take care of their own health problems.

Some evidence points to the differences in the roles men and women have traditionally played in child care, nurture, and participation in the labor force as a factor in health and illness behavior.

Gender roles

Many have suggested that women have a constitutionally based greater resistance to infectious and degenerative disease (for example, Marcus and Seeman, 1981). Reviewing a number of animal studies, Mechanic (1978) points out that with some exceptions the "female advantage" is also found in most animal species. Also, more females than males survive in utero and in the first years of life.

Whatever the role of biological factors, there is no question that many of the differences can be understood in social-psychological terms. For example, most reports of morbidity are based on self-reports of illness or injury. The variations in such reporting have already been discussed.

> Apart from any objective physical symptoms, numerous social and psychological factors can encourage someone to report an illness or injury—or inhibit that report. If males and females differ in these factors, but not in physical symptom rates, a sex differential will exist. and it will have nothing to do with vulnerability to disease or injury (Verbrugge, 1976, p. 388).

Faced once again with the subtle but pervasive differences in the reporting of illness, a number of investigators have sought other means of determining whether women indeed are sicker than men. One approach* has focused on determining differences in the rates of acute versus chronic illness. For 1957 to 1972 it was found that women report more acute health problems than men. Men report more injuries than women do. Women not only report a greater number of acute complaints, but they also spend more time in bed when ill (23% to 44% more than men) or otherwise restrict their activities to a greater extent (12% to 35% more than men).

Verbrugge found that an adult woman is also more likely to have a chronic condition than an adult man. However, men are less likely to be able to carry on their usual activities when experiencing chronic illness than are women. This suggests that chronic conditions in men are more debilitating and severe than those experienced by women.

A number of hypotheses to account for these differences are suggested: (1) men do heavier work than women and thus are less able to carry on when they have a chronic condition; (2) it is more socially acceptable for women to report discomfort, since men are expected to be strong and not show their suffering; (3) women have more stress, thus generating more illness; and (4) women have fewer fixed work obligations and therefore can more readily take time off. The data suggest that even when women are performing work comparable to men's, women still report a greater number of acute conditions. Data are not readily available on the relationship among gender and socialization, gender roles, and illness behavior. It has been suggested that women have a greater variety of obligations, often involving work and family roles. In the view of some, fulfilling nurturant roles leads to fatigue or self-neglect, which in turn lowers resistance to illness.

One important study (Marcus and Seeman, 1981) examined the effect of "fixed role obligations" on health and illness behavior. Fixed role obligations involve (1) the degree of financial responsibility for a family's total income carried by an individual, (2) whether the individual is seen as heading the household, and (3) the employment status outside the home. The findings are instructive. Employment status sharply reduced the male-female differences in restriction of activity. Marcus and Seeman suggest that the work commitments factor helps to clarify the relationship between obligations and reduced activity. However, these differences do not help to explain women's greater tendency to recognize and act on symptoms of illness.

> At present, there is no comprehensive theory to explain sex differences in reports of illness and disability. Instead one encounters a series of hypotheses that include biological explanations, social and psychological factors,

* Much of the following data represents a summary of information presented by Verbrugge, L.M.: Females and illness: recent trends in sex differences in the United States, Journal of Health and Social Behavior **17:**387, Dec. 1976.

and differences in interviewing behavior* (Marcus and Seeman, 1981, p. 181).

Relevance for social work. Clearly these findings permit no clear-cut conclusion; however, a number of factors stand out. If women consistently feel ill more frequently, what is it about the conditions of their lives that generates this feeling? The women's movement has focused attention on the "double role" that women carry now that so many are in the labor force. Participation in the labor force, as we have seen, reduces the option to take time out. If this trend continues, and men do not assume a greater share of nurturant tasks, will women become even more stressed? Or does participation in the work force provide an enhanced sense of identity and self-worth that reduces discomfort? Recent work (Verbrugge, 1983) suggests a positive effect on health. Clearly these factors bear watching by social workers. Those women who head households usually do so with minimal economic wherewithal. Thus supports for this group must be built in.

Because men apparently experience more debilitating chronic illnesses than women and have a shorter life expectancy, the additionally stressful factors of spouse illness, displacement, and young widowhood are of concern. The long-range effects of the women's movement on deeply ingrained beliefs and behaviors about strength and vitality cannot yet be assessed. These findings do suggest that social workers have an obligation to be on the alert for the different kinds of psychological and social support that may be needed by women and men, if each is to have fewer negative illness effects. The stance suggested is one that goes beyond the rhetoric of "female oppression" or "male superiority," and looks for sources of support in family, friendship groups, social networks, and social organizations.

Women and the health care system. The women's movement has identified a number of aspects of health care delivery that appear to reflect a more general pattern of societal oppression of women. Olson (1977) points to those institutional arrangements based on the assumption that women's basic function is to bear and care for children. Marieskind (1975) states:

> Women's principal involvement with the medical system is through those organs uniquely female. Socialization patterns have taught women to regard their reproductive organs and their functions as unclean, a "curse" and secret, yet nonetheless central to their identity as women (p. 219).

Chesler (1972), Olson (1977), and others comment on relationships between women and the mental health system. Chesler suggests that women are victimized by the mental health care system and that they are inappropriately diagnosed or hospitalized. Olson suggests that any deviation from the norms of sex role behavior is viewed as pathological and results in treatment designed to

* Reference here is to possible differences in the way men and women respond to interviews in the annual health interview survey, carried out by the National Center for Health Services Research.

effect conformity with "appropriate" role expectations. Rosenfeld (1982) finds that both women and men are treated negatively by the mental health system when their behavior departs from that expected of the two sexes. Men are disproportionately hospitalized more often for disorders considered feminine (for example, depression, feelings of helplessness) and women for such "male" disorders as substance abuse.

Sex role stereotypes affect other mental health judgments (Broverman and others, 1970). Those traits identified as masculine are equated with mental health and those traits identified as feminine are considered fragile and equivalent to emotional disturbance.

Various medical treatments for women have been questioned. For example, are the number of radical mastectomies performed on women with breast cancer necessary—or does extensive use of this procedure reflect insensitive approaches practiced by a sexist and male-dominated medical profession?

Feminists have expressed concern at the widespread use of oral contraceptives, citing perceived threats to health (for example, increased risk of cancer, heart disease). Because of the immense popularity of these oral contraceptives, drug companies make great profits, and thus some critics view women as victims of the profit motive. Analogously, the use of estrogen therapy for menopausal women came under major attack when early studies suggested their use significantly increased the risk of cancer (*The New York Times,* 1976). Furthermore, the idea that menopause—a natural, biological stage in the life of women—was to be treated like a disease was seen as additional evidence that women were belittled by the health care establishment. The battle for a woman's right to have an abortion was, of course, a further component of this struggle.

There have been many efforts to inform women about the nature of their bodies and such body processes as menstruation, pregnancy, and menopause. A number of books have tried to help women learn about their bodies (for example, *Our Bodies, Ourselves,* 1971).

Women's health centers and health collectives have opened to teach women self-care (for example, to do their own internal examinations) and demystify and "demedicalize" these aspects of health care. In many of these centers women learn breast and cervical self-examination and help to interpret their own pregnancy tests.

There has been a tendency in some of these women's collectives, however, to base advice on limited or incomplete evidence. For example, recent investigation suggests that the risks associated with oral contraceptives are related to age, smoking, and certain other health characteristics (*Physicians' Desk Reference,* 1982). Some sources have failed to compare the risks associated with "the pill" with those incurred by unwanted pregnancies. Furthermore, it has often been ignored that the pill, more than most other contraceptive methods, freed many women to engage in sexual activity as they chose without fear of unwanted pregnancy.

It is quite true that menopause is a natural consequence of aging—and not a physical or psychic state to be bemoaned. Nevertheless, significant numbers of women do experience distressing "hot flashes" that can be minimized by use of estrogen therapy. Recent investigation has strongly and carefully pinpointed and clarified the nature of risks related to such therapy (Bachman and others, 1982; *Physicians' Desk Reference,* 1982).

Such information allows women to make considered choices based on personal and family medical history. The risks can be weighed and compared to the degree of discomfort that some menopausal women experience. As social workers consider these kinds of issues with women—in family planning centers, hospitals, and outreach programs—they need to be able to help women sort out fact from rhetoric.

Much remains to be done to increase the knowledge base needed to identify the differences in illness behavior that are biologically or socially based. Nevertheless, recent developments have served to sensitize social workers to these issues.

ETHNICITY AND ILLNESS BEHAVIOR

It has been suggested that "culture exerts its most fundamental and far-reaching influence through the categories we employ to understand and respond to sickness" (Kleinman, 1978). These culturally based understandings and responses are transmitted in myriad ways. A major vehicle for their persistence through generations is the ethnic group.

In this section I will review an approach to understanding the relationship between ethnicity and health behavior. I will also summarize some of the basic themes that emerge from various ethnic group memberships, how these affect perspectives on health and illness, and their practice applications.

Ethclass and the ethnic reality

One important line of inquiry has focused on the impact of and connections between social class and ethnic group membership in America. Taking the view that social class is a major determinant of chances for a good life, Gordon (1964) suggested that ethnicity might explain major differences among people who occupy similar social class positions. The point at which ethnicity and social class interact he called *ethclass.* At this intersect, identifiable differences in perspective and behavior, including illness behavior, are discerned. Devore and Schlesinger (1981) termed the dispositions that are generated at this intersect *the ethnic reality,* or ethclass in action. The term *ethnic reality* then translates the concept ethclass into behaviors that can be observed, interpreted, and understood in terms of ethnicity and social class.

Dispositions related to illness, pain, and death affect all of human existence and are intimately derived from ethnic and family experiences. These include ritual, prayer, foods that spell comfort, and a basic belief about whether the gods and nature control fate or wheter humans can overcome the threats of illness and forestall death. They relate to the work people do, how that work is evaluated by others, and what the fruits of that work can buy. These behaviors are reinforced by persistent discrimination and negative evaluation by mainstream society. The ethnic reality then buttresses and supports members of an ethnic group against insult and degradation. Lack of power, of course, limits the degree of protection that can be offered. In considering the relationship between ethnicity and illness behavior, it is important to note that much of that behavior is also related to position in the social structure. These factors converge to generate persistent variations in health beliefs and practices of different groups, including (1) views about the cause of illness, (2) perspectives on curing practices, (3) views about the types of facilities and resources consid-

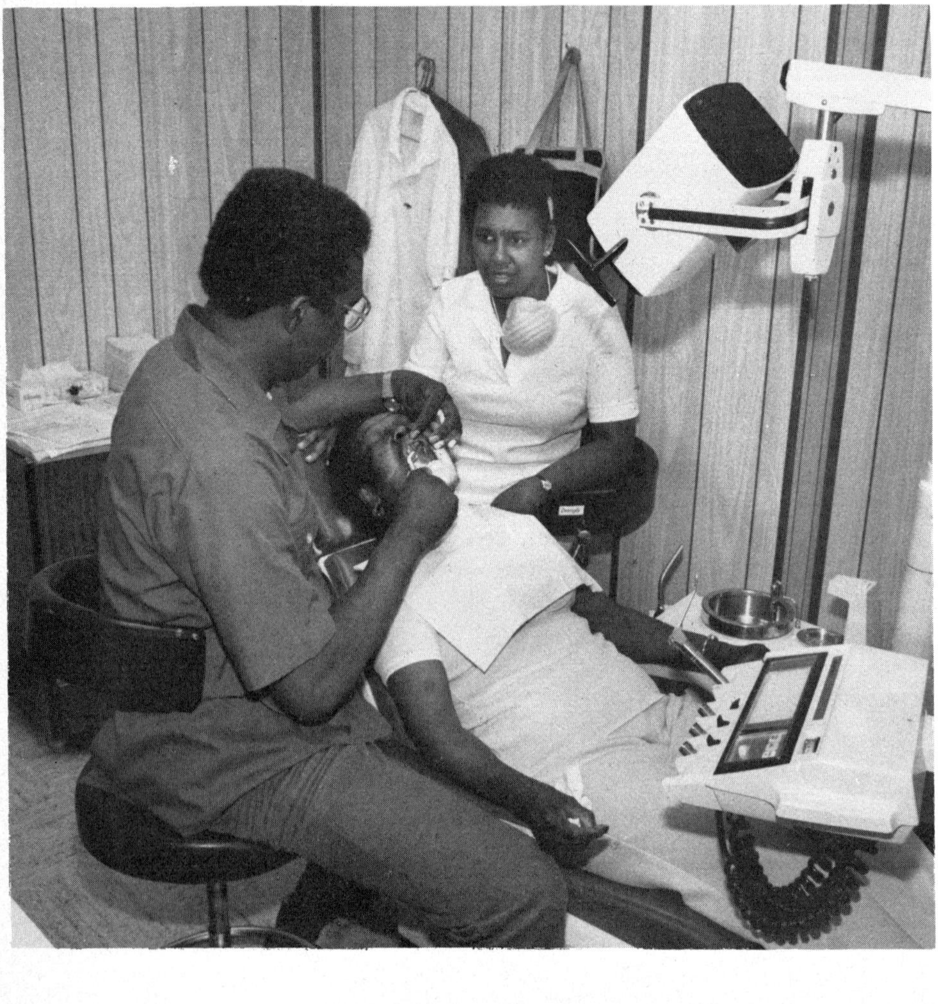

ered to be appropriate healers, and (4) "legitimate" reactions to pain and illness. Also significant are views about the relative importance of the role of formal health systems as contrasted with that played by family, neighborhood, and community in relieving the distress associated with illness (Devore and Schlesinger, 1981).

Views on illness causation

One important difference among ethnic and social groups is the perceived cause of illness. Snow (1974) reviews the health beliefs entrenched in a system of folk medicine, elements of which are shared by such diverse groups as Mexican-Americans, Puerto Ricans, southern whites, and Kansas farmers. Many of those who adhere to these folk beliefs are members of the underclass, or what some term the lower class. Snow's work suggests that many of the health beliefs of this group result from a composite of premodern classic medicine, European folklore, some African traits, modern scientific medicine, fundamentalist Christian views, and the voodoo religion of the West Indies. Illness may be viewed as a result of disharmony or of the actions of a vengeful God or nature. Some people simply view illness as one of many undesirable conditions, much like poverty and unemployment. Some Navajo Indians view illness as indicative of underlying disharmony that may be a reflection of witchcraft, spirits, animal contamination, and disordered relationships (Coulehan, 1980). Many members of Hispanic groups view fate, the gods, spirits, or fellow human beings as the cause of illness (Garrison, 1977; Martínez, 1978).

Fabrega (1974) suggests that some non-Western health belief systems have complex, integrated taxonomies of disease and curing practices. He reviews diverse studies of "folk curing" in preliterate societies that have attempted to analyze problems of illness and medical care in relation to other cultural activities of the group. Some of this work demonstrates that "beliefs about the causes of all types of illness . . . explicitly refer to notions of friendship, rivalry, envy, moral worth, and malevolence" (p. 6).

These views are in sharp contrast to the views of illness causation advanced by mainstream Western society. Contemporary medical theories of causation all derive from the conviction that nature can be understood and mastered.

Healing practices

Most Americans are familiar with and use physicians, hospitals, nurses, and various social services, whether they are upper-middle-class white Protestants in luxurious city apartments, Navajo Indians on a reservation, or working-class Puerto Ricans in a Newark ghetto.

Yet to varying degrees some members of these and other groups will, at some time in their lives, be inclined to use nontraditional healers. I attended a 1978 meeting in Philadelphia on holistic health care at which a number of health practitioners spoke. Psychics and experts on traditional Chinese medical beliefs joined professors of medicine from some of America's most prestigious medical schools in lecturing on or learning about departures from classic Western healing practices. The present focus is on diverse curing practices that derive from ethnic belief systems. That conference underscored the fact that the dominant curing practices are found wanting by many. Recourse to a variety of health care practitioners is much more common than is commonly known.

Consider an anthropologist's definition of the *healer:* "Healers are defined . . . as 'persons who provide counselling, advice or other services directed toward the relief of symptoms or improved functioning for persons with complaints that the modern Western Medical Social/Mental Health care system might define as health, social or mental problems.'" These healers are further classified by whether they are folk or professional healers. From this perspective a wide range of healers have been identified.

Ethnographic study (Garrison, 1979) of a catchment area in Newark, New Jersey, identified a series of folk healers who operate independently of the formal health care system. Most users of these systems are also active users of the formal health care system. In some communities as many as 70% of residents will use both folk and contemporary medical practitioners. They include those who practice "rootwork," a form of folk medicine, and spiritualists. There are "health centers" such as *botanicas* (Spanish religious stores), which may sell various herbs, and *espiritisto centros.*

A number of Catholic churches whose congregants are white members of various ethnic groups sponsor charismatic prayer and healing groups. The increase in faith-healing beliefs and practices of some American charismatic religions is well known because of several television programs emphasizing these beliefs.

The services offered by practitioners in Afro-American religious stores, although referred to as "readings," usually involve talking about problems. Garrison (1979) characterizes these talks as "a lay form of the open-ended interview of psychiatric social work, based on popular knowledge of psychology" (p. 12). Examination of their practices, based on extensive case examples cited, suggests that such things as magic spells and powders are used as strategies to attract or repel people with whom they are involved in problematic relationships.

Espiritismo is firmly grounded in Puerto Rican culture and has its own set of theories about causation: There is an invisible world of spirits consisting of all those who have ever lived, will be born, or are to be reincarnated. Human beings are born with "material impulses" that predominate over spiritual sentiments. Patterns of behavior are attributed to these spiritist forces. Spirits can get out of control.

The essential belief is that any individual jealous of the achievement, advantages or abilities of another, whether in love, business or politics can arrange to have an evil spell cast on the adversary (Wintrob, 1973). In sessions with the *espiritista* these spirits are said to express their feelings to the afflicted "I want you dead"; or the spirit would confess to changing its form into a snake, getting into bed between the afflicted and her husband or causing her to have cesarean deliveries. The treatment procedures focus on exorcising harmful spiritual influences in sessions that extend over considerable time periods (Garrison, 1979).

Lest the reader consider this detailed discussion to be an irrelevant digression, the following observation made by Garrison may dispel that notion:

> Most Puerto Rican psychiatric patients, 66 to 94 percent reported in three different studies have sought the help of spiritists prior to coming to mental health services and may continue to embrace a "spiritual" explanation and understanding of their problem. . . .
>
> It is possible that, with the cultural confusion and misunderstanding of Spanish speaking patients in the mainland mental health services . . . the spiritists are providing more appropriate and effective services. . . . An active working relationship between the *espiritistas* of the catchment area and the community mental health center could serve to improve the quality of care provided in both settings (p. 33).

Mexican-Americans have a similar set of beliefs and practices. The *curanderas* have healing powers believed to be a gift from God; they practice a system of curing known as *curandismo.* Description of the work of *curanderos* (or *curanderas*) suggests an emphasis on counseling, advice, and support. Ritual, confession, massage, and herbal remedies are parts of the treatment. Evidence varies on how successful *curanderos* are in treating emotional problems and on how extensively they are used. In their study in Los Angeles, Edgerton and others (1978) found relatively limited use of such practitioners. On the other hand, they cite Madsen, who finds the work of *curanderos* to be very effective.

Simultaneous use of folk remedies and folk healers continues, despite different findings on the extent of such use.

My own unsystematic explorations give some indication of the tensions as well as the unspoken collaboration that exists between the various healing systems.

On a visit to a neighborhood health center that serves a Chicano community in Denver I asked one of the physicians whether any of the center's patients used "non-Western" approaches to healing. He shrugged off my question and said that on occasion a child was brought with some dried up egg yolk on its chest.* But other than such an occasional experience he thought not.

As my visit through the center progressed I talked with "Anglo" social workers and with community-based Chicano health aides about the same issue.

* Apparently a procedure meant to heal.

Some of the aides were angry with the physician whom I'd interviewed. They thought he did not really understand their people. More important, they thought he could do them harm because, they said, he did not bother to inform himself about such practices as taking herbal teas to reduce agitation. If he also prescribed tranquilizers he might be overdosing people.

And some of the Anglo social workers were quite aware of the fact that some of their patients consulted *curanderos* for such symptoms as "feeling lizards in their stomach." And, importantly, the *curanderos* often seemed to be able to rid people of their affliction, "caused" by the bad will of a relative or a spirit, thus ruling out a diagnosis of severe psychopathology.

Other important folk healers are found among various American Indian nations or tribes. Customs, practices, and beliefs clearly differ among the various groups. The example of the Navajo is instructive. There is little distinction within the culture between religion and medicine, and healing experiences are an integral part of community life. Harmony—of people with each other, with nature, and with gods—is the desired state. The Navajo "sing" is a public event that draws in the entire community on behalf of afflicted persons (Coulehan, 1980). Through such ceremonies, persons suffering from depression that had not responded to modern psychotherapeutic intervention improved and returned to their former activities.

Literature on the disposition to healing of various groups points to a persistent theme. The family and the community are seen as a major source of healing and care:

> The clients of *espiritistas* receive advice about interpersonal relations, support, encouragement, and physical contact such as stroking or massage; treatment typically takes place at public meetings of spiritist groups. The patient's family is often required to be present in the healing process (Devore and Schlesinger, 1981, p. 257).

This emphasis on the healing and caring role of family and community systems is not limited to a group of people who have deeply ingrained beliefs in non-Western healing systems. Many white ethnic groups view the "extended family [as] the front-line resource for intensive advice on emotional problems" (Frandetti and Gelfand, 1978). This has been documented in a three-generation study of Italians, Jews, and Slavs (Krause, 1978) and in a review of the dispositions of diverse ethnic groups (Giordano and Giordano, 1977).

Many Asian-Americans prefer to deal with mental health problems within the confines of the family (Kitano, 1976). To do otherwise brings shame on the family and acknowledges severe emotional problems, which is not consonant with many ingrained belief patterns. Just "being in therapy" may generate such extensive anxiety that the process of verbalization may bring no relief (Toupin, 1980). Members of "blue-collar" white ethnic groups share similar perspectives. To be a client is to be stigmatized (Giordano and Giordano, 1977).

The implications of this kind of understanding for social work practice have been developed into a model of "ethnic-sensitive social work practice"; suggestions for their application in the health arena have been made (Devore and Schlesinger, 1981).

Illness responses

Studies of variation in response to illness have focused on at least two different issues. One relates to the varying conceptions of symptoms, symptom complexes, and disease as these are understood and described by members of many groups, especially those of Hispanic origin. The second centers on the difference in response by various ethnic groups.

Alternative symptom and disease complexes. Martínez and Martin (1978) identify a number of disease concepts prominent among urban Mexican-Americans. *Mal ojo* (evil eye), *empacho* (surfeit), *susto* (magical fright), *caída de mollera* (fallen fontanelle), and *mal puesto* (hex) are all concepts that persist. Some of these (for example, *caída de mollera*) are said to originate from dislocated internal organs; others (for example, *mal ojo*) have magical origin, while *susto* is a disease of emotional origin.

According to Rubel (1978), *susto* is a syndrome that reflects the belief that an individual is composed of "a corporeal being and one or more immaterial souls or spirits which may become detached from the body and wander freely." When the soul leaves the body, a number of symptoms may be present: (1) restless sleep patterns; (2) listlessness, loss of appetite, poor personal hygiene; or (3) loss of weight and strength. *Susto* may manifest itself as a result of emotional distress (for example, a woman's negative reaction to her husband's extramarital affairs). Case studies demonstrate the presence of still more diverse symptoms and circumstances that trigger the appearance of *susto.* Rubel hypothesizes that some Mexican-Americans will identify the presence of *susto* in some forms of self-perceived stressful situations or as a consequence of an experience in which an individual is unable to meet societal role expectations.

Symptoms that in the disease concepts of Western medicine may be attributed to stress are, in this system, linked to magical thinking.

The *ataque,* not uncommon among mainland Puerto Ricans, has been described by Garrison (1977) and other researchers.

> A set of symptoms—which may consist of tearing off one's clothing in public, screaming, and falling into a semiconscious state while twitching—is considered a culturally recognized cry for help when people are experiencing a lot of strain (Devore and Schlesinger, 1981, p. 244).

Clearly this discussion can only touch on a few of the symptom complexes identified for some Mexican and Puerto Rican Americans; however, extensive literature is available on this subject.

The intent of this brief discussion is to sensitize the reader to the existence of folk healing practices. Sufficient evidence exists that many of those who use modern health services may explain and act on their symptoms in the terms described here. Unless the health professional is aware of this possibility, there is great potential for faulty communication with patients.

Response to symptoms. A profile can be constructed of ideal users of health and social services based on prevailing professional standards and typical modes of organization. According to this ideal, patients would behave as follows:

1. *Patients articulate their complaints and symptoms in terms readily recognized by professionals.* A headache is to be described as such, with detail given about location, intensity, and duration. The person experiencing a marital problem should say so and not couch his concerns in other symptoms. (However, wise social workers know that the complaints originally presented are often not those for which people actually seek help.)

2. *In articulating complaints patients are* not *to make a diagnosis.* Diagnosis is the professional's prerogative.

3. *Complaints are to be appropriate to the degree of discomfort or disease present.* Volatile patients who have pain no matter where touched hamper efforts to isolate the true source of difficulty. Stoic patients, although perhaps to be admired for their capacity to suffer in silence, can nevertheless create problems for health care professionals, because failure to envince the cry of pain associated with a particular diagnosis can lead the diagnostician astray.

4. *People are to cooperate with prescribed treatment.*

5. *People should keep appointments, notify health professionals if they cannot be there, and try to avoid getting sick during the night or on week ends.*

Few people, including members of ethnic groups with distinct orientations to care and to how they manifest and worry about symptoms, can meet all of these expectations. However, these expectations are imperceptibly entrenched in the behaviors health care professionals have come to expect. People are not supposed to pay too much attention to illness (at least no more than is "appropriate"); they are supposed to believe physicians when told something is wrong or not; and they are supposed to acknowledge problems when they have them so they can get the proper help.

How close do members of various ethnic groups come to meeting these expectations? A number of studies have shown that as a group Jews have extensive concern with health (Zborowski, 1952); this is believed by some to be related to "the sense of precariousness and fear concerning survival related to centuries of dispersal and persecution" (Howe, 1975). They are thought to behave in general accord with the objectives and methods of modern medicine, make extensive use of physicians, and have great concern about the meaning of symptoms (Greenblum, 1974; Suchman, 1964). In these respects they make "ideal" patients when measured against the ideal patient profile. But their volatile emotional concerns cause "trouble" and extra work. They are said to raise many questions and make many demands. So the Jewish mother who hovers over her child becomes the butt of jokes and in more serious terms is described as overprotective and demanding.

The stoicism of some Slavs (Stein, 1976), Old Americans, or white Anglo-Saxons (Zborowski, 1952), and others has been noted. Greeks worry more about illness than people of Irish or British origin (Pilowsky and Spence, 1977). Italians are also said to be volatile (Zborowski, 1952).

Many American Indians consider efforts to engage them in discussion of emotional issues as "interference" (Goodtracks, 1973). Many Asian Americans refrain from using mental health services, fearing that to do so may mean that one has shamed the family and the community (Lin and Lin, 1978; President's Commission on Mental Health, 1978).

Applications for social workers

I have touched on predominant patterns of ethnically related health and illness behavior repeatedly identified in the behavioral science literature. The discussion illustrates that almost all people can be expected to depart from idealized norms. Sometimes these departures are dramatic and seemingly incongruous with the prevailing, accepted approaches to health care delivery. The use of the *espiritista,* the *curandero,* and the Navajo singer exemplify this group. The more subtle variations or deviations derive from custom, with experience with mainstream society, and from deeply ingrained habitual responses.

Appropriate professional response to these dispositions is crucial—because often these behaviors are manifested at times when people are experiencing major crises. A social worker may not do too much harm in chiding the mother of a healthy infant for her overprotectiveness. By contrast, volatile Jewish stroke victims may be expressing the most profound kind of sorrow in those ways by which they have learned to respond to threats to their well-being. The folk healer is a respected and trusted member of the community whose efforts are too often demeaned. When that happens, patients may conceal the fact that they use them. The consequence may be failure to understand why our ministrations do not work.

Health care social workers can adapt their efforts to ensure greater sensitivity to (1) the ethnic and class roots of illness behavior, (2) the disproportionate prevalence and incidence of health problems found among many minority groups, and (3) the real and perceived barriers in health care delivery.

THE SICK ROLE

The last section emphasized how individual and group characteristics affect a people's sense of whether they are ill or well and what to do if they feel they are not well. As soon as people identify themselves as ill—especially to others—a host of responses is set into play:

You really must go to the doctor, so that you'll feel better.
Come on now, don't let a little thing like a backache get you down.
If I'm really sick, I'll lose my job.

or

I'm really sick enough to take a few days off from work.

These examples of the ways in which people ruminate about being sick reflect some of the responses to the consequences of illness. While these consequences are many, emphasis here is on the socially triggered responses to the disturbances in social life generated by illness. They relate to the rules and norms about how people are expected to behave when they get ill and to the privileges or withdrawal of privileges and obligations associated with being sick.

Sociologists have termed these rules and norms to be those governing the *sick role.* This term, first introduced by Talcott Parsons (1958), focuses on the unspoken rules that social groups develop to govern the behavior of those who are ill and their relationship to those who presumably can help them get better. The concept, though considerably expanded, refined, and critiqued, is nevertheless very important to understanding illness behavior.

According to Parsons, American society does not "blame" people for getting ill and does not hold them responsible for their illness. However, illness is thought of as undesirable and disruptive because it keeps people from fulfilling their obligations. Therefore people have a clear-cut responsibility for doing all possible to regain their health. Basically that involves putting oneself into the hands of experts—usually physicians. Based on these perspectives Parsons outlined four basic components of the sick role:

1. As noted, people are not responsible for illness; however, to be sick is not viewed as a desirable state.
2. For the duration of an illness, people are exempted from their usual responsibilities.
3. While ill, they must demonstrate a willingness to get well.
4. To demonstrate their willingness to get well they are obliged to seek technically competent advice and treatment.

This concept, though brilliant in its simplicity, requires some elaboration, criticism, and examples to highlight strengths and flaws.

Most people learn appropriate spoken and unspoken rules while growing up. Despite the variations in response to symptoms, once these are acknowledged, people are expected and allowed to reduce their normal activities. Being sick means being allowed to stay home from school or work without expecting punishment. By the same token, if people are suspected of feigning illness as an excuse for not fulfilling a responsibility, their behavior is viewed negatively. The child who consistently develops stomachaches in the morning is accused of not wanting to go to school. Workers who are frequently absent because of minor illness are soon viewed with some skepticism.

If people around the sick person believe that some course of action will shorten or cure the illness, they are inclined to badger individuals who do not follow that course:

If you'd gone to the doctor a week ago you'd be better now.

Admonitions to take it easy and not to worry about usual responsibilities are frequently voiced, as is the need to be in shape to work:

> Oh, of course dear, don't come to work today. We can manage. Just be sure to rest and take your medicine so you'll be in tip-top shape when you get back.

Those who carry on their responsibilities despite evident illness are in some sense admired:

> Imagine, he came to work every day with that bad back, and never a word of complaint out of him.

But those who seem to enjoy the benefits of being sick are suspect:

> Seems to me, he's been collecting those disability checks for much longer than he really needed to.
>
> I think he really likes all that pampering he's getting. It's about time he got up and did some work.

Despite the remarkable accuracy of certain components of the sick role concept as outlined by Parsons, major questions have been raised concerning several points, including (1) the contention that the sick are truly relieved of their usual tasks and not blamed for being ill and (2) the implicit assumption that if they do all that is required to get better, they will get better.

Illness as deviance

Thinking about illness as deviance proceeds from the assumption that like criminal behavior, illness is to be avoided because it is disruptive. Any deviance requires control, and society develops mechanisms for controlling and curbing deviance. Freidson (1970) and others have suggested that contemporary society assigns to physicians the role of curbing the deviance associated with illness. Because of their professional expertise, they are the people who determine whether and when someone is "legitimately" ill.

Although this may be an oversimplified idea, examples can readily be cited. Many American industries and schools require a physician's note when people claim they are ill and cannot attend. Lacking this proof, they may be punished by being classified as truant or may not be paid under rules governing payment for workdays lost because of illness. In the Soviet Union plant physicians are said to have the power to determine how many people can legitimately be classified as ill without unduly disrupting production quotas (Field, 1953). Thus people are allowed to take time from their duties only when a "technical expert"—the physician—agrees that they are ill. If they "act sick" nevertheless, they are considered deviant and are deprived of the benefits associated with the sick role.

Also at question is the contention that the sick are not blamed for their illness. There are many conditions under which people are held responsible for being sick. There has always been a tendency to hold people responsible for getting sexually transmitted diseases. At a more simplistic level is the familiar admonition, "If you'd worn a sweater, you wouldn't have caught that cold," Currently, people are held responsible for getting lung cancer if they smoke and heart disease if they do not exercise or adhere to a proper diet. Indeed, many life insurance companies have lowered premiums for nonsmokers.

Stigma and chronicity

Another important consideration for social workers is whether health care providers and the community deal with people *as if* they were responsible for being ill. Freidson (1970) proposes that analysis of the stigma attached to some conditions (for example, stammering, convulsive disorders) and the chronic character of much illness evokes behaviors and feelings akin to those generated when people are held responsible for deviant acts. He contends that the relationship between illness and exemption from ordinary obligations is not as clear-cut as Parsons proposes. Furthermore, the societal reaction imposes burdens beyond those triggered by the illness itself, namely, stigma. For example convulsive disorders are thought to involve a serious deviation from the norm. While those who have such disorders are relieved of some obligations, certain privileges may also be suspended (for example, they may have their drivers' licenses suspended). Even though they do all they can to get well (for example, see a physician regularly, take medication) they do not get better in the clear-cut sense. Using Goffman's idea of equating stigma with "spoiled identity" (1963), one can see that many people do not regain a "normal identity" or get truly better no matter how well they play the sick role.

Yet much of health care is predicated on the assumption that sick people ought to behave in ways such as those outlined by Parsons.

In Freidson's view the perspective presented by Parsons also does not account for what happens to those who are chronically ill or dying. They too do not get better, even if they do all the experts prescribe. Freidson also suggests that much done in the name of health care and rehabilitation is based on this limited perspective on the sick role, in turn generating behavior by health care providers that is designed for the comfort of providers and those who are well. For example, teaching the blind to "face" those to whom they are speaking does not make it easier for the blind to function; it merely makes sighted people more comfortable. Conformity to societal norms is then one dimension of prescribed sick role behavior. The extent to which such conformity serves the needs of the ill must be examined.

Posed this way, the view of illness as deviance to be controlled raises many questions for health care social work. Is the profession's function to help people maximize their capacities despite illness or conform to social expectations? Freidson's questions prod us to examine what we do in the name of helping people to "adapt." The example of blind people who are trained to face their audience pinpoints some issues. It may be said that if the blind can assume ordinary physical stances in social interactions with sighted individuals, people are more likely to react to them based on characteristics other than their blindness—the fact that they have something important to say, or can sing, for example. When sighted individuals are confronted with someone who faces away, the blindness becomes an organizing theme for the social interaction, deflecting attention from the ordinary pleasures and routines of what is going on. Similarly, the stroke victim who regains speech, albeit with some evidence of deficit, has increased opportunity for social interaction.

Are these then undue burdens imposed on the sick by the well in the name of social control, or are they expectations based on the assumption that certain characteristics enhance social functioning? In my view it is only when rehabilitation processes are rigidly imposed, without sensitivity to the strains involved in coping, that they impose undue burdens. Thus social workers and others must take care not to project expectations that are burdensome. For example, there is an expectation (Holden, 1980) that all victims of severe diseases, such as end-stage renal disease, will do all that is possible to remain alive and to function. This involves undergoing treatment that can be physically and psychologically debilitating. Similarly, cancer victims are often expected to take all available chemotherapy; stroke victims may be considered resistive if they do not take advantage of every opportunity for rehabilitation. These considerations are in keeping with the enactment of the sick role as outlined by Parsons. When an atmosphere is generated that leaves people no out, then the sick are being treated in terms that provide comfort and rewards for professionals and those who are well—not for themselves.

A social work perspective makes it imperative that the wishes and dispositions of those needing care be taken into account. Expansions of the sick role concept that acknowledge chronicity are useful, as are perspectives that focus on efforts to enhance coping skills.* These and related ideas all acknowledge diverse ways of enhancing functioning when sickness is relatively permanent. They also relate to the definition of health I proposed in Chapter 3: a state of being that maximizes dynamic involvement in life, even in the presence of illness. Such a state depends on several factors. Pertinent here is the one related to a major component of Parsons' conception of the sick role—the socially derived notion that the dysfunctions and discomforts associated with illness are undesirable. Few would disagree with that contention. Social work is obliged by its professional mandate to try to minimize those discomforts. In that process, social workers must be aware of the additional burdens imposed by stigmatization, by needless requests to play out the sick role in all of its

---

* See Chapter 5 for discussion of coping-adaptation models.

dimensions, and by social control efforts disguised as treatment.

The prevailing criticisms of the sick role concept, the view of illness as deviance, and insight into the process of stigmatization all serve to sensitize health professionals to major issues. When we prod the sick to do all they can to get better, the motivation and process must be clearly examined and understood. Is the action being carried out based on careful assessment of individual or group need? Are the needs and wishes of the client/consumer given priority, or are societal needs paramount? These questions must continually be raised, because they surface when people are prodded to do all they can to regain function related to a disability or when judgments are made about whether disabled individuals are more comfortable living in the community or in an institution.

The issues surrounding institutionalization are a good case in point. In the past many disabled people were institutionalized to protect society from confronting those it stigmatized. Today, in the name of the "benefits of community care," too many are left without adequate protection or nurture. When those unable to care for themselves are left to roam the streets they are doubly stigmatized.

It is doubtful whether the stigma associated with visible disability can ever be totally eliminated. The negative effects of such stigmatization can be minimized for the individual by attention to the resources and coping skills that permit functioning despite disability, chronic illness, and stigma.

STRESS AND ILLNESS

Stress is invariably considered in any discussion of health and illness. These considerations range from Selye's classic physiological conception of the stress mechanism (1956) to television commercials that promise the relief of presumable stress-induced symptoms by use of aspirin and other nonprescription drugs. The wide interest in stress phenomena may indicate the common subjective sense of distress and pressure that is part of modern society.

It is difficult to present a brief, succinct, systematic discussion of the stress phenomenon that helps to clarify the relationship between stress and illness because of the diverse ways in which the concept is used and the essential lack of clarity about the role it plays in inducing illness. For these reasons the discussion here is limited to (1) efforts to clarify some commonly used terminology, (2) a review of some major themes found in the stress literature, (3) identification of some components of the stress process, and (4) a consideration of how social workers might use these concepts in their work.

Definitions

The term *stress* has been used to refer to "disruptions in personal, social and cultural processes that have some relationship to health and disease" (Mechanic, 1978, p. 222). The term is commonly used to refer to distresses that lead to disease or to the state of being that results from some distressing event—a state of stress.

A useful distinction has been made between *stressors* that act on the body and the resultant state of physical stress. For example, Selye (1956) refers to physical agents such as heat, cold, or infection as stressors that lead to maladaptation in hormonal secretions. "Maladaptation occurs when the secretion of [various] hormones is out of balance with the requirements of the organism in adjusting to stressors" (Kosa and Robertson, 1975, p. 45). Disturbance of hormonal secretion can result from the action of physical or psychological stressors. An illustration of the effect of physical stressors is useful*: Consider the victim of an auto accident. The victim is unconscious, suffers brain swelling, broken bones, internal injuries, and bleeding. He is subjected to surgery. The adrenal glands respond, pumping out great amounts of hormones. A positive effect of these hormones is in the brain. However, the hormones of the adrenal gland also cause an increase in the secretions of the stomach. Thus the unconscious victim of an auto accident can develop a bleeding ulcer, which is aptly termed a *stress ulcer*. The battering the body endured as a result of the accident and its treatment affected the hormonal secretions. It is hypothesized that psychological stressors can have effects on the body similar to those generating a stress ulcer.

Another use of the term suggested by Mechanic (1978) conceives stress as the discrepancy between demands made on individuals and their capacity to respond to these demands. The discrepancy is said to generate physiological changes, feelings of discomfort, and concern.

Closely related is a concept of *crisis,* which suggests that crisis is not defined by any particular situation but by whether or not people have the capacity to deal with a given situation. New stimuli or new life situations may be viewed as crises or stress states when people lack the resources to deal with them. Some diseases, illnesses, or injuries are crises by this definition.

This line of reasoning is consistent with the view that new life events, whether these are positive, such as marriage or job promotion, or negative such as divorce, job loss, or illness, are stressors because they call for new coping skills and resources.†

Life events

Substantial evidence supports the view that people who have been exposed to many difficult life events or are isolated are more frequently ill than is ordinarily expected. A few repeatedly noted examples are instructive. Meyer and Haggerty (1962) found that among a group of persons with streptococcal infections, a disproportionately high number had previously experienced cri-

*The example and suggestions concerning the physiological impact of physical and psychic stressors are based on conversations with Richard Schlesinger, M.D.

†This view of stress has generated considerable research using the Social Readjustment Rating Scale. (See, for example, Holmes, T.H., and Rahe, R. H.: The Social Readjustment Rating Scale, Journal of Psychosomatic Research **11:**213, 1967.)

ses such as a death in the family, job loss, unusual job pressures, or change in residence. Of special interest is one study that examined which employees in tuberculosis sanitoriums developed tuberculosis. It was found that employees with extensive stressful experiences in the two years preceding onset were much more likely to get tuberculosis than employees who were not involved in such stressful experiences (Holmes and Masuda, 1970). Holmes (1978) discusses the results of laboratory studies that show clear-cut relationships between psychological and familial stressors and symptom onset.

Personality traits

Many efforts have been made to relate the onset of certain diseases to personality types, or "weakness of personality structure." In reviewing work on personality structure, Kosa and Robertson (1975) suggest that those working from this perspective have not identified the link between various personality structures and the stress that induces illness.

Nevertheless, the relationship between certain personality traits (described as type A) and a disproportionately high rate of coronary heart disease has been well documented. This coronary-prone behavior pattern is said to include excessive striving for achievement, time urgency, and hostility (Glass, 1977).

Environmental situations

Chapter 1 examined the relationship between socioeconomic status and illness; it was seen that more people at the lower rungs of the socioeconomic ladder consistently seem to suffer from any given health problem than those more favorably situated. The processes whereby conditions of low socioeconomic status and disadvantage trigger disease are poorly understood.

The stress process. Cassel's work (1974) is of particular importance. Citing the work of Selye and Wolff, he suggests that they have not identified the nature of "noxious stimuli" that generate the neuroendocrinal changes characteristic of the stress state. Their reasoning, and that of others, he contends, is based on the assumption that psychosocial processes act in the same way as microbiological disease agents, that is, various psychosocial stressors will generate specific diseases. This idea, in Cassel's opinion, is dubious. He proposes that psychosocial processes acting as "conditional stressors" will alter the endocrine balance in the body and increase the body's susceptibility to disease. It is this susceptibility together with people's response to their social environment that is critical; this might be implicated in any disease process. Genetic endowment and experience also play a part.

Focusing on change and dislocation in the social environment, he cites a number of studies that indicate that people who for any reason have been deprived of meaningful social contact are particularly susceptible to disease, injury, and other health problems. Minority status, isolation, and frequent changes in occupation or residence have been implicated.

In Cassel's view this "formulation of the role of psychosocial factors in disease etiology would have important implications from the point of view of both research and intervention strategies" (Cassel, 1974, p. 474). Such an approach would involve efforts to clarify the nature of experiences of people who become ill by particular assessment of the kinds of isolation, negative societal evaluation, or loss they have experienced.

He postulates that two major sets of psychosocial factors may be involved in illness causation. One is the need for positive environmental feedback that their actions are effective and important. Migrants, the elderly, and many poor people do not receive such feedback.

A second includes those factors that cushion or protect individuals from physiological or psychological exposure to stressors. While clear-cut evidence is lacking, some research suggests that people who experience many stressors but have help and support available from family, friends, and community are less subject to illness.

This concept has enormous implications for health care social work. The thesis put forth by Cassel suggests that (1) psychosocial stressors are implicated in the development of illness and disease as these have been defined here; (2) for the most part, it is unlikely that specific psychosocial stressors can be related to the development of specific disease or illness processes; (3) the specific manifestation will vary by heredity, experience, and susceptibility; (4) people who are in marginal or deprived social circumstances are especially susceptible to health problems, as are people who have experienced recent loss or major changes in their life; (5) this is related to the fact that they find themselves in a situation where they do not receive sufficient positive feedback concerning the effect of their action; and (6) such positive feedback is more likely when people are surrounded by family, friends, neighbors, and fellow workers who can provide social support and cushion them against negative psychosocial stressors.

Surely much of what health care social work is all about relates to these concepts. In subsequent chapters discussion will focus on (1) early social work identification of hospitalized people in particular need of supportive care following discharge; (2) working with chronically ill patients and their families to identify sources of support through the illness; and (3) preventive endeavors targeted at the young, the isolated, and others whose own resources may not be sufficient to carry them through the life crises that can generate illness.

SUMMARY

This chapter has focused on variations in response to health and illness, with discussion of how members of different social classes, ages, genders, and ethnic groups respond to illness. Group membership and the availability of health services and resources to pay for those services affect these responses.

The fact that a number of Americans rely on the family and folk healers as well as modern health care delivery services when illness strikes was highlighted. The special needs and concerns of women and the elderly were briefly reviewed.

Two major sociological perspectives on health and illness behavior were presented: the sick role and a view of illness as deviance. Each of these concepts highlights the importance of the contention that illness and the response to illness are social phenomena, not solely guided by physiological processes.

I examined the view that certain efforts to rehabilitate the disabled serve more of a social control than a healing function. Although found wanting from a social work perspective, the view does sensitize social workers to that possibility.

Some possible relationships between stress and illness were explored. The view that some illness represents a crisis or state of stress because it calls for coping resources that may not be present is particularly useful for health care social workers. The same is true for a perspective that implicates lack of positive environmental feedback and social support as causing illness. To the extent this is true, these factors can serve as guides for social work intervention, which seeks to strengthen and locate sources of positive identity and social support.

REFERENCES

Bachman, G., Eskin, A., Speroff, L., and Sarrel, P.M.: A return to estrogen replacement therapy, Sexual Medicine Today (suppl. to Medical Tribune) June 16, 1982.

Boston's Women's Health Collective: Our bodies, ourselves: a book by and for women, New York, 1971, Simon & Schuster, Inc.

Broverman, I.K., Vogal, S.R., Broverman, F.E., and Rosenkrantz, P.S.: Sex role stereotypes and clinical judgment of mental health, Journal of Consulting and Clinical Psychology **34:**1, 1970.

Cassel, J.: Psychosocial processes and "stress": theoretical formulation, International Journal of Health Services **4**(2):471, 1974.

Chesler, P.: Women and madness, New York, 1972, Avon Books.

Coulehan, J.L.: Navajo Indian medicine: implications for healing, Journal of Family Practice **10**(1):55, 1980.

Devore, W., and Schlesinger, E.: Ethnic-sensitive social work practice, St. Louis, 1981, The C.V. Mosby Co.

Edgerton, R.B., Karno, M., and Fernandez, I.: Curanderismo in the metropolis. In Martínez, R.A., editor: Hispanic culture and health care, St. Louis, 1978, The C.V. Mosby Co.

Fabrega, H., Jr.: Disease and social behavior: an interdisciplinary perspective, Cambridge, Mass., 1974, The M.I.T. Press.

Fandetti, D.V., and Gelfand, D.E.: Attitudes towards symptoms and services in the ethnic family neighborhood, American Journal of Orthopsychiatry **48**(3):477, 1978.

Field, M.G.: Structured strain in the role of the Soviet physician, American Journal of Sociology **58:**493, 1953.

Freidson, E.: Profession of medicine, New York, 1970, Dodd, Mead & Co.

Garrison, V.: The Puerto Rican syndrome in psychiatry and espiritismo. In Crapanzano, V., and Garrison, V., editors: Case studies in spirit possession, New York, 1977, John Wiley & Sons, Inc.

Garrison, V.: The inner-city support systems project: an experiment in medical anthropology and community psychiatry: a preliminary report, Newark, N.J., Jan. 1, 1979, College of Medicine and Dentistry of New Jersey (mimeo).

Giordano, J., and Giordano, G.P.: The ethno-cultural factor in mental health: a literature review and bibliography, New York, 1977, American Jewish Committee.

Glass, D.C.: Behavior patterns, stress and coronary disease, New York, 1977, John Wiley & Sons, Inc.

Goffman, E.: Stigma: notes on the management of spoiled identity, Englewood Cliffs, N.J., 1963, Spectrum Books.

Goodtracks, J.G.: Native American noninterference, Social Work **18**(6):30, 1973.

Gordon, M.: Assimilation in American life, New York, 1964, Oxford University Press.

Gove, W.R., editor: The labeling of deviance: evaluating a perspective, New York, 1975, Halsted Press.

Greenblum, J.: Medical and health orientations of American Jews: a case of diminishing distinctiveness, Social Science and Medicine **8:**127 1974.

Health, United States, DHHS Pub. No. (PHS) 83-1232, Washington, D.C., 1982, U.S. Government Printing Office.

Holden, M.O.: Dialysis or death: the ethical alternatives, Health and Social Work **5**(2):18, 1980.

Holmes, T.H.: Life situations, emotions, and disease, Psychosomatics **19**(12):747, 1978.

Holmes, T.H.: and Masuda, M.: Life changes and illness susceptibility. In Dohrenwend, B.S. and Dohrenwend, B.P., editors: Stressful life events: their nature and effects, New York, 1974, Wiley-Interscience.

Holmes, T.H., and Rahe, R.H.: The social readjustment rating scale, Journal of Psychosomatic Research **11:**213, 1967.

Howe, I.: Immigrant Jewish families in New York: the end of the world of our fathers, New York **8**(41), 51, 1975.

Kitano, H.H.L.: Japanese Americans, ed. 2, Englewood Cliffs, N.J., 1976, Prentice-Hall, Inc.

Kleinman, A.: Clinical relevance of anthropological and cross-cultural research: concepts and strategies, American Journal of Psychiatry **135**(4):427, 1978.

Kosa, J., and Robertson, J.S.: The social aspects of health and illness. In Kosa, J., and Zola, I.K., editors: Poverty and health: a sociological analysis, Cambridge, Mass., 1975, Harvard University Press.

Krause, C.A.: Grandmothers, mothers and daughters: an oral history study of ethnicity, mental health and continuity of three generations of Jewish, Italian and Slavic American women, New York, 1978, American Jewish Committee.

Marcus, A.C., and Seeman, T.E.: Sex differences in reports of illness and disability: a preliminary test of the "fixed role obligations" hypothesis, Journal of Health and Social Behavior **22**(2):174, 1981.

Marieskind, H.: The women's health movement, International Journal of Health Services **5**(2):217, 1975.

Martínez, C., and Martin, H.W.: Folk diseases among urban Mexican-Americans. In Martínez, R.A., editor: Hispanic culture and health care, St. Louis, 1978, The C.V. Mosby Co.

Martínez, R.A.: Hispanic culture and health care, St. Louis, 1978, The C.V. Mosby Co.

Mechanic, D.: Medical sociology, ed. 2, New York, 1978, The Free Press.

Meyer, R.J., and Haggerty, R.: Streptoccocal infections in families: factors altering individual susceptibility, Pediatrics **29:**539, 1962.

New York Times, 1976.

Olson, M.M.: Health: women. In Turner, J.B., editor: Encyclopedia of social work, Washington, D.C., 1977, National Association of Social Workers, vol. 1.

Parsons, T.: Definitions of health and illness in light of American values and social structures. In Jaco, G.E., editor: Patients, physicians and illness: a sourcebook in behavioral science and health, New York, 1958, The Free Press.

Physicians' desk reference, ed. 36, Oradell, N.J., 1982, Medical Economics Co., pp. 647–653, 1385, 1393.

Pilowsky, I., and Spence, N.D.: Ethnicity and illness behaviour, Psychological Medicine **7**(3):447, 1977.

President's Commission on Mental Health: Task panel reports no. 3, Washington, D.C., 1978, U.S. Government Printing Office.

Rosenfeld, S.: Sex roles and societal reactions to mental illness: the labeling of "deviant" deviance, Journal of Health and Social Behavior **23**(1):18, 1982.

Rubel, A.J.: The epidemiology of a folk illness: *susto* in Hispanic America. In Martínez, R.A., editor: Hispanic culture and health care, St. Louis, 1978, The C.V. Mosby Co.

Selye, H.: The stress of life, New York, 1956, McGraw-Hill Book Co.

Snow, L.F.: Folk medical beliefs and their implications for care of patients: a review based on studies among black Americans, Annals of Internal Medicine, **81:**82, 1974.

Stein, H.F.: A dialectical model of health and illness attitudes and behavior among Slovak Americans, International Journal of Mental Health **5**(2):117, 1976.

Suchman, E.A.: Sociomedical variations among ethnic groups, American Journal of Sociology **70:**319, 1964.

Toupin, E.S.: Counseling Asians: psychotherapy in the context of racism and Asian-American history, American Journal of Orthopsychiatry **50**(1):76, 1980.

Verbrugge, L.M.: Females and illness: recent trends in sex differences in the United States, Journal of Health and Social Behavior **17**(4):387, 1976.

Verbrugge, L.M.: Multiple roles and physical health of women and men, Journal of Health and Social Behavior **24**(1):16, 1983.

Wintrob, R.: The influence of others: witchcraft and rootwork as explanations of behavior disturbances, Journal of Nervous and Mental Diseases **156:**318, 1973.

Zborowski, M.: Cultural components in response to pain, Journal of Social Issues **4**(8):16, 1952.

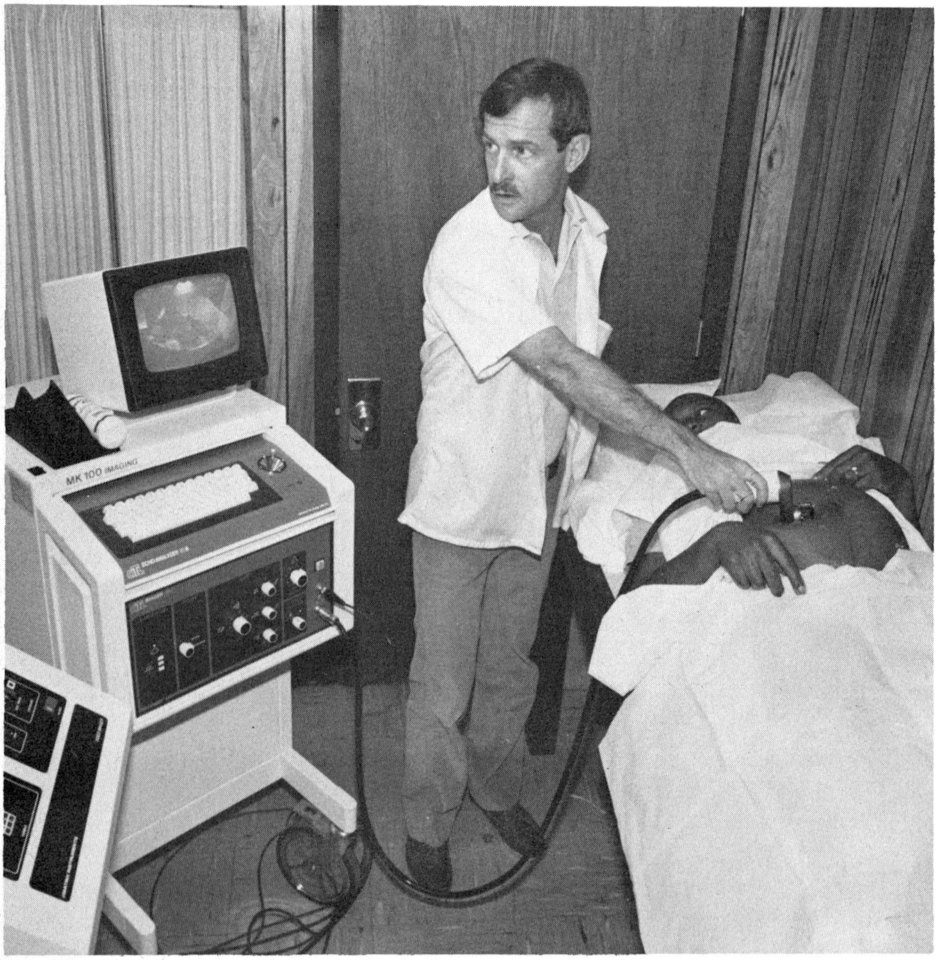
MK 100 IMAGING

Chapter 5

Frameworks for health care social work practice

In the three preceding chapters attention has been focused on the health problems that confront us, the patchwork system of health services financing and delivery that is characteristic of contemporary American society, and on a number of concepts that examine how people respond to the discomforts of illness and disease. This chapter presents a number of conceptual formulations to guide and organize thinking about social work practice in health care.

In her seminal work, *Social Work Practice in the Health Field* (1961), Bartlett suggested that "when social work, medicine and public health are viewed together as social institutions, it becomes important to define the social work contribution in the particular field in broad terms. There is evidence that social work in the health field has not yet provided itself such a framework of thinking" (p. 49). Considerable progress has been made in the intervening 20 years. Nevertheless, no single, integrated framework has emerged yet.

The frameworks presented in this book have been selected and developed because they are consonant with basic social work values, perspectives on social functioning, and the diverse health needs and problems that have been discussed. They include (1) a public health perspective, (2) the concept of "person-environment fit" (Coulton, 1981), (3) the continuum from cure to care, and (4) a social work perspective on illness termed "the careers of illness." Together these formulations suggest how basic social work perspectives, current developments in health care, and understanding the impact of illness converge to provide a conceptual base for practice.

PUBLIC HEALTH PERSPECTIVES

From its beginnings, social work has recognized the relationship between poor housing, poor working conditions, poverty, and high rates of infant mortality, tuberculosis, and other health problems. Reference has already been made (Chapter 1) to social work's early involvement in community-based efforts to study and prevent those conditions thought to be disease related. Since this early beginning, public health principles and methods have been clarified and their scope expanded. In the view of many health care social workers (for example, Bracht, 1978; Insley, 1977; Reichert, 1980; Rice, 1959, 1962; Wittman,

1978), a public health orientation is an essential component of social work practice in health and related areas. Social workers have played a part in this development while the profession has refined and clarified how basic public health and social work perspectives converge to generate a unique contribution.

This section reviews some of the basic public health approaches that cut across the work of various health care professionals. This review is followed by consideration of how these approaches can and have been adapted to various arenas of health care social work practice. In beginning this discussion, it is worth noting that several basic principles governing public health approaches are particularly important to the approach being developed here. One is that "public health activity is characterized predominantly by the principle of preventing disease and disability and promoting positive health" (Solon, 1977, p. 612). A second is that preventive principles can and should govern all levels of intervention. A third focuses on responsibility and accountability for the health of various groups in the population. Many contemporary approaches in health care social work are implicitly or explicitly derived from these basic tenets.

Definitions of public health

Various definitions of public health have been presented. Among the best known is the following one presented by Winslow: Public Health is the Science and Art of (1) preventing disease, (2) prolonging life, and (3) promoting health and efficiency through organized community effort for (1) the sanitation of the environment, (2) the control of communicable infections, (3) the education of the individual in personal hygiene, (4) the organization of medical and nursing services for the early diagnosis and preventive treatment of disease, and (5) the development of the social machinery to insure everyone a standard of living adequate for the maintenance of health so organizing these benefits as to enable every citizen to realize his birthright of health and longevity (cited in Hanlon and Pickett, 1984, p. 4). This definition anticipates the continuous extension of public health boundaries. These boundaries have grown from an initial focus on gross environmental sanitation, to preventive medicine, to a focus on the behavioral aspects surrounding health behavior and care, to assuring the availability of comprehensive health services for all.

Before considering how public health perspectives can serve as a conceptual base for much of health care social work, it is appropriate to define some basic terms commonly used in public health.

Epidemiology and the epidemiological method

> Epidemiology is the study of why and how diseases are distributed within a community. It is concerned with searching out and understanding the factors related to the occurrence and distribution of disease in a population, studying the sick and the well in relation to each other and to their environment (Smith, 1979, p. 17).

Public health is "a social enterprise" with a community orientation; the physician seeks the diagnosis of individual cases. The counterpart of individual diagnosis on a communal scale is epidemiology (Solon, 1977, p. 612). The parallel between this view and social work's attention to problems requiring a community, organizational, and population perspective will concern us throughout this book.

The field of epidemiology was originally limited to identifying the living conditions of people with communicable diseases. It was subsequently expanded to include efforts to study other health problems. The basic principles embodied by this method have been applied to a wide range of problems, including mental health, mental retardation, child abuse, and the vulnerability of young families in the early stages of child rearing.

Epidemiological model of illness. The epidemiological model of illness has been referred to as a *trilogy* involving interaction between the *host* (the individual who can/may develop a health problem), the *agent* (factors capable of inducing health problems), and the *environment,* conducive to generating or preventing health problems. Kosa and Robertson (1975) suggest this traditional model portrays an image whereby a "noxious agent" comes into contact with a tissue and produces pathological changes. Some epidemiological investigation using this model has focused on how social variables function as *agents* to induce health problems. Chapter 4 briefly reviewed the potential etiological role of stress in many contemporary health problems.

The "noxious agents" presumably involved in stress-related illness have not been clearly identified. The postulated relationship between stress and illness discussed earlier may be considered an extension of the epidemiological model because it focuses on genetic predispositions, physical agents, and stress and coping mechanisms that may function to predispose to or avoid health problems (Kosa and Robertson, 1975). This view of epidemiology and stress models has particular relevance for social work, which focuses on environments, their potential to produce disease-stress, and how these environments affect individuals and families.

Another important component of the host/agent/environment trilogy is the view that a change in any one of the three factors can increase or decrease susceptibility to health problems. For example, people who have developed coping skills that serve them well in a crisis may be better able to withstand the threats posed by environmental stressors such as family disruption. Conversely, environments conducive to good family functioning (adequate income and housing) may reduce the susceptibility to disease. This approach can clarify our thinking about those people particularly prone to health problems because of the situations in which they find themselves. It can also help to develop efforts to effect change. A number of additional concepts clarify this relationship.

Population at risk. An important public health concept relates to identifying groups particularly prone to developing certain health problems. An important methodological tool is the concept *population at risk,* which may be defined as all people in a community who may acquire a condition (Smith, 1979, pp. 20-21). For example, when attention is focused on the occurrence of a particular condition in the community, that condition is expressed as a ratio of people having the problem and the population at risk. This ratio is expressed as either a crude or a specific rate. Crude rates are calculated without considering particular population characteristics. Specific rates consider factors such as age, gender, and ethnicity.

The difference between incidence and prevalence is crucial in defining population at risk. *Incidence* refers to the number of "new cases" of a health problem reported in the population within a designated time period. *Prevalence* refers to the total number of known cases of a specific problem in the population within a given time period. Increased or decreased incidence of a problem can give some clue of the environmental or toxic agents affecting the numbers of people subject to a problem. Observed increase in a health problem can, for example, set off a series of actions designed to ascertain the source of the problem.

The incidence of child abuse, suicide, or alcoholism may be higher in certain segments of the population than in others. Investigation can then focus on community problems that may be contributing to this high incidence. There are several cases in point. Most readers are probably familiar with efforts to trace the reason for the outbreak of "legionnaire's disease" in Philadelphia some years ago, or those to identify possible sources of toxic waste because of more than the expected number of cancer cases in a particular area. Social workers, mental health professionals, and other health professionals may try to identify the environmental or social sources of increased suicide and homicide rates, referred to in Chapter 1.

The incidence of hospital admissions for suspected victims of child abuse has been known to rise with an increase in unemployment rates in an area. This kind of information can help to compare the distribution of various problems in different populations and communities and can serve to target preventive efforts.

Prevalence rates, especially in the case of chronic illness, are particularly important in determining the nature and numbers of health services required. A high cancer prevalence rate calls for increasing available medical and supportive services. For example, the prevalence rate of heart disease among men between the ages of 40 and 65 is determined by counting the number of known cases in a community and dividing it by the actual number of men in that age group living in the community.

Together these concepts help to clarify the view of population at risk. For example, women are a population at risk for cervical cancer. Thus any calculation of the population at risk for cervical cancer would not include men. The *population at risk* then includes all people in a community who have the potential for acquiring a condition.*

Prevention. A variety of well-known and extensively used social work interventive methods are identified as preventive measures. Among these are sex education and anticipatory guidance in health and medical care that helps people prepare for the possibility of a traumatic reaction to the experience. Considering levels of prevention is crucial to public health thinking.

There are three levels of prevention: primary, secondary, and tertiary. Smith defines *primary prevention* as those efforts preventing the condition from occurring at all.

> The aim is to reduce the incidence by utilizing established preventive techniques and strengthening the ability of people to cope with stress. It deals with the life conditions of a currently healthy population. It is potentially the most attractive, efficient and effective approach to community health problems. Primary prevention seeks to reduce the intensity of crises in order to increase their chances of adaptation. It also prepares people for crises and helps them during crises so that a health outcome may be more likely (Smith, 1979, p. 225).

To this consideration must be added the view that primary prevention involves efforts to change behaviors and environmental risk factors that trigger disease. Thus nonsmokers can virtually eliminate the risk of getting the type of lung cancer induced by smoking. People who never drink alcoholic beverages will not become alcoholics. A social system that makes it possible for all individuals able to do work in keeping with their interest and ability will reduce or virtually eliminate stress associated with unwanted unemployment.

Secondary prevention involves early detection and treatment. It reduces the duration of infirmity that occurs in spite of primary prevention programs (Smith, 1979, p. 225). Much preventive activity that is carried out by social workers and other health professionals is carried out on the secondary prevention level. Much of the effort involved in social work case finding derives from the idea that secondary prevention can minimize the risks associated with certain problems. Chapter 9, which deals with social work practice in hospitals, describes newly developed high-risk screening mechanisms. These procedures are essentially designed to identify people thought to be at particular risk regarding psychological problems generated by or derived from the conditions that initially brought them to the hospital.

Tertiary prevention has been defined as rehabilitation. It tries to aid the recovered person so that past difficulties will not hamper return to full community participation (Smith, 1979, p. 225). I question whether tertiary prevention as defined here and elsewhere is truly a preventive activity, or whether it is defined more appropriately as treatment.

---

*See Smith (1979) for technical discussion of how incidence and prevalence rates can be calculated.

Social work perspectives of prevention. In a classic work Rice (1962) suggests that social work's long-standing experience in working with people already experiencing a variety of handicapping conditions provides a base of knowledge and skill that can make an explicit contribution to prevention. Using the epidemiological perspective and its application to preventive medicine Rice proposes an adaptation of the basic principles to the field of social work. These principles revolve around conceptions of social functioning and the processes that maximize or hinder such functioning. This early statement of preventive principles applied to social work is succinct and merits detailed examination.

Social functioning is a dynamic process involving people constantly responding to new stimuli and situations. The response to these situations is varied and related to capacity, limitation, and the particular strength of the stimuli requiring response and adaptation. Prevention requires full understanding of individuals, their psychological experiences, and the environments in which they are interacting. Understanding social functioning presupposes a broad understanding of these forces and influences, within both the family and the community, that have an effect on the individual and group in their social functioning, as well as presupposing knowledge of the individual or group psychodynamics (Rice, 1962). Preventing social dysfunction requires early disruption of those processes that threaten social functioning. Alteration in any one of the three areas can disrupt the path to social dysfunctioning. This conception can be related to the basic epidemiological trinity of the host/agent/environment relationship.

Rice stresses that preventive measures are most effective when applied before any dysfunction occurs. This perspective has been applied in maternal and child health fields in which support, clarification, and anticipatory guidance can help to avert resource deficits and foster positive child-rearing experiences. Also important is Rice's view that preventive measures may have greatest value when economically and efficiently targeted to populations thought to be at greatest risk for social dysfunction. Subsequent developments in various aspects of health care social work that focus attention on high-risk populations have drawn heavily on such a view. This conception holds true in the processes of high risk screening referred to previously, social work's involvement in public health programs such as hypertension screening, and identification of populations at greatest risk of abusing their children. However, the risks and ethics of labeling and intervening with groups that do not perceive themselves as having problems are now being raised (for example, Gilbert, 1982). Preventive efforts must be weighed for their potential of generating the problems they aim to prevent, especially in emotionally laden areas.

Rice raises questions about the extent to which the present organization of social work services is geared to using preventive measures. Returning to neighborhood- or community-based practice in which social workers are familiar with the people and the stresses they experience and reach out to offer help and guidance is indicative of preventive activities implicit and explicit in Rice's presentation.

Wittman (1978) suggests that preventive social work is not as well developed as preventive medicine and preventive psychiatry. Reviewing a series of developments in social work that led to an increased interest in prevention, he characterizes preventive social work as "an organized and systematic effort to apply knowledge about social health and pathology in such a manner as to enhance and preserve the social and mental health of the community" (Wittman, pp. 205-206 [citing Parad]). This definition suggests that prevention by social workers is carried out at both the macro and micro levels of practice.

Wittman identifies a number of programs having prevention as their main theme. Secondary prevention is used in abortion and rape counseling to minimize the unhealthy effects of unwanted pregnancy or the traumas experienced by rape victims. Special efforts for prevention of suicide and drug and alcohol abuse are examples of primary or secondary preventive approaches. Social work's involvement in maternal and child health programs that aim to reduce infant mortality and inadequate nutrition during pregnancy and infancy and to impart parenting skills is an example of primary prevention.

Bracht (1978) identifies the spectrum of social work activities and outlines the social worker's role in assessing community health needs and functioning as a community health planner.

> In public health social work, the focus of professional practice is on populations at risk, in the context of their community environment. [This includes] preventive case services, multidisciplinary consultation, epidemiologic studies, community health assessment and the health-planning process (pp. 257-258).

This brief review of public health perspectives and their application to social work has sought to identify the basic preventive, community-oriented thrust of public health. It also has suggested that a public health approach is always governed by (1) efforts to identify the environment and community source of health problems, (2) activity designed to minimize the health hazards generated by these problems, and (3) particular awareness that certain populations are particularly vulnerable or at risk of developing certain problems. This perspective provides one of the major conceptual focuses guiding current social work practice in health care.

THE PERSON-ENVIRONMENT FIT AND COPING/ADAPTATION

In commenting on a series of papers focused on clarifying social work's objectives and purposes, Briar (1981) notes that "a persistent component in the conceptual frameworks of social work since its earliest beginning is that person-environment interaction is the focus of social work. [Regardless of the terms used to characterize that focus] person-environment interaction means that social workers *want* to perceive and analyze persons with their needs and problems in the context of the person's environment" (p. 84).

Coulton (1981) has proposed a framework for viewing the person-environment interaction "as it takes place among the clients of social workers in heath care" (p. 26). Her perspective is based on considerable empirical evidence suggesting that the harmony or "fit between people and their environments can affect and is in turn affected by their health" (p. 20). This fit is often disrupted by changes in physical and coping capacity, environmental resources, and health. Lack of fit can derive from lack of individual capacity to meet environmental demands or from environments incongruous with individual need and capacity. Coulton points to evidence that suggests how various life changes disrupt the equilibrium between individuals and the environments in which they function. A number of investigations relate the onset of illness to stressful life events. The importance of harmony with the environment for promoting health or dysfunction has been demonstrated in a number of investigations.* Studies of nursing home residents suggest that when the homes were congruent with residents' need for privacy, freedom, order, and routine the residents were healthier and more satisfied than when such fit between environment and need did not prevail.

Several dimensions of the person-environment interaction are: (1) physical dimensions of the environment, (2) psychosocial dimensions, and (3) economic dimensions. In respect to physical dimensions, the need of the physically disabled for barrier-free public places and homes adapted to their needs is an obvious case in point. Psychosocial dimensions are complex and varied. Inability to continue carrying out responsibilities in keeping with societal expectations is a problem confronting many people with long-term illness. The stroke patient who can no longer function as bread winner or the dialysis patient who tires too easily to play the accustomed mothering role (Coulton, 1979) exemplify the lack of congruence between individual capacity and social and personal expectations. Disharmony results when significant others in the environment are unable to alter their expectations. Analogously, people having major difficulty in altering their self-perceptions and activities (as they relate to illness) also have difficulty in regaining a state of equilibrium. Also important are those studies showing some tendency by healthy people to avoid those with major disability. Thus environmental supports may be withheld or diminished at a point when illness generates extensive demands for affection, attention, and support.

The relationship between economic dimensions and disability is quite clear. For many people the onset of disability is associated with a decline in income. Simultaneously, costs related to illness may be out of proportion to

*The work drawn on by Coulton is similar to much that was reviewed in Chapter 3 in the section on stress.

available funds. Using these conceptions Coulton suggests that "many . . . actions of social workers that relate to patients may be viewed as attempts to restore, maintain, or enhance congruence between the individual and his or her environment" (p. 29). She presents a typology of social work practice in health care that identifies two overlapping goals for health care social work. One goal focuses on the changes affected individuals must make; the other focuses on effecting needed environmental changes. The typology covers both the goal and the target of intervention. Inherent in the typology is the basic social work perspective that if person-environment fit is to be enhanced, intervention is frequently focused on both the individual and the environment. This perspective helps to focus attention on primary targets and goals as they arise out of assessment.

Crisis, coping, and adaptation

Chapter 4 discussed various views of stress and crisis and their relationship to illness. One view of crisis focused on a discrepancy between the demands of a situation and people's capacity and resources to meet those demands. Major health problems may be construed as crises because they call for skills in coping with pain; disfigurement; and major changes in self-perception, perception by others, and ability to carry out previous responsibilities. Coulton (1981) cites a definition of coping suggested by Monat and Lazarus: "Coping refers to efforts to master conditions of harm, threat or challenge when a routine or automatic response is not readily available" (p. 27).

Mechanic (1977) has drawn on these and related views of crisis and coping to outline the major features of a "coping-adaptation model to improve patient functioning" (p. 83). Adaptation to illness, in his view, calls for five types of resources: (1) economic resources, (2) abilities and skills, (3) defensive techniques, (4) social supports, and (5) motivational impetus.

Suggesting that efforts to modify or alter patients' feeling states have not been shown to be very effective, he proposes alternative intervention focused on the availability of resources, skills, and information. Each type of illness or disability requires specific skills and information. The skills identified are (1) compensating for physical inadequacies, (2) pacing oneself given the new level of functioning, and (3) preparing for and anticipating new embarrassing situations (for example, a cardiac patient who no longer wants to go to the supermarket because he is unable to carry heavy bags may review his own and others' reactions in advance and develop strategies to cope with his own feelings or the disdainful stares of others who cannot imagine why a man would let a woman carry heavy bags). An important point is that now more than ever skillfully dealing with bureaucracies may be important for making necessary resources available because disabled people have frequent contact with hospitals, rehabilitation agencies, and other complex organizations.

Mechanic's explicit attention to the components of adaptation to major illness complements Coulton's conceptualization of the "person-environment fit" and directs attention to the social components of adaptation.

> The social process of adaptation depends on the degree of fit between skills and capacities of individuals and their relevant supporting group structures on the one hand and the types of challenges with which they are confronted on the other (Mechanic, 1977, p. 80).

This perspective suggests that when the individual is viewed as the primary target of change, strategies need not be focused on personality change or development of insight, but rather on skills that enable people to avert the crisis of incapacity to meet environmental demands. Efforts to modify the environment so that new skills may be used or to lessen inappropriate demands are essential. The concept of "person-environment fit" and attention to the social components and skills involved in adaptation to illness will be brought to bear on efforts to illustrate social work practice in a spectrum of health settings.

THE CONTINUUM FROM CURE TO CARE

Morris (1978) points out that social work's original purpose was "to take care to the weak and helpless groups in a new industrializing society; the severely disabled, neglected children, mentally ill, developmentally disabled and the enfeebled aged" (p. 82). He further suggests that along with the physical and social sciences, social work increasingly became imbued by the belief that the new sciences could find solutions for all human needs. This development generated an emphasis on prevention and cure. Social work then simultaneously became involved in both large-scale social reform and intensive clinical work with emotionally disturbed persons presumed "curable." Traditional caring functions including the development and enhancement of social support systems, mutual aid networks, and approaches to care of the most seriously disabled were in some measure neglected.

Recently it has become evident that medicine, social work, and political groups cannot cure all.

> In the last analysis, social work confronts—along with medicine, its central mentor of the past—a serious challenge. Medicine and science are able to keep people alive, but often with severe handicaps, some of which are physical, and some mental and emotional. Social arrangements do not remove those handicaps. A society and a scientific system that keep people alive have an obligation to do something about the conditions in which they live. A redistribution of effort between cure and care is an absolute necessity (Morris, 1978, p. 89).

The preceding chapters have pointed out that at present there is no cure for many of the chronic diseases prevalent in society today. Millions of people live with various degrees of limitation on their physical mobility and with chronic discomfort and dietary restrictions. Cancer is no longer necessarily equated with imminent death. However, for many cancer victims life involves periodic treatment and disfigurement and the pervasive fear of impending death. Using life-maintaining equipment such as dialysis requires massive physical and psychological adaptation. The movement toward deinstitutionalization of the mentally impaired has resulted in a large number of people with minimal capacity for self-care being left in communities in need of constructive activity and protection. Most people who suffer from these various chronic conditions need ongoing, lifetime care beyond that offered by medicine.

There are other people who can benefit from the "miracles of modern medicine" and the practice technologies developed by social work and other health professions to cure or ameliorate major dysfunction. Many recover from major surgical procedures or from delimited episodes of emotional disturbances such as bouts of depression. The efficacy of psychotherapeutic and pharmacological approaches has been demonstrated.

Social workers can meet the challenge posed by Morris while they continue to attend to the curing or ameliorating functions that have become an integral component of social work practice. A framework that highlights the importance of both and recognizes a continuum from cure to care can shed light on many aspects of our practice. The development of such a framework requires a review of the components of cure and care and an analysis of those factors that have served to accord greater importance to curing than to caring functions.

Cure

During the ceremonies dedicating a new medical school teaching hospital the keynote speaker is reported to have made the following comment: "I would hope that before too long, some (medical problems) will yield themselves to investigating and solving problems—not patching up machinery that is not running too well" (*The Home News,* May 17, 1982). The news item then goes on to report that on completion of the dedication ceremonies a number of medical artifacts (hospital documents, stethoscope, pacemaker, intravenous bottle, and thermometer) were placed in a time capsule and buried. It was hoped that if the time capsule is unearthed in 100 years people will know "what health care and education was about on May 16, 1982."

This news item reveals much about a number of prevalent conceptions on current health care and education. It calls attention to the frustration over medical problems not yet amenable to treatment and to the fact that there is a tendency (inappropriate in the view of many) to equate health and medical care. This tendency is reflected in the cited comments and in the objects buried in the time capsule. Patching up is much of what contemporary health care is about. Stethoscopes and thermometers provide diagnostic information but do not cure. Pacemakers are one device for patching up malfunctioning hearts. Intravenous bottles that carry nourishment and medication to ailing bodies may save or restore a life to good functioning. But other components of current health care were omitted. These components are related to cure and care and reflect important advances in modern medicine, the work of other health care providers, and the experience of individuals with health problems.

One wonders why antibiotics or a contemporary surgical scalpel were not buried in the capsule. These items are surely important components of current medical care. One also wonders why a miniature wheelchair, a model of physiotherapy equipment, or an intensive care unit were not buried. A captioned picture of a social worker or physician counseling people about long-term health problems would have revealed much. One hundred years from now people should also know how many babies were or might have been saved if more mothers had adequate nutrition and effective parenting skills.

In short, contemporary health care is "about" more than a few technical medical artifacts. It involves a variety of functions; only a few of these are strictly within the purview of medicine. Much of medicine involves the skillful work of dedicated, brillant physicians who have developed and now use the advances of modern medical technology. Not all of these advances serve to "cure." According to one dictionary cure means "successful remedial treatment." Much that has already been said suggests that many current interventions do not involve successful remedial treatment. Rather, the term has come to encompass a curing thrust focused on extensive use of technology in medicine and an emphasis on intensive clinical work by social workers.

A number of developments in medical and social work education and practice help to explain this thrust. Reference has already been made to the Flexner report that led to dramatic changes in medical school curricula. Among these changes was a strong emphasis on the firm foundation of physical and biological sciences with less attention being paid to the social and psychological aspects of care. Increased specialization meant that physicians spent more and more time in training. Much of this time was spent in in-depth study of one set of skills, such as surgery or developing intensive knowledge about a group of diseases and procedures associated with a particular body system. Thus ophthalmologists focused on diseases of the eye, cardiologists on diseases of the heart, and nephrologists on diseases of the kidney. There was the expectation that this type of focused attention on particular disease processes would do away with much disease. The appearance of the National Institutes of Health (NIH) with their multiple specialty and disease-oriented grant and contract programs further increased the trends toward specialty training (*Interim Report,* 1979, p. 5). These efforts were rewarded with many medical breakthroughs.

Who would have dared to dream just a few short years ago that damaged arteries leading to the heart could be replaced, as in coronary bypass surgery? The work involved in mastering the art of replacing damaged kidneys with healthy ones from a live or dead donor took much vision and courage (Fox and

Swazey, 1974). There is unfathomable skill involved in reattaching severed limbs and developing drug therapies that can slow or reverse the growth of cancerous tumors. The discovery of drugs to quell the hallucinations and anxieties suffered by some schizophrenics is a remarkable feat. When physicians administer antibiotics to rid the body of infection (as in pneumonia) they effect a cure, as does the surgeon who removes a diseased gallbladder. Combined psychotherapeutic and drug treatment of reactive depression can help morose, melancholy, and perhaps suicidal people to cope, experience hope, and go on with their lives.

However, this massive concentration of energy and resources into specialized training based on the biochemical model has had a number of major effects on the character of health care. Early on physicians like Richard Cabot (Chapter 1) recognized that major advances in medical techniques generated a tendency to treat diseased organs without paying attention to the person or persons suffering from the disease. The possible relationship between stress, personal problems, and routine health problems for which people seek care has already been noted. In addition, a significant majority of the problems for which people seek the services of health professionals are relatively mundane and routine. The intense training focused on major disease categories and making sophisticated diagnoses does not, for the most part, prepare physicians to deal with more benign discomforts. Physicians trained to diagnose and excise a brain tumor may well lack the patience or knowledge to deal with a headache induced by persistent daily irritation. Furthermore, those same physicians may find the vague postoperative complaints of patients whose tumors have been successfully excised irritating and not worth their attention. Certainly, the needs of those individuals whose neurosurgical problems leave them totally or partially disabled are not met by physicians.

Much current medical education is focused on finding and curing major diseases. One medical student poses the problem this way:

> There's a conflict for a medical student . . . We should be most concerned with learning how to manage and deal with the most common situations, with things that are going to happen 90 percent of the time. But the excitement of medicine is the differential diagnosis, solving the puzzle of what the patient is suffering from (Black, 1982).

Specialized, disease-focused medical education, extensive reliance on complex medical technology, and use of various measures to sustain the lives of those with major impairments are all examples of current approaches to medical care that extend the traditional view of cure as successful remedial treatment. Current perspectives on cure, or curing, have been identified by using various sophisticated means to make diagnostic assessments and by skillfully using the range of elaborate technology such as chemotherapy, renal dialysis, and complex surgical procedures.

Thus much contemporary medical education is focused on cure. But the perspective as currently used goes beyond successful remedial treatment. Given available knowledge and the emphasis on diagnosis and treatment of disease, the terms *curing* or *cure* have come to be identified with the "technology of the healing arts" (Spiegel and Backhaut, 1980) and the use of sophisticated means to keep people alive. The point that the use of such means is frequently not equated with cure in the traditional sense of that term has been made repeatedly. Yet the quest for cure goes on. Excited by medical innovations, both students and graduate physicians expect modern medicine to "produce wonders." Citing the perspective of one medical student, Black (1982) comments:

> And he seemed to assume that the gaps still left in medical technology would eventually be filled. Medicine is almost unlimited in what it can do, Aaron believed. Doctors may not be able to help people live much longer than they do now, but more and more, they will help people stay healthier right up to the end (p. 35).

Social work, like contemporary medicine, developed in a period of population growth and of faith and hope in progress generated by modernization and the growth of new sciences. Leiby (1977) suggests that the professionalization of social work was one of a number of developments that shared a hope for change aimed at the protection of the vulnerable and disadvantaged. In the early 1900s it was recognized that good intentions and motivation were not sufficient to carry on the work of the evolving field of social work. Therefore early in the century the first school of social work opened its doors. This step acknowledged the need for systematic understanding of human behavior and the helping process.

Like medicine, "the leadership of the emerging profession of social work was caught up in the promise of science welcoming its intellectual power to influence guided social change" (Lewis, 1981, p. 1). The early leaders of the profession became active in pursuing facts, convinced that "from description would come explanation" without which remedies for the social ills they hoped to eliminate would be less than adequate (Lewis, 1981, pp. 1-2). These early leaders set about studying statistics and engaging in action-oriented fact-finding.

Much of this early work lacked a clear-cut conceptual base or theoretical foundation designed to explain human behavior. In 1915 Abraham Flexner, whose report had served to catapult American medicine into the scientific age, made a penetrating analysis of social work entitled "Is Social Work a Profession" (Flexner, 1961). Using a number of criteria of professions, he suggested that social work was not a profession like medicine or engineering. He thought social workers were mediators with such diverse functions that "no compact, purposefully organized educational discipline is feasible" (cited in Pumphrey and Pumphrey, 1961, p. 394). These observations had a profound influence on subsequent thrusts of social work—education, practice, and theoretical developments. Their particular impact on social work in health care was profound.

Some viewed Flexner's work as a challenge to systematize practice theory and forge toward the identification and development of a theoretical base. Partially in response to Flexner's view social work turned to the developing theories of Freud as a way of interpreting human response, thus providing the first theoretical system used by social workers (Specht, 1981). The emerging work of Freud generated the hope that trained persons could alter and cure personality dysfunction. Some viewed this emphasis, focused as it was on instinctual drives and distortions in psychosexual development, as deflecting attention from the social and environmental pressures that generated emotional, health, and economic problems.

The thrust toward professionalism had major consequences for social work education. One consequence involved the effort to clarify and synthesize the distinct body of skills characteristic of the several intervention methods that social work had begun to develop. During the 1950s and 1960s schools of social work put increasing emphasis on educating caseworkers, group workers, community organizers, social work administrators, and social work researchers. For some social workers terms such as *medical* or *psychiatric social work* implied a lack of independent, autonomous, professional function. These terms were seen as symbolic of a "handmaiden" or secondary role carried out in host settings such as hospitals. There was greater attention to research and documenting the effectiveness of social work intervention. This increased attention led to an emphasis on "effective practice" (for example, Fisher, 1978) and the effort to evolve clear-cut strategies designed to deal quickly with the massive problems brought to social workers.

These are significant developments that have galvanized the profession. The resulting advances in practice theory and technology have brought the profession closer to achieving its original objectives. However, these developments, like those in medicine that have focused on "curing," as we have used that term, have had some unanticipated and unintended consequences.

Armed with theories designed to explain and alter personality functioning, social workers were eager to put these to use in working with individuals and families in emotional turmoil. Aware of new technologies of behavior modification, many sought to apply these techniques across a range of problems, from helping "latent" homosexuals acknowledge and cope with their sexual identification (for example, Fisher, 1978) to involvement in techniques of biofeedback designed to minimize pain. Knowledge about the relationship between the stresses on family life posed by early child-rearing years and the availability of economic and social resources led many to develop approaches to preventive intervention (for example, Geismar, 1969). The political ferment of the 1960s generated a renewed emphasis on the skills of developing mechanisms that would allow the poor to gain greater control of their personal and social destiny.

These and related developments promised that social work would at last develop the autonomous professional base and role that seemed for so long to have eluded the profession. Less attention was paid to refining and expanding those technologies and approaches focused on care. The dictionary defines care as "solicitude" and "the making of suitable arrangements." Earlier reference was made to Morris' suggestion (1978) that social work like medicine became imbued with a "curing" orientation.

Care

Howell (1976) and her colleagues suggest that *caring* is distinguished from *curing* by the psychosocial, patient-centered components of health services. Spiegel and Backhaut (1980) refer to caring as the art of medicine, while Fuchs (1974) proposes that caring involves the opportunity to "share troubles" and to obtain sympathy and encouragement. Review of diverse studies, subsumed by Spiegel and Backhaut under the category of *caring,* indicates that care involves attention to the way health services are organized, the inequity associated with differential access of the poor and minorities, and the acceptability and accessibility of services. Salber (1975) identifies caring with consumer participation in health planning and delivery and recognition of the part played by social factors in causing illness. Morris (1978) and Morris and Anderson (1975) are more focused in their deliberations, concentrating on the range of social services required by individuals left permanently or temporarily disabled by illness.

How do these definitions and uses of the term *care* serve social work's purpose in conceptualizing health care practice? The fact that the term has been used in so many different ways underscores a point made by Morris and Anderson (1975). Briefly they suggest that modern society has generated a set of social and psychological needs that cluster around health issues. These social needs are multifaceted and include (1) the desire for human attention when complex medical care is being given; (2) the availability of patient, sympathetic health providers who "listen and hear" when troubled people tell about their health problems or those affecting loved ones; (such "listening and hearing" may take time and depart from the rigorous, scientific stance so often used by health providers trying to make a clear-cut differential diagnosis); (3) services rendered in keeping with one's ethnic traditions, even when these run counter to mainstream perceptions of health and illness; (4) services that are available and accessible, regardless of ability to pay or geographical location; (5) services that contribute to recovery or maintenance and comfort related to illness, such as home health care, homes that are physically adapted to the needs of the handicapped, counseling to cope with new life roles and changing life-styles engendered by illness; and (7) recognition of the part played by environmental, social, and psychological factors in illness causation and recovery.

The reader will note that the discussion of *care* revolves around issues that have always involved health care social workers. Yet, focusing their attention on people needing extensive long-term care, Morris and Anderson (1975) contend that neither social work nor other professions or social institutions have developed appropriate organizational forms or practice technologies that begin to take an integrated view of the complex care needs of various populations. The set of social and psychological needs that cluster around health issues requires an expanded definition of care and the associated social work tasks generated by this definition.

Expanded definition of care. The definition of health proposed in Chapter 3 identified health as active involvement and social functioning, even in the presence of disease or illness. That definition is consonant with basic social work perspectives. Based on these considerations, care can now be defined as:

> The range of perspectives and practice technology thought to contribute to "wellness," to prevention of disease and illness and to the reduction of the economic, social and psychological burdens related to illness and disease.

This definition is compatible with the tasks health care social workers carry out and facilitates efforts to further delineate and refine the varying levels and nature of activity in social work. It is also consistent with the various needs of people experiencing the diverse health problems identified in this book. Some of these needs require curing efforts in the traditional sense of the term. For the most part they involve attention to a continuum of caring and curing activities.

A TYPOLOGY OF CARING

Given (1) the social functioning orientation to health and disease presented earlier and (2) the current level of development of social work practice technology, emphasis perforce is on the caring component of the continuum. Recognizing this, a typology of caring is presented.

Social work goals, purposes, and tasks have been delineated in a number of ways. Lurie (1977) suggests that health care social work is focused on curing, preventing, and caring. Lowy (1979) identifies curative, ameliorative, preventive, promotional, and enhancing goals. The typology presented in this chapter draws and expands on these conceptions, using *care* as an umbrella term to highlight the need for focused, systematic attention to caring that has been defined.

Development of the typology. Efforts to conceptualize social work activity can present difficulty because they involve decisions about whether task, client need, or professional method forms the major basis of the conceptual scheme (Berkman and Rehr, 1972). The typology presented here attempts to conceptualize caring tasks as they are derived from the definition of care presented, professional values, and current health needs. The typology is based on the assumption that the bulk of health care social work involves *preventive, curative-ameliorative,* and *maintenance tasks.* As this discussion will suggest, the tasks encompass various social work roles, practice technologies, methods, organizational contexts in which social work is carried out, and research efforts to enhance and refine social work knowledge and skill.

Definition of major terms. Although much health care social work can be subsumed under the rubric of prevention (Germain, 1982), the term does not fully specify the range of caring tasks. Therefore I will define prevention, curing-amelioration, and maintenance.

Prevention. At the beginning of this chapter there was a detailed discussion of prevention. As pointed out, prevention can involve efforts to avert or reduce (1) the incidence of problems, (2) infirmity by early detection and treatment, and (3) the amount and extent of defect related to infirmity.

Cure-amelioration. In both medicine and social work a *curing stance* was identified not only with successful remedial treatment but also with an emphasis on using all available theory and skill. Implicit in the foregoing discussion was some skepticism about the extensive emphasis on curing because contemporary health care has a more limited curing capacity than desired. It was also suggested that in social work the focus on cure may have deflected attention from systematic efforts to refine caring tasks.

The terms *cure* and *curing* when applied to social work tasks have a number of other limitations. One limitation is the association of these terms with a clinical, medical orientation focused on diagnosis and treatment in the narrow sense. As early as 1961 Bartlett suggested that the clinical conceptualization to which health care social work had long been tied was useful though insufficient as a base for social work practice in health. In commenting on the increased emphasis on demonstrating "effective" outcomes of intervention Lewis (1981) implicitly suggests that in social work these outcomes are not necessarily identified with curing.

There is another sense in which the identification of health care social work tasks with curing is problematic. The social work research literature of the last 20 years has shown that it is difficult to demonstrate clear-cut evidence of the effectiveness of intervention when focus is on showing clear-cut, measurable improvements. Experimental studies of intervention in family functioning, delinquency prevention, and other areas suggest that the goals and tasks exceeded social work's capacity to effect basic changes in human functioning (for example, Mullen and Dumpson, 1972). Fanshel (1980) comments on this finding, suggesting

> It is foolish and unseemly to become excessively defensive in the face of adverse findings. Given the severe nature of the problems targeted for inter-

> vention, it may well be unreal to expect more promising outcomes.
>
> The social work profession may have matured so that it will no longer blithely claim a capacity to transform people or eliminate problems which are rooted in pernicious social circumstances (p. 13).

Many of the problems with which health care social workers deal have diverse roots and involve the intervention of multiple professionals. Indeed there have been virtually no studies of outcome, cure, or effectiveness in health care social work analogous to those carried out in other fields of social work practice. More attention has been paid to describing patterns of service delivery (Coulton, 1980).

These and related factors suggest that a curing stance does not suffice as a conceptual base for health care social work practice. An important exception related to the component of curing is using and developing all possible skills and strategies in efforts to remedy individual, group, or systemic malfunction.

In the conceptualization being developed in this book many social work tasks are more appropriately termed ameliorative. To ameliorate is to make better or improve. Much that is involved in health care social work, at varying levels of practice, can be characterized as efforts to ameliorate.

Maintenance. Various data have been presented to suggest that substantial segments of the population have health problems that have reached the point of limited, if any, hope for effecting *substantial* improvement in their social, psychological, or physical functioning. Morris and Anderson (1975) estimate that as much as 25% of the population is in a situation in which the attention and care of adults (other than parents) is required for some part of the day. When the estimates are limited to people receiving such services under the broad rubric of social work (for example, hospitals, probation, and public assistance), they suggest that 10% of the population requires close supervision and monitoring. Another estimate suggests that the pool of "resourceless" people (those with long-term disability and handicap who require emotional support and help with the tasks of daily living) may be increasing at the rate of 5% every 5 years. Social work must find a way of conceptualizing the tasks that relate to this segment of the population. These tasks should be differentiated from those involving prevention or curing-amelioration.

The concept of maintenance—defined as *preserving* and keeping in *existence or continuance*—envelopes the wide range of care needs required by the most disabled groups in the population. An expansion of the concept includes a view of maintenance that is carried out in a humane, concerned manner and is attentive to physical and psychological comfort. Clearly no conceptualization of tasks is exhaustive, nor are the distinctions between them ironclad. In most instances intervention takes place at all levels. Extensive skill is required in each of these areas.

The goals related to the tasks needed differ. Recognizing these differences (1) minimizes the diversion of energy into efforts to effect major change in social functioning where such potential is most limited; (2) facilitates efforts to develop organizational mechanisms and practice technologies that are variously focused on prevention, amelioration, and maintenance; and (3) serves to clarify efforts to identify the most appropriate loci of intervention.

• • •

The basic elements of the typology of caring have now been presented. The social and psychological needs that cluster around health issues and generate caring tasks were presented earlier. These needs can be grouped into those revolving around

1. The way health care is rendered, including the emphasis on technology, a certain degree of depersonalization, and the tendency

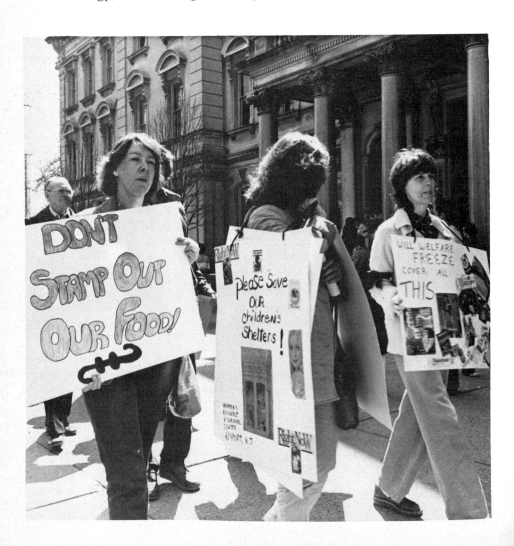

to expect patients to conform to the language, values, and stance of the medical care system regardless of their ethnic and religious dispositions

2. The diverse health and welfare services required by many, particularly the chronically ill, the elderly, and the handicapped
3. Consumers' input into decisions around their own care
4. The financial and geographical availability and accessibility of care

These four categories of need are now used to suggest related preventive, cure-ameliorative, and maintenance tasks.

The reader should note the congruence between this typology and the concept of person-environment fit. The chart on pp. 147-149 outlines the major components of the typology and shows if the target of change is the environment, the individual or small group, or both.

A TYPOLOGY OF CARING TASKS

I. Tasks related to prevailing medical care approaches

Target of change	**A.** *Preventive tasks*
Environment	**1.** Minimizing depersonalizing, and dehumanizing aspects of care through education and interpretation
Environment	**2.** Interpreting varied dispositions to caring for different classes and ethnic groups
Environment	**3.** Humanizing health care environments
	B. *Ameliorative tasks*
Individual and group	**1.** Counseling people to help them cooperate and comply with practitioners performing complex medical procedures
Individual, group, and environment	**2.** Providing the opportunity to decide about participating and/or continuing in complex medical treatment
	C. *Maintenance tasks*
Individual	**1.** Helping patients and families cope with the situation when limited or no improvement can be expected
Individual	**2.** Helping patients and families decide about further care

Continued.

A TYPOLOGY OF CARING TASKS—*cont'd*

II. Tasks related to the needs of the severely ill and disabled

	A. *Preventive tasks*
Individual, group, and environment	**1.** Averting family disorganization while caring for people with severe illness or disability (for example, counseling and/or resource provision)
Individual	**2.** Helping family members identify their own risk of similar and/or related health problems by seeking preventive measures (for example, screening)
	B. *Ameliorative tasks*
Environment	**1.** Coordinating and developing resources
Individual	**2.** Providing opportunities for socializing
Environment	**3.** Involving volunteers in service provision
Environment and individual	**4.** Promoting adaptation to illness
Environment, individual, and group	**5.** Developing patient/client networks
	C. *Maintenance tasks*
Environment	**1.** Participating in coordination and resource development
Environment	**2.** Developing integrated service systems or networks
Environment	**3.** Ensuring humane care is rendered
Environment	**4.** Providing concrete resources

III. Tasks related to consumer input about care decisions

	A. *Preventive tasks*
Environment	**1.** Participating and/or providing leadership in organizing to reduce work-related health hazards
Environment	**2.** Highlighting the futility of planning for health needs in the event of a nuclear threat
Environment	**3.** Interacting with consumers to identify populations at risk for particular health problems
Target of change	**B.** *Ameliorative tasks*
Environment	**1.** Helping consumers in particular geographical or work areas identify health services needs
Environment	**2.** Helping consumers identify and work for service delivery changes

	C. *Maintenance tasks*
Environment	**1.** Ensuring provision of adequate resources to people wanting to "take care of their own"
Environment/ individual	**2.** Providing help and/or information to connect people with various resources and skills to others needing those various resources and skills

IV. Tasks related to problems involving availability and accessibility of care

	A. *Preventive tasks*
Environment	**1.** Participating in individual and collective activity (for example professional organizations) to lobby for development of programs and/or adequate funding
Environment	**2.** Documenting need and preventive potential of adequate health and/or financing programs
	B. *Ameliorative tasks*
Environment	**1.** Creatively using and developing resources in cases of inequity
Environment	**2.** Developing familiarity with regulations and entitlements to fully use them
Individual	**3.** Helping people feel comfortable about using available resources
Environment	**4.** Securing, organizing, and coordinating services and funds from volunteers
	C. *Maintenance tasks*
	Not applicable

The typology of caring presented represents an effort to conceptualize major social work tasks in four areas: (1) caring needs generated by the manner in which health care is rendered, with an emphasis on the level of technology, degree of depersonalization, and expected adherence to prevailing standards; (2) the diverse nonmedical needs of the chronically ill, handicapped, and elderly; (3) consumer input for making decisions about health services; and (4) problems related to availability and accessibility of care. Three major types of tasks were conceptualized: (1) preventive tasks, (2) ameliorative tasks, and (3) maintenance tasks.

I do not claim that the typology is exhaustive, but it does suggest an approach to systematic delineation of social work activity as generated by social work values, the prevailing level of medical practice technology, social work practice technology, and definitions of health focused on social functioning.

CAREERS OF ILLNESS*

The concept careers of illness has been used by a number of sociologists to identify the various phases and stages involved in the course of illness (for example, Davis, 1963; Freidson, 1970; Goffman, 1968; Roth, 1963). *Career* may be defined as progress or general course of action through life or through some phase of life. When this concept is applied to illness and its social and psychological consequences, it focuses attention on the fact that these consequences vary with the nature of the disease or illness; the different stages that can be expected; and the medical, social, and psychological interventions that need to be used at different stages. Dinerman, Schlesinger, and Wood (1980) have proposed that this concept or framework

> Facilitates social work efforts to organize a vast body of knowledge about illness and the varied tasks of consumers and providers that are engendered by different courses of illness and preventive endeavors (p. 17).

This view helps identify the recurrent or typical sequences of events that are an integral part of the illness experience. Focusing on sequences or stages highlights the fact that responses and needs typically evident in an earlier phase are likely to be supplemented or replaced by those of a different nature at a later stage.

The concept differs from the medical approach to the natural history of a disease, which tends to be limited to the predictable physical changes related to identified disease processes. Instead the framework encompasses the range of consumer and provider experiences and tasks generated by illness over a protracted period of time. The view of illness as a career calls attention to (1) the fact that most illness is not time limited but is extended over time; (2) the variation in the biological, social, and psychological impact of various types of

*Abstracted from Dinerman, M., Schlesinger, E., and Wood, K.: Social work roles in health care: an educational framework, Health and Social Work **5**(4):13, 1980.

illness at different points in time; (3) the different resources and coping capacities required at different phases of the illness process; (4) the role of significant others, including family, community, and health care providers; and (5) the part played by health policies and provisions in affecting the career or course of illness.

Most illness, except that of a very transient nature, necessitates a series of psychosocial transitions in role and self-perception, involving learning new roles and self-concepts. These changes call for marked alteration in coping habits and skills. The concept of careers of illness encompasses these changes in self-definition, the effort to learn new coping strategies, and the required and available sociopsychological resources and other care needs. The concept also helps specify the paths experienced by ill people and those with whom their lives are intimately intertwined, while recognizing that different patterns are observed for the same illness because illness produces different identifiable experiences in different people. In addition, it emphasizes the contrast with clinical definitions, which tend to concentrate on one point in time when rehabilitation processes are said to have been successfully or unsuccessfully applied.

The response to illness of all people involved, including patients, their family and community networks, and caretakers, as well as the response of the social system, including prevalent health care social policy and provision, will vary by the nature and facts of the illness as well as by a variety of personal, social, demographic, and political factors.

Illness may manifest itself suddenly, unexpectedly, and dramatically, as exemplified by stroke, heart attack, or quadriplegia following an accident. Or the onset may be slow and insidious, as is often the case with diabetes or mild schizophrenia. Recognizing developmental lag in children may be delayed and acknowledging the presence of a lump in the breast is often drawn out or resisted.

These and other health problems have various outcomes. In the case of some health problems such as pneumonia, gall bladder disease, or adolescent adjustment reactions, it is usually expected that the problem is relatively self-limited and will require no long-range changes in life's plans, hopes, or dreams. Nevertheless, these problems call for adaptation and coping skill. Many health problems on which I have focused thus far call for massive adaptation in ways of living, working, and loving.

In many instances the nature of the illness is such that the required adaptations are lifelong and ever changing. For example, a diagnosis of diabetes may initially require minor adaptations of customary eating patterns. Should the disease progress and entail complications, impotence related to circulatory difficulties, blurring of vision, gangrene of the limbs, or kidney failure are possible problems. These kinds of problems may or may not surface over time. Unless or until they do, diabetics and people with other chronic health problems that may entail different complications expect to live and function for extended periods of time without massive disruption. Yet life and self-perception are never quite the same as before the onset of this type of illness.

Other health problems that may also begin slowly and in a seemingly insidious manner involve more deterioration and greater discomfort following onset. The change in life-style triggered by the illness may be more dramatic, and long-term prognosis is almost always poor. Chronic schizophrenia that severely limits functioning, some types of multiple sclerosis, advanced stages of emphysema, and some forms of rheumatoid arthritis are examples of this type of health problem. These types of illnesses require marked alterations in life-style and major, daily attention to the illness and its consequences. Other health problems not only surface rapidly and unexpectedly but also have a poor prognosis. Some cancers, for example, do not yield to treatment and lead rapidly to death.

Whatever the nature of the disease or illness, or the character of the onset and expected course, there is an indication that much illness is more than a fleeting, time-limited event. Viewed in these terms disease or illness may be more profitably understood as a process involving recurring or typical problems and needs faced by those individuals who are ill and those with whom they are involved.

Although each individual and family experiences illness in a unique and personal manner, it is nevertheless possible to identify the particular types of stresses and concerns that tend to accompany various categories of illness. A number of illness careers have been identified. Their major organizing focuses are (1) the nature of onset, whether sudden or slow and insidious; (2) the expected outcome, in terms of the disease process and in relation to social and psychological functioning; and (3) the degree of role change, adaption to the sick role, and changes in life-style related to the nature of the illness. An infinite number of health problems can potentially be subsumed under each career. These problems have been grouped into the following categories:

1. Sudden onset and predictable positive outcome (for example, acute pneumonia or adolescent adjustment reaction)
2. Illness with gradual onset and long duration requiring changes in life-style and adaptation to the role of being sick (for example, diabetes or mild developmental disabilities)
3. Slow onset with poor long-term prognosis requiring a marked alteration in life-style (for example, emphysema, advanced aging, chronic schizophrenia, and multiple sclerosis)
4. Sudden onset with predictable adequate long-range functioning (for example, mild heart attacks and acute situational depression)
5. Sudden onset with a predictable, rapid, negative outcome (for example, liver cancer and Tay-Sachs disease)

While this is clearly not an exhaustive classification, the substantive nature of the problems and the order in which they are presented suggest that they include common acute illnesses both of a physical and emotional nature as well as chronic and/or severe maladies leading to marked alteration in feeling and life-style, discomfort, and sometimes premature death.

Applying the career of illness concept in social work practice

How can the view of illness as a career serve the social worker at varying levels of practice and in different types of organizational contexts? The concept focuses on the fact that each of the identified careers tends to be characterized by certain similar issues and problems, although the substance may vary significantly. Therefore it can, for example, serve to organize thinking about coping tasks and interventive skills generated by the type of long-term illness that is not totally disruptive of accustomed life-styles. These tasks and skills are in contrast to those confronting people whose every move may be governed by their particular problem.

There are points in any illness experience when interventive and caring tasks become paramount. To identify those times when social work intervention is particularly important, a number of areas of knowledge and skill about careers of illness can be specified.

Dinerman, Schlesinger, and Wood (1980) have suggested that for all illness careers (and/or specific health problems) social workers require thorough familiarity with the following three points:

1. Understanding of the disease or illness from a medical standpoint, including the usual nature of onset and the usual prognosis or expected outcome. Brengarth (1981) points out that all health care social workers need an understanding of biomedical issues and their impact on human development. However, "sickness impact" varies by disease and by the stage of the disease. Social workers assigned to a coronary care unit need particular familiarity with the usual nature of onset of a heart attack, the expected course of treatment, and the usual recovery rates. The worker involved in planning for stroke victims must be familiar with the impact a stroke can have on verbal and physical functioning. Knowledge of how physiotherapy and speech therapy are used in the rehabilitative process is essential.

It is crucial that social workers become familiar with the physiological and psychological aspects often associated with certain medical procedures or drug therapies. For example, many women experience some feeling of depression following a hysterectomy, perhaps partially related to hormonal changes. Cardiac patients often experience anxiety about having another attack. Knowing about these kinds of reactions can forestall an inappropriate or premature diagnosis of psychopathology. Without such knowledge social workers will be limited in their ability to understand client experiences and concerns. As health care team members their contribution will not be respected unless they demonstrate understanding of minimal basic information. Clearly social workers are not required to have mastery of medical information. However, they are expected to "learn how to learn" the information required to fulfill their unique tasks.

2. Understanding of the population at risk and the prevalence and incidence of the particular problem. Considerable attention has already been paid to public health concepts and their implications for preventive intervention in social work. These concepts are important not only for social workers whose major activities involve planning, but for all health care social workers needing to organize their work and their inevitably limited resources to ensure care for particularly vulnerable people.

3. Understanding the recurrent or typical contingencies awaiting people with different health problems or careers. This knowledge involves in-depth understanding of the experiences and coping tasks likely to be generated by various problems. This type of understanding is derived from researching the daily problems of people enduring different illnesses and from the practitioner's work experience.

Social workers are responsible for familiarizing themselves with research focused on these kinds of issues. Some of that work is organized and planned to facilitate insight into the shifting problems occurring over time. Strauss and Glaser (1975) presented a series of papers focusing on the long-term problems of individuals with rheumatoid arthritis (Weiner, 1975), ulcerative colitis (Reif, 1975), childhood diabetes (Benoliel, 1975), and emphysema (Fagerhaugh, 1975). Croog and Levine and Finlayson and McEwen (1977) studied the experiences of a group of men for extensive periods following a heart attack. Other work has focused on different stages of the illness experience (for example, in the hospital or at certain other critical points). Examining this kind of work facilitates constructing the illness career by piecing together various elements of research and clinical experience.

Strauss and Glaser (1975) identify a series of needs and coping strategies commonly experienced by people with chronic problems. This series includes (1) preventing and managing medical crises; (2) contending with complex medical regimens; (3) learning to cope with symptoms; (4) learning to cope with time; (5) coping with terminal illness—for some there is a predictable downward course while others have an uneven course with periods of remission, decline, and greater discomfort; and (6) handling the social isolation, socially or self-imposed, frequently accompanying severe illness. A review of other studies (Strauss and Glaser, 1975) suggests that the problems and strategies identified by Strauss and Glaser are recurrent among individuals experiencing major chronic illness.

Coping with complex medical regimens. Many chronic conditions entail the potential for difficulty. A diabetic may go into a coma as a result of taking too much or too little insulin. A person with epilepsy may live in constant fear of having a convulsion. A person with asthma may unexpectedly be exposed to allergens and have a severe attack. Life must be organized to deal with such persistent threats. The patient and family must know what the warning signs are, what emergency measures are available, and how to use these measures. Strauss and Glaser stress that in the context of family and community, "nonmedical organization" of effort is involved in management of such crises. The implications for the social worker when working with affected persons and their families are clear; efforts need to be focused on anticipating, rehearsing, and helping people organize their daily lives around such strains.

Dealing with symptoms. The symptom experience is vividly described by Strauss and Glaser (1975) in the following quote:

> Whatever sophisticated technical references there may be for his symptoms, the person who has symptoms will be concerned primarily with whether he hurts, faints, trembles visibly, loses energy suddenly, runs short of breath, has had his mobility or his speech impaired, or is evidencing some kind of disfigurement. Aside from what these may signify to him about his disease or his life-span, such symptoms can interfere with his life and his social relationships. How much they interfere depends on whether they are permanent or temporary, frequent or occasional, predictable or unpredictable, and publicly visible or invisible; upon their degree (as of pain), their meaning to bystanders (as of disfigurement), and the nature of the regimen called for to control the symptom; and upon the kinds of life-style and social relations that the sufferer has hitherto sustained (p. 35).

The impact of symptoms on the daily life of sick persons and their families is an area requiring further research.

Individuals with major mobility impairment must anticipate their every physical move. The stroke patient who forgets something important upstairs before leaving the house may go through various contortions and discomfort to retrieve an important item. People with arthritis or multiple sclerosis who are unable to carry out physical activities because they are painful may need to rely on an extensive network of family and friends to help them care for the simplest daily needs.

Learning to cope with time. Some people prevented from carrying on their routine activities feel "roleless," having little else to do but manage their symptoms. Others who go on with customary activities may find that the combination of those activities with managing the illness leaves little time for rest or relaxation. Diabetics, asthmatics, and cystic fibrosis patients and their families may find the routines totally engulfing. For example, asthmatics need pollen- and dust-free rooms and regular medication, and activities need to be planned around potential threats. Cystic fibrosis patients require postural drainage to assure excursion of mucus.

Coping with terminal illness. Often symptoms and their expected courses are not predictable. This unpredictability is vividly illustrated in the lives of people with terminal illness whose progression is not steadily downward. People with life-threatening health problems may no longer be able to "take life for granted." Much has been written about helping people to cope with imminent death or the fear of dying. For many of the major health problems identified, impending death and the struggles involved are part of the illness career, Moos (1977) identifies a few coping tasks that a dying person encounters: maintaining self-esteem, dealing with anxiety, and mourning for a nonexistent future.

Death is often preceded by protracted periods of gradual decline and withdrawal from the routines of life. The effects on others close to the dying person, such as the family, have been investigated by many researchers. Goldberg (1977) identifies the need to "allow mourning to occur," to relinquish the deceased as a force in family activities, and to alter family tasks and roles. These tasks, which are already emotionally draining, are made more difficult when, in the words of Strauss and Glaser, there is a "pattern of decline-reprieve-decline-reprieve-decline to death" (p. 48). Terminally ill patients, whether experiencing steady or delayed decline, are likely to be socially isolated.

Handling social isolation. Isolation frequently occurs at a time when discomfort and fear are paramount in a patient's life. This isolation can take place for several reasons. Reduced activity can minimize social interaction potential. Many researchers (for example, Strauss and Glaser, 1975; Weiner, 1975) point out that the healthy feel uncomfortable in and too often withdraw from the presence of persons with visible disability. These individuals must use their already depleted energy to cope with isolation or to develop strategies to diminish it. These selected and brief references to typical contingencies and coping tasks merely begin to give some indication of the scope and depth of the impact of sickness. How an understanding of the chronically ill patient's problems can guide social work practice shall concern us throughout this book.

Awareness of resource needs. The review of certain components of daily life experiences of people with major chronic health problems readily leads to the identification of resource needs. Individuals who regularly experience life-threatening medical crises require continuous medical care. Symptom control not only requires medication but also help in organizing life to manage symptoms. Parents of children with chronic problems need relief. This includes "sitters" trained to deal with health problems that may arise. Those patients who can no longer carry out their accustomed work require retraining, retooling, and obtaining alternative employment.

The careers of illness concept is illustrated by some typical problems and suggested points for social work intervention in two health problems—mild diabetes and mild developmental disability. The daily management tasks and long-term negative impact tend not to be as severe as the kinds of difficulties discussed previously. Nevertheless, the reader will recall that large numbers of people are affected by these kinds of problems.

The medical definitions and courses of mild diabetes and mild developmental disability are quite different. Nevertheless, both share certain features. They are both illustrative of health problems with gradual onset, of long duration, with a likely positive outcome, and requiring changes in life-style. The social worker needs to be aware that these problems are ongoing and require continuous attention.

When working with diabetics and developmentally disabled people, the social worker needs extensive familiarity with medical and educational definitions and interventions and with the kind of crises that may occur. People with mild diabetes should be continually concerned with diet, weight control, and blood sugar levels. Developmentally disabled individuals and their families are constantly worried about accomplishing learning tasks and overcoming mild physical handicaps. Both types of patients need to be in regular contact with health providers and both need supportive families helping with health needs or learning tasks.

These clients may worry about their futures, but they are able to work, go to school, and engage in ordinary social life without major disruption. Both types of persons require certain essential resources and need readily available health providers. Lacking financial resources diabetics may need help obtaining adequate food. Special educational needs are usually essential for persons with developmental disability. These individuals and their families may become discouraged and fearful.

Social workers can identify points along the spectrum where intervention may be particularly essential.

1. *The point at which a health problem is suspected and/or confirmed.* At this time there may be extensive need for information about the problem and resources to deal with it. People will vary in the extent to which they can cope with and integrate the information and in the extent to which they deny the total impact. Decisions about how much information, guidance, and counseling is offered at this point will depend on expressed client need and professional judgment.

2. *The point(s) when there appears to be a lack of adherence to recommended regimen or intervention.* Initial enthusiastic compliance may give way to discouragement. For example, diabetics may adhere to their diets only to find that their blood sugar levels do not drop the way they expected or hoped. Figuring "it doesn't matter anyway" they may go on a binge of eating prohibited foods such as candy or liquor. The mothers of developmentally disabled youngsters may decide that the children are not learning to read as they had hoped and withdraw them from special programs. With these and related problems, it is often essential to review the situation and attempt to discuss whether emotional turmoil or lack of understanding is contributing to the difficulty.

3. *The point(s) when major life changes are contemplated or essential.* For example, the diabetic may be considering taking a new job and may be fearful that the demands are too rigorous. Or the family of a developmentally

disabled child may be contemplating a move to another community and may have questions and fears about the effect of the change or the availability of resources in the new community.

4. *The point(s) at which complications develop.* Diabetics previously able to control their blood sugar levels with diet may need to shift to insulin. This entails major changes in daily routine and need for help with the routine and generates much fear. The developmentally disabled child may begin to go to school and find that he or she is taunted by peers or that the particular learning deficit is not understood by teachers.

Health promotion, when defined as social functioning in the face of illness, must always involve the social worker in attempts to clarify the medical and psychosocial meaning of different phases in the illness process. These phases may be exacerbated by stressful life events unrelated to the illness for example, (the death of a parent or spouse). The relationship between the onset of symptoms in disorders long considered psychosomatic and life stressors is well established (for example, Holmes, 1978). These and like experiences become part of the dynamic with which social workers deal as they organize their thinking and intervention within the career concept.

SUMMARY

A number of conceptual frameworks were presented in this chapter. They are (1) public health perspectives, (2) the concept of "person-environment fit", (3) the continuum from cure to care, (4) a typology of caring, and (5) the careers of illness. Taken as a whole the materials presented link basic social work perspectives, current developments in health care, and understanding of the illness experience and further develop a conceptual base for social work practice in health care. Public health perspectives focus on the collective conditions of life that minimize or intensify illness. Classic public health and epidemiological models are consonant with social work's focus on the person-environment interaction. The concept *person-environment fit* serves to specify how the illness experience has an impact on individuals and points to areas of intervention variously focused on individuals and their environments. Efforts to intervene at either level are enhanced by making distinctions between the curing and caring components of contemporary health care delivery. The typology of caring identifies a series of tasks for health care social work that are derived from analyzing current health needs. The illness careers concept identifies the major problems related to typical illness patterns. The concept facilitates identification of recurrent events integral to the illness experience and suggests a framework for integrating knowledge of these events with the tasks confronting consumers and providers at various points in the illness experience.

REFERENCES

Bartlett, H.M.: Social work practice in the health field, Washington, D.C., 1961, National Association of Social Workers.

Benoliel, J.Q.: Childhood diabetes: the commonplace in living becomes uncommon. In Strauss, A.L. and Glaser, B.G.: Chronic illness and the quality of life, St. Louis, 1975, The C.V. Mosby Co.

Berkman, G.B., and Rehr, H.: Social needs of the hospitalized elderly, Social Work **17**(4):80, 1972.

Black, D.: The making of a doctor, Part 2, The New York Times Magazine, May 30, 1982.

Bracht, N.F.: Public health social work: a community focus. In Bracht, N.F.: Social work in health care, New York, 1978, The Haworth Press.

Brengarth, J.A.: What is "special" about specialization?, Health and Social Work (Suppl.) **6**(4):915, 1981.

Briar, S.: Needed: a simple definition of social work, Social Work **26**(1):83, 1981.

Butt, E.: Family and social network roles, norms and external relationships in ordinary urban families, New York, 1971, The Free Press.

Cassel, J.: Psychosocial processes and "stress": theoretical formulation. In Garfield, C.A., editor: Stress and survival: the emotional realities of life-threatening illness, St. Louis, 1979, The C.V. Mosby Co.

Coulton, C.: Person-environment fit as the focus in health care, Social Work **26**(1):26, 1981.

Coulton, C.: Research on social work in health care: progress and future directions. In Fanshel, D., editor: Future of social work research, Washington, D.C., 1980, National Association of Social Workers.

Croog, S.H., and Levine, S.: The heart patient recovers, New York, 1977, Human Sciences Press, Inc.

Davis, F.: Passage through crisis, Indianapolis, 1963, Bobbs-Merrill Co., Inc.

Dinerman, M., Schlesinger, E.G., and Wood, K.: Social work roles in health care: an educational framework, Health and Social Work **5**(4):13, 1980.

Fagerhaugh, S.: Getting around with emphysema. In Strauss, A.L. and Glaser, B.G.: Chronic illness and the quality of life, St. Louis, 1975, The C.V. Mosby Co.

Fanshel, D.: The future of social work research: strategies for the coming years. In Fanshel, D., editor: Future of social work research, Washington, D.C., 1980, National Association of Social Workers, p. 13.

Finlayson, A., and McEwen, J.: Coronary heart disease and patterns of living, New York, 1977, Prodist.

Fischer, J.: Effective casework practice: an eclectic approach, New York, 1978, McGraw-Hill Book Co.

Fisher, D.: The hospitalized terminally ill patient: an ecological perspective. In Germain, C.B., editor: Social work practice: people and environments, New York, 1979, Columbia University Press.

Flexner, A.: Is social work a profession? In Pumphrey, R.E., and Pumphrey, M.W., editors: The heritage of American social work, New York, 1961, Columbia University Press.

Fox, R.C., and Swazey, J.P.: The courage to fail: a social view of organ transplants and dialysis, Chicago, 1974, University of Chicago Press.

Freidson, E.: Profession of medicine, New York, 1970, Dodd, Mead & Co.

Fuchs, V.R.: Who shall live? health economics and social choice, New York, 1974, Basic Books, Inc., Publishers.

Geiger, J.: Foreword. In Salber, E.J.: Caring and curing: community participation in health services, New York, 1975, Prodist.

Geismar, L.W.: Preventive intervention in social work, Metuchen, N.J., 1969, Scarecrow Press, Inc.

Germain, C.B.: Teaching primary prevention in social work: an ecological perspective, Journal of Education for Social Work **18**(1):20, 1982.

Gilbert, N.: Policy issues in primary prevention, Social Work **27**(4):293, 1982.

Goffman, E.: Asylums, Middlesex, England, 1968, Penguin Books, Ltd.

Goldberg, J.B.: Family tasks and reactions in the crisis of death. In Moos, R.N., editor: Coping with physical illness, New York, 1977, Plenum Medical Book Co.

Hanlon, J.J., and Pickett, G.E.: Public health: administration and practice, ed. 8, St. Louis, 1984, The C.V. Mosby Co.

Healthy people: the Surgeon General's report on health promotion and disease prevention, DHEW Pub. No. (PHS) 79-55071, Washington, D.C., 1979, U.S. Government Printing Office.

Holden, M.O.: Dialysis or death: the ethical alternatives, Health and Social Work **5**(2):18, 1980.

Holmes, T.H.: Life situations, emotions, and disease, Psychosomatics **19**(12):747, 1978.

Howell, J.R., Osterweis, M., and Huntley, R.R.: Curing and caring—a proposed method for self assessment in primary care organizations, Journal of Community Health **1**(4):256, 1976.

Insley, V.: Health services: maternal and child health. In Turner, J.B., editor: Encyclopedia of social work, Washington, D.C., 1977, National Association of Social Workers, vol. 1, p. 602.

Interim report of the graduate medical educational national advisory committee to the secretary, Department of Health, Education and Welfare, DHEW Pub. No. (HRA) 79-633, Washington, D.C., 1979, U.S. Government Printing Office.

Kavanaugh, R.E.: Humane treatment of the terminally ill. In Moos, R.N., editor: Coping with physical illness, New York, 1977, Plenum Medical Book Co.

Kosa, J., and Robertson, L.S.: The social aspects of health and illness. In Kosa, J., Zola, I.K.: Poverty and health: a sociological analysis, Cambridge, Mass., 1975, Harvard University Press.

LaRocco, J.M., House, J., and French, J.R.P.: Social support, occupational stress and health, Journal of Health and Social Behavior **21**(3):202, 1980.

Leiby, J.: Social welfare: history of basic ideas. In Turner, J.B., editor: Encyclopedia of social work, Washington D.C., 1977, National Association of Social Workers, vol. 2, p. 1512.

Lewis, H.: The emergence of social work as a profession in health care: significant influences and persistent issues, Paper presented at the Third Doris Siegel Memorial Colloquium (Health care concepts: developmental milestones in social work and medicine) at the Mt. Sinai Medical Center, New York, April 9, 1981.

Lorber, J.: Good patients and problem patients: conformity and deviance in a general hospital, Journal of Health and Social Behavior **16**(2):213, 1975.

Lowy, L.: Social work with the aging, New York, 1979, Harper & Row, Publishers, Inc.

Lurie, A.: Social work in health care in the next ten years, Social Work in Health Care **2**(4):419, 1977.

Mechanic, D.: Illness behavior, social adaptation and the management of illness, The Journal of Nervous and Mental Disease **165**(2):79, 1977.

Middleman, R., and Goldberg, G.: Social service delivery: a structural approach to social work practice, New York, 1974, Columbia University Press.

Moos, R.N., editor: Coping with physical illness, New York, 1977, Plenum Medical Book Co.

Morris, R.: Caring for vs. caring about people, Social Work **22**(5):353, 1977.

Morris, R.: Social work function in a caring society: abstract value, professional preference and the real world, Journal of Education for Social Work **14**(2):82, 1978.

Morris, R., and Anderson, D.: Personal care services: an identity for social work, Social Service Review **49**(2):157, 1975.

Mullen, E.J., and Dumpson, J.R., editors: Evaluation of social intervention, San Francisco, 1972, Jossey-Bass, Inc., Publishers.

Pilisuk, M., and Froland, C.: Kinship, social networks, social support and health, Social Science and Medicine, Medical Psychology and Medical Sociology, **12B:**273, 1978.

Pumphrey, R.E., and Pumphrey, M.W., editors: The heritage of American social work, New York, 1961, Columbia University Press.

Reichert, K.: Essentials of social work practice in public health programs. In Watkins, E.L., editor: social work in a state based system of child health care, based on the proceedings of the 1980 Tri-Regional Workshop for Social Workers in Maternal and Child Health Services, sponsored by Department of Maternal and Child Health, School of Public Health, University of North Carolina and The Office for Maternal and Child Health, Department of Health and Human Services.

Reinhold, R.: Economics of life and death arises in debate over kidney therapy, Science Times, The New York Times, May 25, 1982.

Rice, E.: social work in public health, Social Work **4**(1):82, 1959.

Rice, E.: Concepts of prevention as applied to the practice of social work, American Journal of Public Health **52**(2):266, 1962.

Rief, L.: Ulcerative colitis: strategies for managing life. In Strauss, A.L. and Glaser, B.G.: Chronic illness and the quality of life, St. Louis, 1975, The C.V. Mosby Co.

Riska, E., and Vinter-Johansen, P.: The involvement of the behavioral sciences in American medicine: a national perspective, International Journal of Health Services **11**(4):583, 1981.

Ross, J.W.: Ethical conflicts in medical social work: pediatric cancer care as prototype, Health and Social Work **7**(2):95, 1982.

Roth, J.: Timetables, Indianapolis, 1963, Bobbs-Merrill Co., Inc.

Salber, E.J.: Caring and curing: community participation in health services, New York, 1975, Prodist.

Sabik, C.: $65 million medical facility links health care, education, New Brunswick, N.J., May 17, 1982, The Home News.

Schlesinger, E.G., and Devore, W.: Ethnic networks: conceptual formulations and interventive strategies, Paper presented at the annual meeting, American Public Health Association, Los Angeles, Nov. 3, 1981.

Smith, B.C.: Community health: an epidemiological approach, New York, 1979, The Macmillan Co., Publishers.

Solon, J.A.: Health services: public health programs. In Turner, J.B., editor: Encyclopedia of social work, Washington, D.C., 1977, National Association of Social Workers, vol. 1, p. 611.

Specht, H.: Origins of the profession. In Gilbert, N., and Specht, H., editors: The emergence of social welfare and social work, ed. 2, Itasca, Ill., 1981, F.E. Peacock Publishers, Inc.

Spiegel, A.D., and Backhaut, B.: Curing and caring, New York, 1980, Spectrum Publications.

Stein, H.F.: A dialectical model of health and illness attitudes and behavior among Slovak Americans, International Journal of Mental Health **5**(2): 117, 1976.

Strauss, A.L. and Glaser, B.G.: Chronic illness and the quality of life, St. Louis, 1975, The C.V. Mosby Co.

Task panel reports, submitted to the President's Commission on Mental Health, Washington, D.C., 1978, U.S. Government Printing Office, vol. 11, Appendix.

Vance, E.T.: Social disability, American Psychologist **28**:498, June 1973.

Wiener, C.L.: The burden of rheumatoid arthritis. In Strauss, A.L. and Glaser, B.G.: Chronic illness and the quality of life, St. Louis, 1975, The C.V. Mosby Co.

Wittman, M.: Application of knowledge about prevention to health and mental health practice. In Bracht, N.F., editor: Social work in health care, New York, 1978, The Haworth Press.

Zborowski, M.: Cultural components in response to pain, Journal of Social Issues **4**(8):16, 1952.

LA
PLACITA
GROCERY
ONE WAY

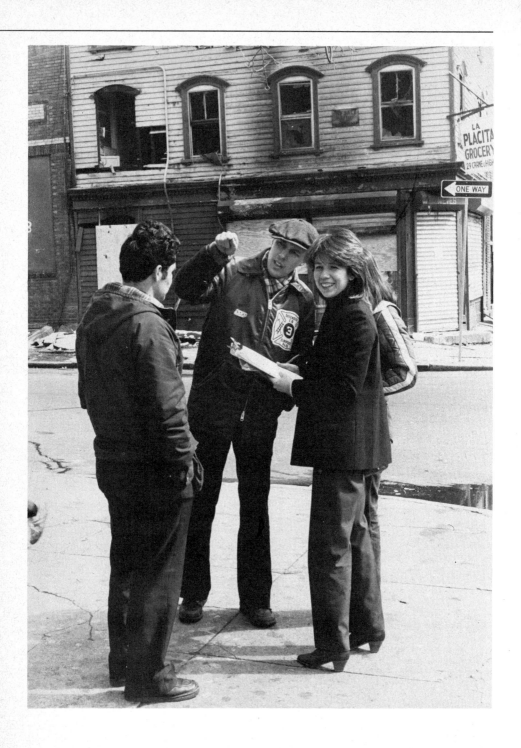

Chapter 6

Principles for health care social work practice

Much of the preceding material has focused on several specialized areas of knowledge and conceptual formulations that need to be understood by social workers whose practice is concentrated in health settings or on health issues. This chapter presents a series of practice principles for health care social work.* These principles are derived from the following:

1. Social work values
2. Analysis of the nature and scope of contemporary health problems
3. Prevailing characteristics of the health services delivery system and social work's role in that system
4. Formulations from the social and behavioral sciences concerning the social, psychological, and structural factors that affect the behavior of health care consumers and providers
5. Approaches to social work practice congruent with the major types of health problems with which social workers deal
6. The view of health care social work as a problem-solving endeavor

When social workers approach any practice task they do so by drawing on the body of knowledge and skills on which these principles are based. This body of values, knowledge, and skills may be viewed as the components of a professional perspective that guides action. One useful way of identifying these components has been termed the "layers of understanding" for social work practice (Devore and Schlesinger, 1981).

THE LAYERS OF UNDERSTANDING FOR HEALTH CARE SOCIAL WORK PRACTICE: COMPONENTS OF A PROFESSIONAL PERSPECTIVE

The layers of understanding consist of (1) core social work values, knowledge, and skills and (2) the specialized body of knowledge pertaining to a particular area of practice. Based on the material presented in earlier chapters and on assessment of a number of prevailing approaches to social work prac-

* Webster has defined *principles* as "generalizations that provide a basis for reasoning or a guide for conduct or procedure."

tice, the following factors are considered the essential layers of understanding for health care social work practice and the principles guiding practice:

1. Social work values
2. Knowledge of human behavior and social welfare policy and services
3. Self-awareness with emphasis on understanding how one's own dispositions to disease, illness, and death affect practice
4. Assumptions concerning the relationship between social life, health problems, and recurrent, typical individual and social responses
5. Knowledge of the prevailing approaches to social work practice and how these may need to be adapted to or modified for the needs of health care social work clients
6. Knowledge of the characteristics of the organizations and communities in which practice is carried out
7. Adaptation of social work practice technology to the health field
8. Appreciation of the social worker's role in knowledge building and developing stances on accountability congruent with professional perspectives

Points 1 through 5 are discussed in detail in this chapter. Points 6 through 8 are covered in subsequent chapters.

SOCIAL WORK VALUES

Basic to all social work practice are the values that guide and inform practice. In health care social work values form the basis for making judgments about prevailing health policies, the health system, and human needs generated by health problems. Levy's formulations (1973) of social work's value base is useful and facilitates considering value issues encountered in health care. In his discussion Levy views values as (1) preferred conceptions of people, (2) preferred outcomes for people, and (3) preferred instrumentalities for dealing with people. The first focuses on orientations about the relationships between people and their environment; the second concentrates on the quality of life and beliefs about social provision and policy designed to enhance that quality; and the third on how people should be treated.

In respect to the first, emphasis is on viewing people as intrinsically valuable with the capacity to change and grow. This consideration involves reaching out beyond the narrow boundaries of one's daily life into the larger society where the need for community, succor, and comfort may be met. This aspect of the social work value system has far-reaching implications for health care social workers. It affects the stance social workers take on the quality of life that is likely to generate health or illness and on how individuals affected by health problems are viewed. A professional stance that recognizes and seeks to foster growth compels actions that enhance the capacity for growth.

At all levels social workers aim to modify conditions inimical to such growth. For example, research on nursing homes suggests that the capacity for growth and change can be enhanced by organizational arrangements that facilitate self-direction and decision making among persons with severe health problems (Mercer and Kane, 1979). Many clients of health care social workers have suffered seemingly insurmountable physical and psychological trauma. The restrictions on movement imposed by major illness can generate severe doubt about the potential for change or improvement. The disorganization of feeling and thought associated with much mental dysfunction can alter the fundamental character of important social relationships. When the commitment to the value of individuals and their capacity to grow, even under the most adverse circumstances, can be conveyed by feeling, tone, and action, the potential for enhanced functioning is increased considerably.

Much of social work practice is informed by this value dimension. The sense that all individuals are important is conveyed by a fundamental stance of acceptance and reinforcement of people's continuing value to the human community, no matter how disabled. That community includes their immediate familial and social networks and health providers who use skill and knowledge to enhance the person-environment interaction.

Levy's second dimension points to the perspective familiar to social workers about the importance of self-realization and self-actualization and their relationship to equal opportunity, health status, and access to health care. Inadequate standards of living, unemployment, and negative societal evaluation related to social class and minority group membership have been documented repeatedly. Poor health minimizes the potential for self-realization. Social work's position that health care is a right and not a privilege is derived from this value stance.

The final category focuses on the importance of treating people in a way that maximizes the opportunity for self-direction. As health care social workers face the choices and options made possible by contemporary health care the translation of this value stance into guidelines for action generates a number of questions having major ethical consequences. The introduction of lifesaving and life-maintaining technology such as respirators, renal dialysis, and extensive chemotherapy confronts people with choices about whether or not they want to live with the conditions imposed by these methods of medical intervention. There is some evidence that experts in the administration of such treatment often act as if people have no choice about whether or not to consent to its use (for example, Holden, 1980; Ross, 1982). These experts may fear that some people will refuse to undergo complex treatment. Such refusal may (in some people's minds) slow the pace of knowledge development and keep persons skilled in carrying out such treatment from doing all they deem appropriate.

When social workers are collaborators in interdisciplinary endeavors in which such choices are constantly at issue they have a particular obligation to adhere to professional tenets of self-direction. This may pose value conflicts as social workers weigh their commitments to clients, fellow health professionals, and the organizations employing them. It is not easy for social workers to make the "right" decisions when working with clients having to make choices in this area. Ross (1982) cites a number of situations that arise in a cancer research center when patients or their families are not given thorough information by the medical staff about the likely consequences of various treatment approaches. I stress the social worker's obligation to function in a manner that ensures all possible information is available before decisions are made.

Each of these value perspectives has important implications for the way social workers view issues related to policy, organization, personnel, financing, and access to health care services. The importance attached to person-environment relations affects judgments about how those relationships serve to facilitate or constrain healthy growth and development. Social work assessments of health care delivery mechanisms must therefore be guided by the extent to which they foster such growth.

Arrangements that minimize the opportunity to identify and correct remediable difficulties are evaluated from this perspective. If, for example, children of poor families do not have ready access to screening for possible deficits of hearing or vision, social work values compel a negative assessment of the policies and practices that limit such access. This assessment is closely related to the assumption that the provision for basic human needs is an intrinsic responsibility of modern industrial society and must be built into the basic institutional structure (Wilensky and Lebeaux, 1958). This assumption translates into support for policy positions that endorse equal access to health care, independent of ability to pay. This position is reflected in the official professional endorsement by the National Association of Social Workers of a national health service that would provide for such access. Equally important are the values concerning how people should be treated. In health care these values lead to continuing examination of financing; the manner in which health services are organized; and the attention paid by health care providers to concerns about dignity, privacy, and ethnically derived dispositions to care.

HUMAN BEHAVIOR AND SOCIAL WELFARE POLICIES AND SERVICES

Human behavior and the social environment

From its inception the profession of social work has considered thorough grounding in the theories and knowledge of human behavior a major prerequisite for practice. The new Curriculum Policy Statement of the Council on Social Work Education* points to the following areas of needed knowledge:

*Curriculum policy for the master's degree and baccalaureate degree programs in social work education, adopted by the Board of Directors, Council on Social Work Education, May 1982 and effective July 1, 1984.

> In keeping with social work's person-in-environment focus, students need knowledge of individuals as they develop over the life span and have membership in families, groups, organizations, and communities; of the relationships among biological, social, psychological, and cultural systems as they affect and are affected by human behavior; and of the consequences of diversity in ethnic background, race, class, sexual orientation, and culture in a pluralistic society (p. 10).

How such fundamental knowledge is intertwined with the understandings needed for health care is readily illustrated. Social workers with thorough knowledge of the theories and research that deal with the cycle of human development will use such knowledge to understand how illness and critical life-cycle stages interact to create a unique configuration. For example, when adolescents are stricken with a chronic health problem they confront a series of tasks associated with managing the illness. Often these tasks involve increased dependence at the very time in life when thrusts for developing autonomy and independence are paramount.

Concepts of social role can facilitate the development of insight into the disruption of role expectations related to illness. The turmoil associated with being unable to carry out expected role performance can be as great as that connected with the illness itself. Expectations that men support their families or that women care for their children are deeply ingrained. Personality theory contributes major insights into how people do or do not cope with illness-related stress. Strategies designed to effect institutional change will be enhanced when workers understand the dynamics of community and organizational behavior.

Chapters 3 and 4 reviewed a number of concepts related to health and illness behavior and to how ethnicity and social class affect these behaviors. These and other areas of knowledge aid health care social workers' efforts to understand the complex problems with which they deal.

A vast body of theory seeks to explain human behavior. The sociological and psychological theories that have developed contribute to social workers' understanding of behavior. How they select those theories that best serve their need to understand has been the subject of much debate. Given the fluid, ever-expanding knowledge base, an eclectic stance that draws selectively from diverse bodies of thought seems most appropriate for health care social work. Therefore, health care social workers will want to use insights from psychoanalytical theories, behaviorist theories, existential perspectives, interactionist theories, and diverse sociological, political, and economic theories seeking to explain social change.

Social welfare policies and services

The new Curriculum Policy Statement previously referred to is explicit in asserting the importance of this area of study and practice. Students are expected to learn how to provide service and to become "committed participants in efforts to achieve change in social policies and programs." Knowledge and skill "in these areas should prepare them to exert leadership and influence as legislative and social advocates, lobbyists, and expert advisors to policymakers and administrators" (p. 10). Understanding and use of political processes in the effort to further social work goals is also emphasized.

SELF-AWARENESS

According to Bartlett (1958) social workers need to develop an understanding of themselves which enables them to be aware of and take responsibility for their own emotions and attitudes as they affect professional function. This awareness includes the capacity to develop insights into one's own dispositions—both those that generate empathy and those that have the potential for destructive actions. Only such insight can help to hold destructive impulses in check.

For all social workers this process involves insight and awareness of attitudes toward those who are different from oneself, whether they are of a different gender, class, or ethnic group. In health care there is a particular obligation to sensitize oneself to feelings that erupt in the face of physical or emotional disability, prolonged dependency, disfigurement, or limited mental capacity. The impulse to reach out and "do" for those who can do little for themselves must be tempered by a respect for effort to grow and surmount obstacles.

Many of the problems encountered by health care social workers are close to home. Young women who work with developmentally disabled children and their families worry if children they may bear will be without defect. Middle-aged workers who help clients their own age with a decision to institutionalize an elderly parent must be careful not to project their own feelings. However, personal experience with a similar situation can facilitate understanding. This assertion especially holds true for social workers who have surmounted their own handicaps. However, workers who have overcome a handicap or other difficulties similar to those faced by their clients must guard against assuming a stance of "I've made it, why can't you?" In short, thinking and feeling through one's own experiences with and reactions to health problems can facilitate a self-aware but disciplined empathic stance.

ASSUMPTIONS FOR HEALTH CARE SOCIAL WORK PRACTICE

Rapid change in health care technology, the quality of life, and the policies and organizational arrangements involving health care is an ongoing facet of contemporary life. Nevertheless, as has been suggested by the discussion in preceding chapters, a number of themes can be identified concerning the relationships between social life, health problems, and typical responses persisting over time. The following assumptions bear on these relationships.* They syn-

*As used here, *assumptions* are defined as matters taken for granted.

thesize and integrate much of the material reviewed in earlier chapters and suggest how that material can guide social work action in health care.

Disease and illness generate discomfort, disruption, and fear

Illness, except that of a passing, fleeting nature, strikes at the fundamental core of human existence. Although illness is a universal phenomenon all social groups seek ways to stave off its occurrence and minimize its disruptive effects. Social workers, along with other health professionals and consumers, have a major obligation to participate in efforts that will reduce illness and disease and to carry out curative/ameliorative functions as well as efforts that primarily serve to maintain or sustain individuals whose level of social functioning has become severely impaired. Opportunities to engage in preventive, curative/ameliorative, and maintenance tasks must be sought out and identified at all levels of health care social work practice and in the diverse organizational contexts that employ health care social workers. Whenever feasible, preventive tasks have the highest order of priority.

Disease and illness are not equivalent to deviance

Considerable analysis has suggested that when people become ill and their ordinary role performance is impaired a number of predictable social and psychological processes are triggered. The alteration in physical and psychological state may generate fundamental changes in self-image and perceptions by others. Common among these changes is negative evaluation by others by which the sick can become stigmatized and negatively labeled. Such labeling can become internalized, thus reinforcing a sense of stigma and isolation. Persons subject to such negative evaluation often develop a "deviant" identity. That is, individuals with severe visible impairment are treated in ways similar to those who have violated major social norms and values. The altered self-image, which is inevitably triggered by permanent disability, is thus negatively reinforced.

When professionals wittingly or unwittingly collude in these processes they contribute to further self-denigration. This in turn can minimize the potential for developing functional coping strategies. Social work strategies designed to help enhance the delicate fit between person and environment must be guided by sensitivity to these issues. Efforts to help people "normalize" despite disability must always be accompanied by mechanisms that translate the value of individual self-worth into action. A social functioning, as contrasted with a disease orientation (Chapter 3), can focus on capacity and self-worth. The process of equating illness with deviance is minimized when strategies of intervention are derived from the perspective that some people have impairments requiring adaptation of accustomed routines. This perspective is in contrast to the view that disease or illness has generated a lesser or deviant person.

The sick role calls for joint problem-solving efforts by consumers and providers

Parsons' formulation (1958) of the sick role concept was derived from societal tenets concerning people's obligation to do all they can to resume expected role functioning. Implicit in that formulation is the view that individuals with health problems and other problems are obliged to turn themselves over to experts. Subsequent criticism of that formulation has pointed to its inadequacy in identifying the consumer's role in problem definition and resolution. Adaptation of these considerations to health care social work suggests that the sick role concept, although useful, requires modification. The view of the sick, the client, or the health care consumer as presented here stresses the fact that diverse coping strategies are needed when people have health problems. These strategies include, but are not limited to seeking the services of health care experts. These experts, social workers or physicians, or others, must take into account the consumer's perception of the problem. The greater the degree of dependence on expert knowledge, the greater is the likelihood that the expert will play a major role in problem definition and suggested paths to resolution. For these reasons social work has a particular obligation to focus on client need and perception. The initial perspective of the sick-role is inadequate to describe, explain, and guide the reciprocal provider/consumer interactions between health care social workers and their clients.

Many health care clients are involuntary clients

The "route to the social worker" (Devore and Schlesinger, 1981, 1983) can be mapped on a continuum from "totally coercive" to "totally voluntary." Much of health practice falls in the "somewhat coercive" segment of the continuum. If the social worker is a member of the team in a rehabilitation center the patients usually have limited options about whether or not to become engaged with the social worker. High-risk hospital patients usually lack the physical or economic resources to refuse service. Some social workers view such efforts to provide unsolicited service as intrusive and at variance with values placing a premium on self-direction and self-determination. Yet it is precisely these high-risk types of clients who are in greatest need of the service available. To withdraw or hold back may be an abrogation of professional responsibility.

As health care social workers consider the implications of the fact that many of their clients are not voluntary clients, in the strict sense of the word, they need to be clear about (1) professional judgments derived from values about the right to care that legitimate intervention, (2) administrative mandates that sanction social workers' intervention, and (3) the need to strike a balance between providing an unsolicited service and respecting self-direction. The view of clients or patients as participants in a problem-solving endeavor, contrasted with the view of clients as people who because of illness turn themselves over to experts, is important in considering the three issues previously mentioned. A social work perspective on client self-direction can mitigate the coercive implications of involuntarily assuming the client role.

A number of other assumptions need to be mentioned at this time. These assumptions relate to the ever-present interaction between poverty, low socioeconomic status, and poor health. They also relate to practices that demean people because of gender, minority status, or sexual preference. Social workers have an obligation to be sensitive to the impact of these factors. When these assumptions converge with social work values and practice approaches they can provide direction for intervention and help to shape practice technology.

CURRENT APPROACHES TO SOCIAL WORK PRACTICE: APPLICATION TO HEALTH CARE

A review of the recent social work practice literature generates a sense of excitement and ferment. Extensive efforts have been made to refine and deepen the profession's knowledge base and approaches to practice (for example, Compton and Galaway, 1979; Epstein, 1980; Fischer, 1978; Germain and Gitterman, 1980; Hasenfeld, 1983; Middleman and Goldberg, 1974; Pincus and Minahan, 1973; Reid, 1978; Reid and Epstein, 1972; Rothman, 1979; Siporin, 1975). Systematic research on the process and outcome of intervention is increasing (for example, Epstein, 1977; Reid, 1978), as are findings suggesting that intervention is effective (for example, Reid and Hanrahan, 1982).

Even the most cursory review of this literature suggests that current approaches to social work are characterized by diversity, both in the concepts on which they are based and in the practice strategies they emphasize. Although there is general agreement that social work's focus is on the interaction between person and environment, substantial differences remain on the relative attention paid to *person* or *environment* and "how intervention should be directed to the interaction between them" (Minahan, 1981, pp. 5-6). To date no single, unified approach to practice has evolved. This statement is true in respect to those theories thought to explain the problems of living with which social workers aim to help and in respect to the practice principles and strategies used in interventive efforts. Therefore much practice is eclectic and draws on a range of approaches presented in social work literature. As health care social workers draw on this rich body of materials they need to identify the perspectives that are most congruent with the needs of health care clients—those that are manifest at the individual, systemic, organizational, or community level.

The view of health and illness presented here has consistently identified the multiple factors that generate health problems. The conceptual formulations in Chapter 5 stressed the continuous interplay between the way individuals experience problems, their diverse origins, and the multiple approaches used in efforts to minimize difficulties. The typology of caring identified a series of interventive tasks variously focused on efforts to effect individual or environmental change. For example, clients who face a life-threatening illness need extensive support as they experience fear and pain. Massive systems change efforts will have minimal effect on terminally ill patients. However, social workers and others who draw on their experiences in working with the terminally ill have identified the need for hospice care and are mindful of the long-range importance of organizational change efforts as a way of minimizing many people's suffering.

This is but one example that can be cited suggesting that health care social workers need to select those elements of practice approaches that facilitate the capacity to focus on the person, the environment, and the interaction between the two. Stated another way, the present health problems call for practice approaches that are sensitive to and congruent with the simultaneous need for attention to individual concerns and systemic issues.

With these considerations as a backdrop, I will identify a few key elements of contemporary practice approaches that can aid health care social workers as they identify and respond to multiple health problems. I will first focus on problem solving as a fundamental tenet of all levels of practice. Next I will review the importance of attention to the immediate and pressing difficulties that clients are experiencing and some of the fundamental tenets of crisis intervention. I will then discuss the role of the client as the key decision maker in the problem-solving effort. After that discussion I will cover the major elements of what has been termed the structural approach to practice. This approach facilitates implementing a perspective simultaneously focused on individual and systemic change efforts. Much that I have said thus far suggests that if the principles presented here are to be implemented, workers need to be familiar with some of the fundamental themes informing "macro practice" or institutional change efforts. Therefore I will review some basic formulations from this area also.

Health care social work is a problem-solving endeavor

One theme that runs through most of the current approaches in social work is that social work aims to bring professional values and skills to bear in efforts to help people mobilize their problem-solving capacities. This is true whether problems are presented at the individual, group, community, or organizational level. Central to this perspective is the assumption developed by Helen Harris Perlman in her classic work *Social Casework* (1957) in which she states that all human beings develop problem-solving capacities as part of the normal growth cycle. In her view, life itself is a problem-solving process. Devore and Schlesinger (1981) suggest this process may be impaired as a consequence of excessive stress, crisis, or inadequate environmental resources.

> Past experiences, present perceptions and reactions to the problem, as well as future aspirations join together to form the person with a problem. Of primary importance is today's reality. Knowledge of current living situations

> by which persons are "being molded and battered" provide the facts necessary for the problem-solving process to be activated (p. 110).

Understanding current circumstances sets the stage and is the starting point for problem-solving efforts. The work of Reid and Epstein (1972) builds on these formulations. They stress the human capacity for autonomous problem solving and the ability to carry out action to obtain desired ends. Problem-solving efforts proceed from dissatisfaction with oneself, others, or an all-consuming, problematic life situation. Many health care social work clients face such life situations. Chronic disability, life-threatening illness, or inadequate nutrition call for mobilizing the client's problem-solving capacity as well as the worker's effort to help marshall client resources and other resources.

Perlman and Reid and Epstein have focused their analyses on the prob-

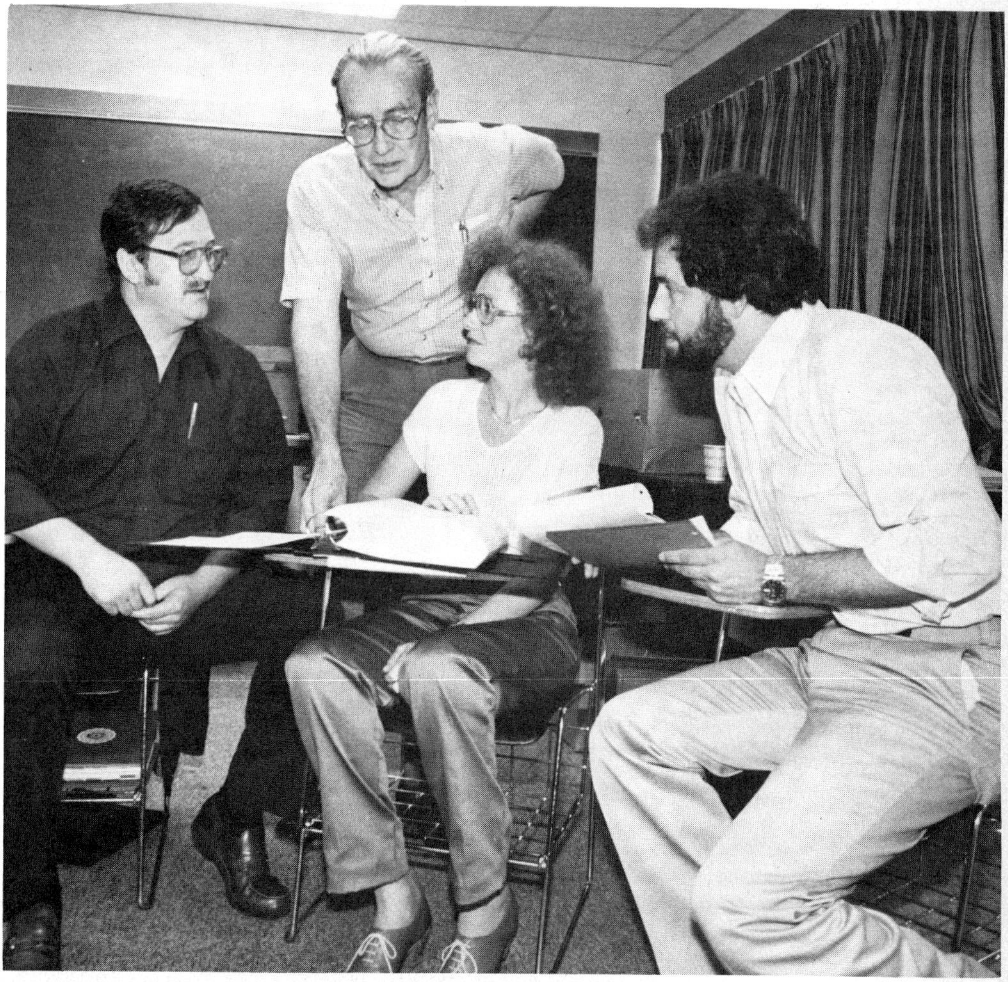

lem-solving capacities of individuals and on the view that these capacities can be activated even under the most difficult circumstances. Closely parallel to these conceptions are those that define social planning and community organization as "a problem solving approach in which a professional change agent helps a community action system composed of individuals, groups or organizations to deal with social problems" (Gilbert and Specht, 1977, p. 1412). For both levels of practice the underlying and common theme is that social workers use professional expertise to identify, unravel, and alter problematic situations, whether encountered by individuals or groups.

Health care social work is focused on current problems

Emphasizing the resolution of current difficulties and how these difficulties are experienced in the present by people with health problems is a major thrust of much health practice. The relationship between past history, unconscious motivation, and the problems presenting themselves now has been and continues to be a matter of inquiry by social workers and other behavioral scientists. Whatever the origin of the health problems people are experiencing, the search for relief, succor, and solutions is usually focused on the "here and now." Intervention may call for help in reducing environmental stressors, making environmental modifications, effecting life-style changes, making massive adaptions to severe physical disability, or facing death with as much ease and comfort as possible. Whatever the case these problems are usually immediate and pressing and call for the greatest possible effort to mobilize currently available energy and resources.

For example, on asthmatic child, a young adult with ulcerative colitis, and newly diagnosed schizophrenic adolescents and their families are all facing difficult current realities. Asthmatic attacks may be triggered by excess dust or pollen or tension-riddled situations. Persons with ulcerative colitis must cope with pain, the unpleasant odors often associated with the disease, and the need to adapt daily routines to manifestations of the disease process. The parents of a newly diagnosed schizophrenic adolescent may be "reeling" under the impact of their child's bizarre behavior or withdrawal from interaction.

Focusing on current reality highlights the need to find ways of reducing dust and pollen in the asthmatic child's environment. Attention to the daily trauma posed by ulcerative colitis may trigger efforts to concentrate on strategies designed to minimize the difficulty. Young schizophrenics and their parents may obtain considerable relief if they locate a day hospital. These factors as well as the emotional strain, guilt, or search for explanations in past life experiences constitute the problems with which client and worker presently engage. Often such efforts require exploration of past developmental patterns and how they may have contributed to the difficulty.

Concentrating on the present and how it is inevitably shaped by both the distant and recent past is congruent with the view of illness as a career that changes over time. Functional coping mechanisms and required environmental resources shift in response to the path taken by illness. Immediately following an accident resulting in quadriplegia, patients and their families may not be able to address the long-range implications of the injury. The real threat to life may be paramount. Only later as the dramatic limitations become visible and real may efforts to cope with the changing and new reality begin. Closely related are those principles focused on working on problems in the terms defined by clients.

Social workers need to be attuned to the client's perspective of problems

One of the major contributions of the task-centered system is the perspective of working on problems in the terms identified by the client. Action taken on behalf of clients in relation to problems not acknowledged by them constitutes a violation of values. Considerable attention is given to involuntary clients.

Health care social workers frequently find themselves working with people who have not sought their services. The basis for social work intervention may be defined by the health services system and social work's definition of what constitutes a psychosocial problem. The social work role in hospital discharge planning is a case in point, as is recognizing the psychosocial components of renal dialysis treatment in which social work services are mandated. These and related services are progressive and patient oriented. Nevertheless, many people when offered these services may view the social worker as simply another person who has arrived on the scene to do something to them. Thus the physician examines, operates, or prescribes drugs; the nurse administers medical treatment; and the social worker talks to the patients about their plans for home care or their feelings about a traumatic turn of events. Most clients have not chosen to be patients; instead unwelcome discomfort or a threat to life has forced them into a state of "patienthood." Fewer still consider the services of the social worker to be an intrinsic element of their efforts to get better.

Professional responsibility and institutional mandates usually do not make it possible to work only with people who have acknowledged a problem in terms suggested by Reid and Epstein (1972). However, sensitivity to the issue posed can focus attention on the meaning and process involved in becoming a social work client. At times social workers may need to acknowledge that intervention, although sound and based on competent professional judgment, is authoritative precisely because the client has limited choice about whether to participate. Recognizing this possibility generates efforts to minimize the coercive component of health care social work practice. Client right to self-determination takes on a special meaning when issues of choice about life and death are involved as in the client's decision about whether to consent to certain treatment. A number of issues arise when long-term institutional care seems the only feasible option, as is the case for many frail elderly people or seriously mentally handicapped persons. Who is the client who must acknowledge a problem? Are they individuals facing lifelong institutional care? Or are they the family members who may need relief from the burden of trying to sustain these persons at home after protracted periods? Or is it the hospital that because of cost considerations, limits the time and process available to "think and feel through" such important decisions?

The principle that social workers should work only on problems in the terms defined by clients is often necessarily violated in health care social work practice. Because of this, social workers have a particular obligation to work toward framing problems in terms the client can manage. Epstein's comments (1980) concerning the centrality of "target problems" as articulated by clients are pertinent in the present context.

> The target problem is what a client thinks is the problem: what should be alleviated, what should be worked on to get a problem cut down. . . People are generally able to make a coherent statement in words defining their target problem. When they cannot do so, practitioners can help clients in various ways to develop a target problem statement. Practitioners can also collect the opinions of important other people to identify these problems with and for the client (p. 11).

This focus on clients' distress, how they perceive that distress, and their own view of a proposed solution often distinguishes the health care social worker's intervention from that of other health professionals.

Health care social workers need knowledge and skills to intervene at points of crisis

Closely related to the view that social workers have a responsibility to respond to the immediate, pressing problems presented by clients is the view that social workers need to be able to respond when people are confronting a crisis situation. Crisis has been variously defined (Chapter 4). The term *crisis intervention* is used both to refer to the body of theory about the life events that precipitate a crisis response and to the interventive strategies that have evolved to help people deal with crises. Golan (1978) defines crisis as an "upset in a steady state" (p. 61). Five components of a crisis are identified: (1) a hazardous event; (2) a vulnerable state; (3) the precipitating factor; (4) the state of active crisis; and (5) the stage of crisis resolution, or reintegration.

A hazardous event or a stressful occurrence may be compounded by several difficult life experiences; it is a "blow." The crises experienced by health care social work clients are often sudden and involve unexpected illness or loss, death, accidents, or the birth of a severely handicapped child. The vulnerable state is "the subjective reaction of the individual to the initial blow" (Golan, 1978, p. 65). The crisis may evoke tension or a sense of challenge. Many workers and people who have experienced crises can describe the sense of anxiety, devastation, depression, and hopelessness felt at the time of loss or threat. For the most part, the person in a crisis state is unable to function.

The precipitating factor may be self-evident, the accident itself, or being told about a severe illness; a minor factor may trigger a crisis response. It is not uncommon for a crisis response to be observed long after an accident or other difficult experience. Golan (1978) points out that

> The state of active or acute crisis describes the individual's subjective condition, once his homeostatic mechanisms have broken down, tension has topped and disequilibrium has set in (p. 68).

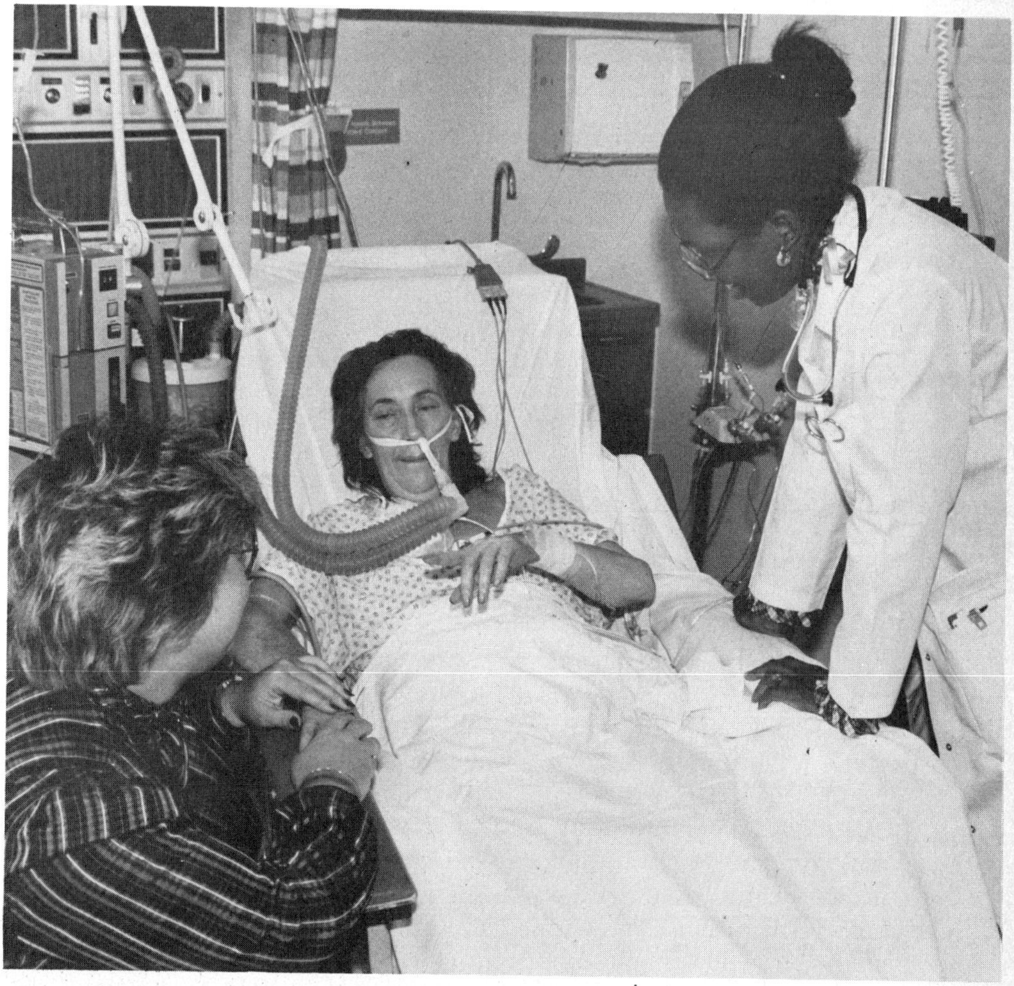

The disequilibrium is of such a nature that individuals are usually unable to carry on.

Whether or not the strategies of crisis intervention should be used depends on an accurate assessment of whether a crisis state is indeed present. The despair, immobilization, and agitation must be differentiated from more permanent pathological states. The key component is the assumption that the crisis state is self-limited and, according to Caplan (1964), likely to last about 4 to 6 weeks. A number of writers (for example, Aquilera and Messick, 1978; Caplan, 1964; Parad, 1965) suggest that during the crisis state people are likely to be receptive to help and ready to change. This contention requires further systematic scrutiny (for example, Ewalt, 1979). Nevertheless, many years of effort by a number of workers suggest that the strategies of time-limited intervention, responsive to the components of the crisis, can be extremely helpful to individuals responding to difficult life events. Many health care social work clients fall into this category.

Several elements of crisis intervention are similar to short-term intervention in that they concentrate on the pressing problem. Intervention is focused on achieving limited goals, usually those related to dealing with the current life problems that have triggered the crisis response. A task orientation is vital. Reintegration, or the capacity to regain functioning, must be sought. An adaptive resolution helps people who have lost loved ones or who are facing devastating diagnoses or other turmoils to go on with their lives.

The problem-solving framework, the emphasis on the present and on client identification of problems, and the approach to people experiencing crisis are all applied within the context of a basic social work perspective that looks for systemic as well as individual sources of stress. The structural framework to be considered next pays particular attention to the multiple sources of stress and to possible paths of problem resolution.

THE STRUCTURAL FRAMEWORK

Almost all approaches to social work practice are based on the assumption that social work has an obligation to be mindful of and responsive to individual and systemic sources of difficulty. The structural approach identifies and delineates practice approaches that are responsive to difficulties at both levels. Key features of the structural model are illustrated in the "four quadrant" concept of practice. As Figure 3 illustrates, each quadrant calls attention to the various types of people or situations with whom social workers engage in efforts to resolve problems. These may be clients or others associated with the clients.

Quadrant 1 identifies work with patients and people close to them on a specific problem. Quadrant 2 points to efforts focused on working in a collective manner with people sharing similar problems. An important aspect of this level of work is recognizing the significant role that people who are experiencing similar problems can play in helping each other. The growth of various self-help groups and support groups is illustrative of this need. Often such groups rely on the work of professionals to help provide direction in mobilizing the energies and capacities they have so they may be of assistance to each other. Quadrants 3 and 4 are ways of conceptualizing a long-held tenet of practice that social workers engage persons who are not experiencing difficulties to help those who are. Quadrant 3 centers on attempts to engage the help of nonaffected persons to ease life for affected individuals. Quadrant 4 focuses on advocacy, policy change, and research to document need. Examples include working with schoolteachers to enlist their cooperation in adapting school routines for the physically handicapped and efforts to alter hospital ward routines to make them more consonant with client preference.

Figure 3 illustrates the components of the framework. The circular arrows

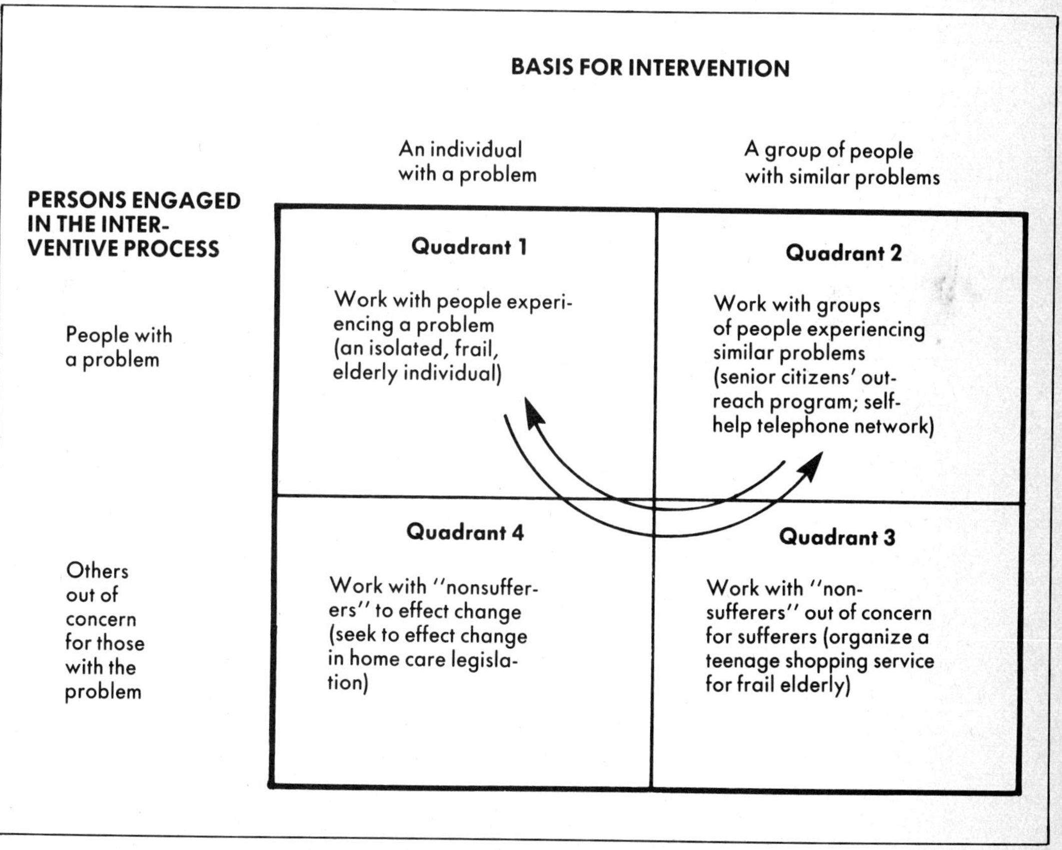

Figure 3. The structural framework. (Adapted from Middleman, R., and Goldberg, G.: Social service delivery: a structural approach to social work practice, New York, 1974, Columbia University Press, pp. 19–22, 29.)

suggest that most of the difficulties experienced by social work clients call for activity in all four quadrants. Depending on the social worker's job responsibilities or location in the delivery system, activity may begin in any quadrant. For example, many hospitals and community health centers are basically organized to work with individuals on the problems they are experiencing. In the course of that effort environmental deficits frequently surface that minimize the likelihood of the problems presented being solved at the one-to-one level. Additional elements of the conceptualization point to the social worker's responsibility to try to close resource gaps.

One principle of the structural framework (Middleman and Goldberg, 1974) termed "following the demands of the client task," is based on the view that workers have the obligation to be ever aware of the multiple sources of client difficulty and the varying ways in which resolution may be sought. In practice this principle entails identifying the various sources of client difficulty or potential resolution of the problem. For example, in working with elderly hospitalized people who are to be discharged to their homes, workers are likely to note some problems unique to the individual, while other problems consistently recur and are shared by all clients. Each person is likely to have a set of private and unique concerns about her or his illness and what the future portends. To respond appropriately at this level, work with individuals and those close to them is usually indicated. Simultaneously, people are likely to share common difficulties. If they are alone and sick they will surely worry about how they can get help if it is needed. Or perhaps they simply feel the need to have someone check on them. Part of the worker's task is to seek collective sources of resolution as well as to maximize people's capacity for helping themselves and others.

Any number of strategies may facilitate this effort. Perhaps the worker can help organize a telephone network in which a group of elderly patients will check on each other after they go home. Elderly people alone may have additional shared problems. If their economic resources are limited and they rely on Medicaid programs for such services as home health care, they may experience inadequate funding for such services. Therefore workers should be aware of the need to work for such policy changes that can minimize some of the major problems of any population.

Another important component of "following the demands of the client task" (Quadrant 3 activity) can be discerned. It involves drawing on or creating resources by using the services of people concerned about a particular population. For example, when working with frail elderly clients who are to be discharged to their homes workers may refer to or think about organizing a shopping service to be run by dedicated teenagers. Thus the client's difficulty rather than the worker's skill or adherence to a particular method of intervention determines what is to be done. Consultation and collaboration between workers with various skills are vital to implementing this approach. Flexibility in learning new methods is most important.

Another component of the structural approach (Middleman and Goldberg, 1974) is termed "the principle of maximizing potential supports in the client's environment." This principle embodies the essential thrust of the structural approach. It points to the importance of using, modifying, or creating structures needed to cope with present difficulties. Existing family and community networks available to support the terminally ill should be used, encouraged, and helped in any way. In the absence of these networks, churches, neighborhoods, or formal agency structures are called on to lend assistance. Policy change efforts are essential.

The elements of the structural approach that have been presented here serve to focus the health care social worker's attention on (1) individual needs; (2) environmental, organizational, and community change efforts that may facilitate problem solving; and (3) the potential of self-help and mutual aid.

APPROACHES TO INSTITUTIONAL CHANGE

The practice approaches focused on work at the community and organizational level are based on a number of developments that reflect diverse perspectives on (1) how communities and organizations are organized, (2) the dynamics that generate change, and (3) the role of social work in effecting change at this level.

The preceding discussion pointed to the view that life is a problem-solving process and that much of one-to-one or small group intervention is viewed as help with problem solving. As various tenets of practice in community organization, planning, and social work administration are reviewed it will become evident that a similar theme pervades much of this work. Fundamental to work at this level is the fact that it involves efforts to effect change in complex, aggregate systems. Considerable work has been done to clarify the processes and goals sought at this level of practice.

Social work administration essentially refers to the administration and management of human service organizations (Sarri, 1977) in a manner congruent with social work values. Social work's major concerns are the efforts to increase the responsiveness of the bureaucracies in which health and social services are rendered to the population. Social policy may be viewed as a set of principles that determines the distribution of societal resources and shapes the quality of life (Baumheier and Schorr, 1977). Social policy formulation derives from the state's right to promote the welfare of the population. Social services are the major ingredients of social policy. The process of policy formulation involves the selection of goals derived from value assumptions and planning for the means of attaining these goals.

Although there are important differences in emphasis among community organization, administration, and social policy analysis that bear on daily work, some common themes can be identified. Basic sociological theory suggests that when individuals interact in large complex units the sum is greater than and different from the parts. This fundamental sociological tenet has generated a considerable literature intended to identify the characteristic functioning of such social units, the social forces that maintain their stability, and those forces that are susceptible to change. Social work has drawn on this literature in its attempt to cull the type of understanding that would further social change goals.

One central question in the efforts to manage human service organizations, shape social policy, or effect community change has focused on the degree to which change takes place as a result of rational consideration of alternative goals, as contrasted with the role of power, influence, and psychological factors. Perlman (1977) suggests that careful analysis of planning practice points to power, influence, and psychological factors as the major sources of change. The viability of "rational planning" approaches has been questioned on the basis of studies of factors that actually impinge on the planning process. The traditions that affect planning practice have their counterparts in theories of administration. Thus rationality was stressed in early scientific management perspectives and remains a feature of current systems approaches. However, social psychological approaches focused on morale, leadership, and small group behavior in organizations remain important.

Community organization and planning

Rothman (1979) identifies three models of community organization practice: locality development, social planning, and social action. The first model emphasizes self-help and community integration. It stresses involving broad sections of the community in self-help processes. Problems are thought to be related to poor relationships among residents. The second model stresses planning targeted at alleviating specific health problems. The third model seeks to effect basic change in the distribution of power and resources.

Different views of the prevailing power structure characterize each of these approaches. In locality development members of the power structure are viewed as "collaborators in a common venture" (p. 30); in the planning model those in power are perceived as sponsors of change efforts and employ change agents like social workers; in the social action model those in power are perceived as oppressors "to be coerced or overturned" (p. 30).

Consumer cooperatives and community health associations are among the sites where locality development takes place. Social planning activities take place in health planning bodies, welfare councils, and regional planning groups. Social movements involving minorities, women, or consumer groups are often the locus of social change activities. They involve broad sections of the community in self-help processes. This involvement may manifest itself in joint efforts by residents to alter practices not conducive to health, join together in reducing community tensions, or develop consumer cooperatives. For example, "swapping networks" among the poor have been identified in which residents share food, babysitting, and other services (for example, Stack,

1974). Professionals can work with such networks in a manner designed to extend scarce resources.

Social planning is a process in which effort is made to target and alleviate identified health and mental problems. The social action models focus on changing the distribution of power and resources.

Social work administration

Drawing on Parsons' formulations (1958), Sarri (1977) identifies several levels of administrative practice, including the institutional and managerial levels. The first level concentrates on implementing social goals. It emphasizes translating societal mandates and problems to be addressed by the organization into agency action. The managerial level centers on tasks involved in obtaining needed resources.

Reflections on institutional change

These different perspectives may appear to be straightforward and self-evident, but further reflection suggests that there are important distinctions to be made if health care social workers are to follow the practice principles outlined here. Often health care social workers are employees of a wide variety of organizations. In principle the goal of these organizations is to deliver quality health care services. Nevertheless, considerable literature as well as day-to-day practice experience attests to the fact that these complex organizations have multiple goals. Sources of power vary by the institutional mandates, sources of funding, and interpersonal dynamics at play in any particular organization.

For example, Chapter 9, which deals with social work in hospitals, discusses the source and nature of the physician's authority in hospitals. Boards of trustees and funding sources also have considerable authority over and influence on how hospitals serve people. Given these multiple sources of authority, the hospital social worker who is interested in effecting a change in an aspect of the hospital's health care delivery system will first want to identify who or what the sources of power are in relation to the particular issue of concern. The experience of many hospital social work directors in attempting to institute an open access system are instructive. In this type of system social work develops its own criteria for determining which patients are to be screened for social work services and does so independent of physician referral. Some hospital medical personnel resisted extensively. Such resistance was thought to derive from physicians' concern that in this process their control over what happens to patients would be diminished. When exploration showed this to be the primary source of resistance, the source of power over this activity was clearly the physicians. The medical board was usually the vehicle for exercising power to prevent social work from instituting an open access system.

Do social work departments view the medical board as an "oppressor" or as a collaborator in the common venture of good patient care? It is likely that a strategy proceeding from the former assumption would be counterproductive; planning approaches in which data were made available were more successful than those in which data were not made available. Data that demonstrate to administrators and physicians that patient care is enhanced and hospital days shortened by social work intervention can help gain support for implementing an open access system.

The stance on sources of power and authority encountered in the effort to obtain high-risk screening is different from that taken when conditions that are hazardous to health and that can be traced to certain power sources are identified. For example, landlords who in the past persistently defied regulations concerning dangerous lead levels in paints they used were a hazard to children at risk for lead poisoning.* When those landlords were protected by the prevailing political power structure, social action was necessary. The extent to which social workers take such action as representatives of their agencies, as members of their professional organization, or as individuals should be considered carefully.

In practice the three prevailing perspectives on power are often blurred. Social workers may proceed from a collaborative stance in situations such as those facing elderly nursing home residents whose personal care allowances are too small or in those situations facing handicapped persons who seek greater physical access in public places. When working directly with these kinds of concerns or with efforts to organize people working for change, seemingly intransigent, oppressive sources of power may surface. Some public figures may be yielding to pressures not to increase costs to the levels needed for making public buildings accessible. Strategies designed to put pressure on persons resisting these changes often develop.

How social workers approach any particular organizational community change or legislative issue is dependent on the analysis of the forces operative in any particular situation and on whether or not the worker's role as employee is congruent with a particular action stance. At times social workers confront situations that conflict with their personal or with social work's principles. For example, convinced that only a strong stand by the hospital would stop the practice of using too much lead in paint, individual workers may have been disturbed if hospital administration refused to take a strong stand. Administration may seek to prevent workers from speaking out and using such methods as using hospital stationery. Whether the social workers view the issue to be of sufficient importance to risk their jobs or whether they will continue to work using less adversary stances is a matter not easily resolved.

---

*Lead poisoning caused by lead-based paint was a causative factor in some types of retardation. Public Law 91-695, The Lead Based Paint Poisoning Prevention Act, has minimized some of these risks.

Middleman and Goldberg's discussion (1974) of "the principle of least contest" is helpful to workers confronting issues that call for varying levels of institutional change. According to this principle workers should exert the least possible amount of pressure to achieve certain valued objectives. Their rationale is as follows: the greater the amount of pressure used the more likely there is to be a negative response and resistance. Thus low-pressure interventions are more likely to result in successful task accomplishment. If these interventions are not initially successful, more pressure can be exerted. For example, efforts to persuade physicians of the need for an open access system by open discussion are more likely to be successful than strident demands of the medical board and administrator. If or when demands are made they should only take place after other avenues have been exhausted. The same kind of thrust or flow of change-focused activities is likely to be the most productive approach in many of the institutional change activities coming from the worker's ongoing effort to meet client need. Many unique configurations of factors may emerge and necessitate departure from this principle.

SUMMARY

In this chapter a series of principles for health care social work practice was presented. These principles guide action in the health field. One way of viewing the components of a professional perspective for health care social work is to conceptualize these as "the layers of understanding." These layers consist of values and a knowledge of human behavior and social policy. Self-awareness is an important component, as are the specialized concepts and knowledge for health care practice. A series of assumptions was also presented. They were derived from analysis of prevailing health needs, dispositions to health and illness, and social work's role in relation to these factors.

Key elements of several approaches to social work were reviewed. All the elements selected are consonant with health care social workers' need to be simultaneously attuned to individual and system change activity. These include the view of social work as a problem-solving endeavor, emphasis on the current reality and on problems as perceived by clients, and crisis intervention. These approaches combined with the structural framework serve to focus attention on client need, the importance of support networks, and efforts to reduce the gap between resource availability and need. Some major tenets of institutional change effort were also reviewed.

REFERENCES

Aquilera, D.C., and Messick, J.M.: Crisis intervention: theory and methodology, St. Louis, 1978, The C.V. Mosby Co.

Bartlett, H.M.: Working definition of social work practice, Social Work **3**(2): 5, 1958.

Baumheier, E.C., and Schorr, A.L.: Social policy. In Turner, J.B., editor: Encyclopedia of social work, ed. 3, Washington, D.C., 1977, National Association of Social Workers, vol. 2, p. 1453.

Caplan, G.: Principles of preventive psychiatry, New York, 1964, Basic Books, Inc., Publishers.

Compton, B.R., and Galaway, B.: Social work processes, Homewood, Ill., 1979, The Dorsey Press.

Devore, W., and Schlesinger, E.: Ethnic-sensitive social work practice, St. Louis, 1981, The C.V. Mosby Co.

Devore, W., and Schlesinger, E.G.: The route to the social worker: a framework for teaching direct practice, Paper presented at the annual program meeting of the Council on Social Work Education, Fort Worth, Texas, March 1983.

Epstein, L.J.: How to provide social services with task-centered methods: report of the task-centered service project, vol. 1, Chicago, 1977, The School of Social Service Administration, University of Chicago Press.

Epstein, L.J.: Helping people: the task-centered approach, St. Louis, 1980, The C.V. Mosby Co.

Ewalt, P.L.: Crisis intervention as social work, Health and Social Work **4**(2):164, 1979.

Fischer, J.: Effective casework practice: an eclectic approach, New York, 1978, McGraw-Hill Book Co.

Germain, C.B., and Gitterman, A.: The life model of social work practice, New York, 1980, Columbia University Press.

Gilbert, N., and Specht, H.: Social planning and community organization: approaches. In Turner, J.B., editor: Encyclopedia of social work, ed. 3, Washington, D.C., 1977, National Association of Social Workers, vol. 2, p. 1412.

Golan, N.: Treatment in crisis situations, New York, 1978, The Free Press.

Hasenfeld, Y.: Human service organizations, Englewood Cliffs, N.J., 1983, Prentice-Hall, Inc.

Holden, M.O.: Dialysis or death: the ethical alternatives, Health and Social Work **5**(2):18 1980.

Levy, C.: The value base of social work, Journal of Education for Social Work **9**(1):34, 1973.

Mercer, S., and Kane, R.: Helplessness and hopelessness among the institutionalized aged: an experiment, Health and Social Work **4**(1):90, 1979.

Middleman, R., and Goldberg, G.: Social service delivery: a structural approach to social work practice, New York, 1974, Columbia University Press.

Minahan, A.: Purpose and objectives of social work revisited, Social Work **26**(1):5, 1981.

Parad, N.W.: Crisis intervention: selected readings, New York, 1965, Family Service Association of America.

Parsons, T.: Definitions of health and illness in the light of American values and social structure. In Jaco, E.G., editor: Patients, physicians and illness, New York, 1958, The Free Press.

Perlman, H.: Social casework, Chicago, 1957, University of Chicago Press.

Perlman, R.: Social planning and community organization. In Turner, J.B., editor: Encyclopedia of social work, ed. 3, Washington, D.C., 1977, National Association of Social Workers, vol. 2, p. 1404.

Pincus, A., and Minahan, A.: Social work practice: model and method, Itasca, Ill., 1973, F.E. Peacock Publishers, Inc.

Reid, W.J.: The task-centered system, New York, 1978, Columbia University Press.

Reid, W.J., and Epstein, E.L.: Task-centered casework, New York, 1972, Columbia University Press.

Reid, W.J., and Hanrahan, P.: Recent evaluations of social work: grounds for optimism, Social Work **27**(4):328, 1982.

Ross, J.W.: Ethical conflicts in medical social work: pediatric cancer care as a prototype, Health and Social Work **7**(2):95, 1982.

Rothman, J.: Three models of community organization practice, their mixing and phasing. In Cox, F.M., Erlich, J.L., Rothman, J., and Tropman, J.E.: Strategies of community organization, ed. 3, Itasca, Ill., 1979, F.E. Peacock Publishers, Inc.

Sarri, R.C.: Administration in social welfare. In Turner, J.B., editor: Encyclopedia of social work, ed. 3, Washington, D.C., 1977, National Association of Social Workers, vol. 2, p. 42.

Siporin, M.: Introduction to social work practice, New York, 1975, Macmillan Publishing Co., Inc.

Stack, C.B.: All our kin—strategies for survival in a Black community, New York, 1974, Harper & Row, Publishers.

Wilensky, N.L., and Lebeaux, C.: Industrial society and social welfare, New York, 1958, Russell Sage Foundation.

Part Two

Strategies for health care social work practice

Part Two draws on the conceptions developed in Part One and focuses on practice in the health field. Chapter 7 covers skills and procedures, and Chapter 8 reviews interdisciplinary practice. Chapter 9 discusses the hospital social worker's role. Special attention is given to discharge planning and high-risk screening. Chapter 10 concentrates on social work in long-term care, and Chapter 11 highlights the potential for social work in primary care. Chapter 12 reviews the needs for research and quality assurance.

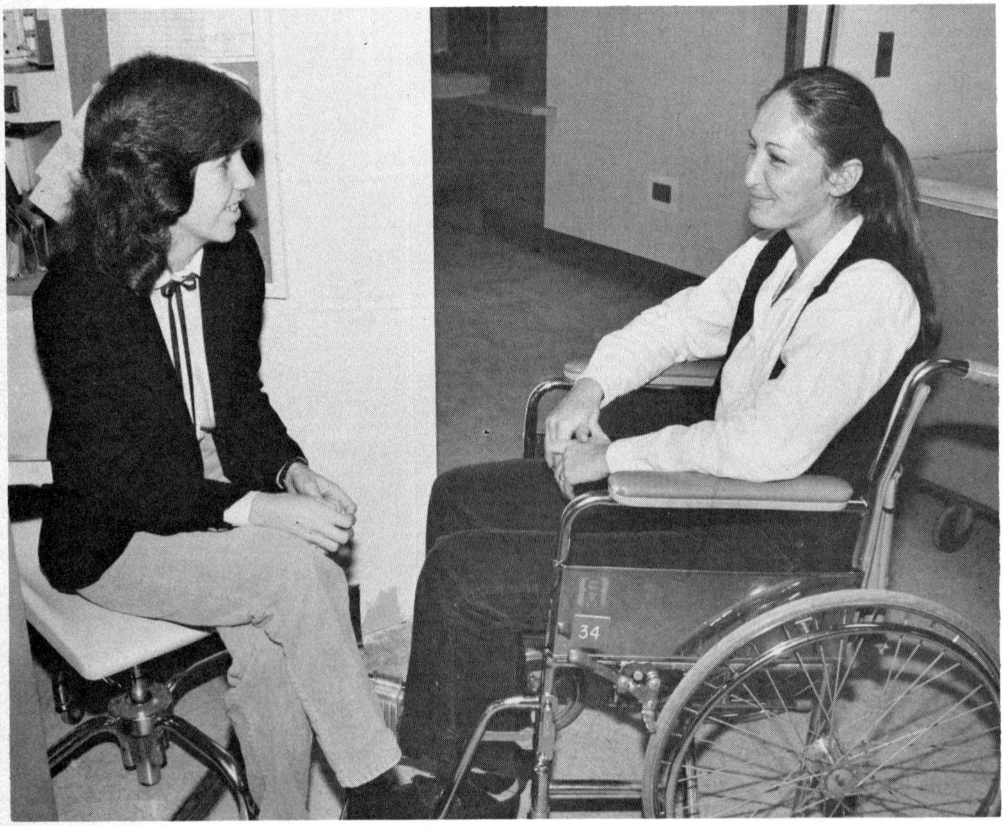
34

Chapter 7

Adaptations of strategies and skills for health care social work practice

This chapter emphasizes the strategies and skills most commonly used by social workers and how these strategies may be adapted to the special types of problems encountered in a variety of health settings. There is now a rich body of literature that has focused on the strategies and skills needed for practice. This was not always the case. For some years considerably less attention was paid to the "what and how" of practice than to the theories and philosophies of intervention. Efforts to guide students and experienced practitioners in mastering the daily intricacies of the helping process have increased substantially. Egan (1975), Epstein (1980), Fischer (1978), Golan (1978), Middleman and Goldberg (1974), and Shulman (1979) are but a few of those who have described important strategies and skills.

In beginning this discussion it is important to make a distinction between the principles for health care practice considered in the preceding chapter and the strategies and skills emphasized in this chapter. *Principles* provide a guide for proper conduct. Golan (1978) identifies *strategy* as a set of procedures involving a planned line of action. "Procedures involve task-oriented interventive actions" (p. 97). *Skill* is "the ability that comes from knowledge, practice, and aptitude to do something well." It refers to "competent excellence in performance."

Most discussions of intervention identify several stages of the process and its associated skills. These include (1) a beginning point, (2) the attempt to discern the nature of the present difficulty, (3) the effort to resolve the problem, and (4) the closing or termination point. Health care social work practice is congruent with this view of the intervention process. In keeping with much that is found in the social work practice literature, the interventive or problem-solving process is broken down into assessment, intervention, and termination. It should be noted, however, that many current health problems are never totally resolved. Although responsibility for ongoing care may shift from one facility to the other, often service is never truly terminated. For example, continuity of care is one of the major tenets of modern long-term and primary care. Therefore particular attention is paid to the concepts of referral, transfer, and "intermittent attention."

A number of other factors warrant consideration. One is the importance of remaining abreast of developments in social policy and health care regulations and having thorough knowledge of the community in which the health service system is located. Understanding the organizational features of the particular setting is crucial, as is keeping abreast of knowledge developments in those disciplines with which social work collaborates. Attention to these matters needs to be ongoing. They usually require "work" before beginning practice in a particular setting. In addition, efforts to intervene in any particular situation should be preceded by attempts to learn as much as possible about the situation before engaging with an individual client or client system.

The dimensions of the interventive or problem-solving process identified pertain, with few exceptions, to all levels of intervention. The practice principles presented in Chapter 6 suggest that health care social workers whose major responsibility is direct practice have an obligation to be familiar with and draw on some of the strategies used in organizational and community change efforts. Therefore examples are drawn from several levels of health practice.

Before considering the various stages of the intervention process, I will focus on what is termed "work before and parallel to intervention." This term refers to the type of knowledge about the setting, medical problems encountered, community, human behavior, and self-awareness that needs to be brought to bear in practice in different health settings.

WORK BEFORE AND PARALLEL TO INTERVENTION

Health care social work is practiced in a variety of settings. Although these settings vary by their major functions, populations served, and locale, the following features are characteristic:

1. Social work services are often viewed as ancillary or complimentary to the major functions carried out.
2. People come seeking relief from disabling physical or emotional disturbances that have often but not always assumed crisis proportions.
3. Settings are complex in their administrative structure, funding sources, and diverse public and professional interests that affect them.
4. When the services they offer are highly specialized (for example, psychiatric hospitals, physical rehabilitation institutes, or cancer research centers), most staff members need to develop extensive expert knowledge pertaining to the specialty.
5. Most workers need to acquire familiarity with a wide range of physical and psychological disorders when people with diverse problems are served (for example, in the emergency room of an acute care general hospital or in a family practice center).
6. Familiarity with the interplay between daily routines, health, and the potential for prevention becomes particularly crucial when

health care is delivered as part of other resource systems (as in a children's day-care center, school, or senior citizens' center).

7. Outreach and health planning activities, originated by federal or state bodies, and community groups presuppose understanding of the health problems that affect community life, as well as the relative priorities accorded to health problems as contrasted with other problems.

Social workers unfamiliar with the particular dynamics operative in their organization will not be effective in their efforts to put "hard-learned" interventive strategies to use. Subsequent chapters will deal with organizational attributes that are likely to characterize specific types of settings. As a general rule social workers are obligated to familiarize themselves with the recurrent medical and psychosocial problems seen in a setting, the prevailing administrative structure and authority system, and the major functions of the setting. Thus specialized teaching hospitals that have major research and educational objectives will take these factors into account when selecting individuals to be served. Medical dominance is prominent in most health delivery settings. Ongoing efforts to understand how that dominance is used and past successful efforts to introduce psychosocial care with greater social work participation can facilitate the social workers' efforts.

The social worker who has gained sufficient understanding of the medical problems that are most commonly treated, the typical care regimens, and what impact these problems have on psychological and physical functioning has made great strides toward becoming a knowledgeable member of the interdisciplinary team. This understanding does not come easily or instantaneously. It is an ongoing component of work in the health care setting. The process of mastering these and related factors is part of the challenge and excitement of health care social work.

Mastering needed medical information

Understandably social workers often feel overwhelmed by the amount of medical information they are expected to master if they are to understand the problems that confront their clients and are to communicate effectively with other disciplines. "Getting on top" of such information is not an easy task. Some health care social workers speak jokingly about carrying a *Merck Manual* or some other handy reference book in their back pockets. Others lament that they did not have a course that included medical information while they were in school. These and other methods of obtaining information are useful. However, a more systematic way to understand and appreciate core medical concepts, how they are used, and how they change is needed.

Appendix A of this book provides (1) guidelines to help social workers learn about how physicians and other medical personnel are trained to think, (2) some familiarity with medical terminology, and (3) an approach to learning about various diseases. Health care social workers are strongly encouraged to use the appendix to help them begin to master the knowledge necessary for their area of work. The reader will note that this appendix is not a mini medical text. It is designed to help organize social workers' search for information and to help them understand the information acquired, both from reading and from consulting with medical personnel. Used in conjunction with the careers of illness concept introduced in Chapter 5, the appendix should help social workers gain the understanding they need of the medical problems they encounter and how these problems generate, intensify, or are triggered by psychosocial problems.

Knowing the community

Also important is understanding the community within which the health service delivery system is located. The term *community* has many meanings beyond those associated with geographical locale. Nevertheless, most health care settings have a specific geographical base and are located in communities that have particular population characteristics, service structures, and needs. Some are intended to serve all the people of the community in which the health setting is located. Others, because of their specialized nature, serve people who come from far and wide. Whatever the case the geographical locale has an impact on the way service is rendered.

Social work is often the only profession charged with the responsibility of linking health care institutions with other service structures in the local community and elsewhere. Health care social workers must take a systematic approach to understanding the community in which they work. Appendix D should help social workers develop this approach. It suggests how documents and discussions with those immersed in the community can help social work departments and individual workers to get a sense of the community's ambience and the important facts about that community. Included in the appendix are suggestions for obtaining important data about population size and characteristics related to age, gender, employment, and ethnicity. The characteristics of other health and welfare systems in the community are also important.

A systematic approach to understanding the community will alert workers to informal community networks, such as those that exist in neighborhoods, churches, union groups, and benevolent societies. Where there are large concentrations of particular ethnic groups it is important to know how they view the health services system, whether they are informally or formally organized to provide support for people in need, and if there are many unmet needs in the ethnic community. Chapter 4 referred to the extensive use that some groups make of traditional healers. Health care social workers not only need to know about their existence, but they will, as part of their effort of getting to know the community, want to determine what the potential for collaborative or cooperative effort is.

Once attuned to the importance of knowing the community, workers will keep abreast of major changes and how they affect health. For example, rising unemployment, the closing of a plant, the infusion of new industry, or change in the racial, ethnic, or age composition of a community will ultimately be reflected in the problems coming to the social workers' attention. Thus while the new worker has a particular obligation to master understanding of the community, all workers need to maintain ongoing involvement.

Understanding policy and provision

Health care social workers who are not always aware of shifting eligibility requirements for various entitlement programs do their clients a great disservice. These requirements are complicated and ever changing and involve a great deal of bureaucratic detail. The elderly and the chronically ill have difficulty understanding and working with these intricacies. While some social workers may resent the tedium involved in such efforts, many health professionals look to social workers for expertise in this area. The social worker who is familiar with regulations concerning Medicare, Medicaid, provisions for the developmentally disabled, and health insurance mechanisms can help clients make use of health services and engage in creative problem solving. Constantly observing these matters also highlights the inadequacies and gaps in health care. When social workers confront these matters in their preparatory and daily work they will be more aware of the need to document the negative impact and to advocate for change when necessary.

Drawing on knowledge of human behavior

Chapter 6 referred to the "layers of understanding" for social work practice. Included as one important component of a professional social work perspective was knowledge of psychological and sociological theories and concepts and how they can help social workers understand their client's behavior, feelings, and needs.

In preparing for work in a particular area of health care practice, social workers need to review that basic knowledge base, and attempt to integrate it into their knowledge of the kinds of behaviors most likely to be evident. For example, in a nursing home or other setting where social workers work with the chronically ill elderly and their families, knowledge about how people experience the last stage of the life cycle is particularly important. Some people approach old age and declining vigor with reasonable comfort. In looking back over their lives they judge them to have been fruitful and satisfying. Others seek to come to grips with a past that, in their view, was marked by failures and disappointments. Those in the latter group may show signs of depression, as may those elderly who have experienced loss of vision, or hearing, or of loved ones.

For the adult children of the elderly, the approaching death of a parent intensifies their own sense of mortality. The following comment made by a 60-

year-old man after his 87-year-old mother died expresses this feeling: "We're next in line." The elderly and their loved ones may experience this feeling or one similar to it. Social workers in this area of work need to sharpen their knowledge of this stage in the life cycle. People working with chronically or terminally ill children and their families will want to expand their knowledge of child development by incorporating more specialized understanding of the impact illness has on the usual developmental stages. Chronic illness can affect the opportunity to engage in experiences that test a growing sense of independence. Customary interactions with peers are affected when pain or disability prevent children from moving about freely. Education also may be disrupted.

Chapter 4 discussed the different ways in which members of various social class and ethnic groups respond to illness. When approaching a new assignment social workers must familiarize themselves with the types of health and illness behaviors that are characteristic of the groups typically served in the setting. Reviewing concepts used to explain and understand such behavior will help the social worker incorporate new understanding and information. As social workers prepare for work in a particular setting or with a specific population they constantly need to use their knowledge of human behavior to help them understand the people with whom they work. That knowledge may come from past experience, reading, talking with other social workers, and observing various situations.

Developing self-awareness

The problems encountered in health settings can be overwhelming. Chapter 6 discussed the critical components of "the aware self." These components include insight into one's feelings about pain, disability, and disfigurement. As social workers encounter any group they must examine their feelings about the problems experienced by the group. Social workers who were quite comfortable in a medical-surgical service where they worked with many elderly people may become uncomfortable if they work with young, physically disabled persons. They may identify with their clients too strongly. Some identification is essential for empathic practice, but young workers may become overwhelmed and immobilized and lose their capacity to help if they are not aware of this possibility.

Just as workers need to be knowledgeable of the health and illness behaviors of the different ethnic groups they serve, they also must sensitize themselves to any biases or stereotypes they may harbor. For example, workers whose backgrounds generate stoicism when confronted with pain need to be sure they do not apply their own stance to people from a different background. Social workers need to think and feel through their views of people who use folk healers, "somaticize" emotional problems, and tend to become dependent when they experience illness.

Workers may be repelled by certain problems, such as ulcerated legs, smells accompanying some disease processes, and physical disfigurement. To experience such revulsion does not make them unworthy. They must recognize the feeling and use it as a basis of empathy for individuals directly suffering from such problems. Such efforts at increasing self-awareness can help to overcome negative feelings and serve as a springboard for an empathic attitude.

The work that is done before intervention is also applicable to what may be termed *ongoing work*. Thus efforts to master medical information, understand the community, develop familiarity with policies, incorporate knowledge of human behavior, and develop self-awareness are ongoing. Such work aids a social worker in the problem-solving process.

ASSESSMENT

Work at any level of social work practice needs be guided by an assessment of the present problem. Assessment is an ongoing process that continues once intervention has begun. It involves trying to discern the difficulty as the client perceives it and integrating the client's perception with the worker's professional judgment. In any interdisciplinary setting assessment also involves taking the expert judgment of other professionals into account.

Assessment, problem definition, and beginning intervention are closely intertwined and often occur simultaneously. For example, the social worker talking about what will happen as a result of the illness can begin to reduce tension for many people. Although assessment is an ongoing process, I will emphasize the strategies and skills needed in the beginning stages of intervention. Some of this assessment takes place before meeting with the client system. In many health settings there is limited opportunity to gather information before meeting the client. Therefore I will review the skills involved in making an initial assessment of frequently encountered situations in health settings.

Obtaining information before the encounter with the client system

Before beginning work with any particular client or group workers are obliged to gather as much data as can be obtained, summon their knowledge of the problem involved, and anticipate their own as well as possible client reactions. This means drawing on the body of knowledge reviewed in this book. What is the medical problem? If the patient has had a heart attack, how severe was it? How does it affect future functioning? What is the family constellation? What have the patient and family been told about the situation? How are they responding? What are the resource needs? What ethnic-related illness behavior may be encountered?

Once familiar with the setting, workers are likely to know the routines of the particular service or other work situation. They are also likely to be familiar with other health care personnel and how they approach people with certain kinds of problems.

In most health settings the information about a particular situation available before involvement varies by setting, route to the social worker, and whether intervention is on a crisis or emergency basis or is part of a planned process. Increasingly health care social workers reach out to people in emergency settings via high-risk screening procedures designed to bring immediate help or to engage them in community action. Often there is limited time to gather important information before beginning direct work with the client or client system. This does not change if the client is referred or is seen because of outreach and screening procedures. The following discussion is focused on a few different situations and on how workers can prepare themselves for the initial assessment process before meeting with clients.

The case of outreach and high-risk screening. Outreach and screening procedures are based on the assumption that people to whom service is offered at the worker's initiative are at particular risk for psychosocial crises or problems related to illness or could profitably engage in preventive behavior. Thus isolated elderly persons admitted to the hospital with a hip fracture can be expected to have problems caring for themselves when they are discharged. Teenage mothers with low socioeconomic status are known to be at high risk for having premature infants. Outreach may compel them to seek needed prenatal care. This type of general information needs to be used in conjunction with how an individual or group is experiencing the problem or has responded to past interventive efforts.

The worker's observations, the observations noted on the chart, and the information given to the worker by the ward clerk or cleaning personnel can help individualize the approach to persons who fall into a high-risk category. The following questions are examples of those the worker may ask: Does the elderly person look despondent and fearful? Is he or she talking to the patient in the next bed? Have there been visitors? Has he or she had many outbursts of crying? Has the neglecting mother visited her child? Are her interactions with the child abrupt or does she demonstrate affection? Does the admission slip provide data about available family or other resources? How does the worker feel about an elderly chronic alcoholic for whom no address could be discerned on admission? What is the worker's reaction to "skid row types"? How does the worker feel about having to conduct an interview with the help of an interpreter?

Similar preparatory work also is essential at the community level. In addition to getting to know the community, workers need to learn as much as possible about the details of a situation, such as the following: Do the women who have asked for help in organizing a program for battered women really trust social workers? Do the members of the senior citizens' center who are said to be depressed respond to traditional psychotherapeutic approaches? Are these members basically concerned about how to get to the stores to shop? Do they fear getting mugged? Workers in this stage of the effort need to know as many facts as possible and anticipate their client's possible feelings. These few examples point out that a large element of the preparatory work needed in outreach efforts involves anticipating by thinking about facts and emotions that will make it possible to individualize the encounter.

The case of the referred client or client system. For many years and in many settings, especially those focused on direct services, health care social workers saw people only on referrals often made by physicians or nurses. There is evidence (Wolock, Nicholas, and Russell, 1982) that many people who are referred to social workers are either not informed of that fact or are given scanty information about how the social worker might help. Workers need to try to find out what people have been told or what their referral sources think the clients know about the social work service. The process of seeking information also can serve to clarify for other professionals what the social worker can contribute. The following questions exemplify this process:

> Dr. Smith, is Mrs. Brown experiencing the usual distortion seen in people with this type of stroke?
>
> Miss Jones, does Mrs. Bernstein understand that there might be a long wait for a nursing home?
>
> Does Mr. Chin understand that you've asked him to see me so he and I might talk about the tensions that trigger his headaches? Does he seem ready to engage in that kind of process?
>
> You said that the kids at the youth center could use a social worker to come and talk to them about drugs. Have you told them how I usually approach these kinds of matters?

Whether the initial contact is from referral or because outreach seems indicated, the type of preparatory work suggested here can facilitate the encounter with the client.

Engaging the client

The most critical part of the early stages of the assessment process is engaging the client(s) in a manner conducive to developing a professional relationship. Such a relationship facilitates efforts to discern what the difficulties are and helps the worker and client agree on how they may work together. Several writers have identified the skills required at this stage. The skills and strategies involved in what has been termed "launching the interaction process" (Middleman and Goldberg, 1974) involve considerable thought and planning. Often termed *entry skills* they include stage setting (Middleman and Goldberg, 1974), tuning in (Shulman, 1979), and attending (Egan, 1975).

Stage setting. Stage setting focuses on the physical setting where interaction takes place and on the physical position workers and clients assume when they interact. There are many settings in which health care social workers meet their clients and others with whom they work. Common places are the patient's bedside, where a barely drawn curtain provides the only semblance of privacy for consideration of pressing, intimate matters; a hospital floor lounge; or an intensive care unit waiting room where anxious relatives wait. Community health centers in low-income areas are busy meeting places in which children clamber about as their parents wait to be seen. Emergency room atmospheres alternate between periods of calm and a most hectic pace.

In a dialysis center people sit hooked up to complex machinery for many hours, during which time they may chat, doze, or read. The nursing home may appear physically cheerful, but observing some of the residents reveals a sense of an impending loss, or disengagement, or a loss of contact with time and place. A lounge, an empty patient room, or a conference room provides a meeting place for groups of people sharing common problems. Wives soon to lose husbands to cancer may meet with the social worker. Individuals who recently had heart attacks may share their concerns about what they will be able to do, and how they will feel when they return home.

Social workers' offices where doors can readily be closed and uninterrupted scheduled discussions can be held are also common meeting places. Conference rooms set aside for interdisciplinary meetings and nurses' stations also are places where information is exchanged. Increasingly health social workers meet people in their homes; elderly patients may wait eagerly for the social worker's home health visits, as may the parents of newborn children recently discharged from neonatal intensive care units. Health planners and consumers also may spend several days in a hotel debating how limited resources for health care should be allocated.

Social workers' need for meeting in private with their clients and providing a comfortable place where anonymity, if desired, can be provided is often honored in the breach in health settings. This very fact compels attention to efforts to enhance comfort and communication. I offer several general guidelines for making the client comfortable and aiding communication.

1. *Create as much privacy as possible, whatever the setting.*

In the hospital room the curtain can be drawn and strategies should be developed to avoid interruptions. Knowing the visiting hours, the usual time when physicians see their patients, and when treatments are administered can guide workers in developing their own schedules. Good working relationships with other staff members make it possible for workers to assert their need for time with patients. Workers who feel their work is of less consequence than that of other health providers will unwittingly convey this feeling to other staff members and experience frequent interruptions. Emergency procedures and visits by loved ones clearly take precedence over the social worker's scheduled time.

Some people, by dint of personality or cultural disposition, may not be concerned about privacy; some may even reject it. To some individuals efforts to ensure privacy (like drawing the curtain around the bed) may be a signal to other people that they are talking about intimate matters with a stranger. This is a source of some concern to members of many ethnic groups. Clients may prefer to have people believe that the social worker is a relative or neighbor. A conversation held in the lounge or without the curtain drawn may avoid the patient's sense of shame or being stigmatized.*

2. *Make creative use of the available space and setting.*

Social work's health care role is focused on health, coping, and social functioning. Many social workers see people in a medical setting where treatment is being rendered. Working with people in this situation can convey empathy and a sense of sharing in the process.

The mother of a sick newborn in the intensive care nursery may be loathe to give up precious time with her child in order to go to the worker's office. After hours spent in a dialysis center the patient may be physically and psychologically exhausted and need to go home. Caring, attentive conversations can be held amidst much hustle and bustle. At other times the worker's office may offer a retreat or haven from the ever-present reminder of sickness.

A community group concerned about drug addicts who loiter in hallways will trust workers who risk themselves and come to observe and participate in meetings in the group's neighborhood. As trust is developed a meeting held in more comfortable quarters, perhaps in those of the local health council or legislator, can contribute to a growing sense of accomplishment and power to control the environment. Home visits are costly but can, if judiciously used, provide the worker with understanding and a sense that the worker cares.

Perhaps the most important guideline is the one that calls for flexibility. The old social work dictum of "starting where the client is" can also be interpreted to mean working with the client in whatever physical locales are available and adapting these locales to emerging needs.

Tuning in. Tuning in may be defined as "development of the worker's preparatory empathy" (Shulman, 1979). The term refers to anticipating the needs, feelings, and opinions that may emerge in the encounter. For example, a social work health planner is preparing to chair a meeting called to consider recommendations that have been made for closing an "underused hospital." Data show that there are many empty beds and a declining number of visits to the outpatient facilities. At the meeting there will be experts who know how costly and inefficient the hospital is and who will suggest that a nearby facility is better equipped. There will also be personnel present who have always used this hospital and think the other one is too far away, especially for emergency use. The community residents are likely to be poor or members of minority groups. The planners, as is often the case, may be white, able to manipulate data well, and prepared with myriad charts.

Tuning in to the conflicting perspectives of the people who will be at the meeting may compel social workers to review experiences when they were in a position to plead for the humane rather than the rational course of action. In an interdisciplinary staff meeting they may have had feelings of powerlessness like

*For more detailed consideration of these issues see Devore, W., and Schlesinger, E.: Ethnic-sensitive social work practice, St. Louis, 1981, The C.V. Mosby Co., pp. 168-170.

those experienced by the community residents. At other times the workers may have used data to back a plan of action, such as confronting irate residents of a neighborhood where there are plans to locate a community home for the mentally disabled. These and related situations suggest how the development of preparatory empathy may facilitate subsequent encounters.

Attending. Attending involves purposeful behavior that conveys to the listener a message of respect and an understanding of the discussion's importance. Simultaneous attention to cognitive, emotional, and nonverbal behavior is often needed.

At some level most people want to know what is wrong. They may ask, "Do my headaches mean I have a tumor?" or "Why doesn't Johnny talk, even though he's four years old?" The level of anxiety expressed in the tone of voice or facial expression gives some clues about how much information is actually wanted. These clues may suggest how quickly or slowly to proceed. Detailed medical explanations about the various types of possible tumors may not yet be appropriate if the thought has newly surfaced and denial processes are helping people to mobilize themselves. The worker may say, "These symptoms can mean many things. Let's see about getting you scheduled for tests." If their anxiety seems diminished by telling them this, they may not be ready to hear any more at this point. Parents first confronting the possibility that their child may have a lifelong handicap usually want to discuss what they can do *now* and often not "hear" when given detailed recitals of the expected long-term course (Drayer and Schlesinger, 1960).

Body language. Egan (1975) identifies certain aspects of "physical attending": face the other person squarely, maintain an open posture, and lean toward the other person. These actions convey a sense of active involvement and aid in active listening. As a general rule these aspects of attending are most important. But workers must always be alert to exceptions. Many patients have been questioned, poked by needles, and "invaded" by surgery or by x-rays. Whether the active, open, touching stance is comforting or implies another invasive procedure must be considered. If someone holds back or physically tries to move away, a more formal stance may be appropriate. Eye contact means intrusion and disrespect in many cultures, especially when practitioners are viewed as authority figures (Devore and Schlesinger, 1981).

Attending involves constantly observing the client's response to the worker's verbal and physical behavior and adapting that behavior accordingly.

• • •

The skills used in stage setting, tuning in, and attending are all designed to set the tone for the initial and ongoing process of assessing the difficulties and determining if and how workers and clients will proceed with prevention, amelioration, or maintenance efforts.

Specifying the problem

A major component of the assessment process is specifying the problem. Problems often seem overwhelming and multifaceted. If efforts to resolve problems are to be at all successful, it is important to identify their component parts as a way of beginning work. Epstein (1980) provides a useful orientation to problem specification, which she terms "general orientation to the elements of a problem" (p. 167). She identifies several orienting perspectives: needs, lack of skills, and classifying a problem by naming or labeling it. Needs focus on deficits in personal and social resources. Skills are those "needed for carrying out a reasonable life-style." Problem classification concentrates on capturing "salient features of problems, conditions, and behaviors" (p. 170).

Closely related to these perspectives is Golan's discussion (1978) of the stresses to which sick people are subjected. She points to (1) the loss of functional ability, debilitation, pain, and threatening procedures; (2) enforced dependency and passivity; and (3) separation, both spatial and psychological, from supportive social networks. Although these stresses and how they are experienced by sick individuals are discussed separately for analytical purposes, they are in fact usually part of the total configuration.

Mrs. Jones

Mrs. Jones, a single mother of three, awakens in the emergency room, suddenly realizing that she is there because of injuries sustained in a car accident. She is immobilized, and tests are being carried out to ascertain the extent of her injuries. Although she is still groggy, she is beginning to feel pain as the effect of pain-relieving drugs wears off.

She needs to be admitted to the hospital. When informed of this she cries and looks around distractedly as she asks where her children are. She cries again when she looks at the bandages on her legs and says, "But I have to work to feed those kids."

Mrs. Jones has suddenly become an involuntary patient of the hospital. When the social worker arrives to talk with her about her fears and concerns for her children, she is also an involuntary social work client. The accident has, for the time being, generated resource deficits because she can neither work nor care for her children. She also cannot use her everyday skills. She is experiencing debilitation, pain, and separation. Mrs. Jones' situation differs only in its details and timing from that of elderly persons who are gradually but irrevocably losing the ability to care for their own needs, or the diabetic patient in a coma, or the mother whose negligent and abusive behavior has led to her child's hospitalization. Although at one level the problems are self-evident, the process of specifying those problems with which the health care social worker might help and distinguishing between the social worker's role and that of others is not as easy.

Epstein's formulation (1980) of "the problem search" by which the "target problems" for intervention are specified is useful. These problems are ones that clients perceive, understand, and want to care for. (p. 3). Together these concepts indicate the need to identify and particularize problems in manageable terms. These terms contrast with the broad, global terms in which problems are often described. In health settings particularizing problems often entails translating the meaning and consequences of medical diagnoses and procedures into explicit psychosocial and behavioral terms around which action must be taken.

A social worker involved with Mrs. Jones would find in early contact that as yet no medical diagnosis exists beyond the need for further exploration. However, the exploration of psychosocial tasks quickly reveals two target problems: (1) finding out where and with whom the children are now and (2) communicating with Mrs. Jones within the limits of her immediate impairment to let her know what action can be taken. Is there a relative who can take charge? If not, should a child welfare worker be called? Her wishes and resources, to the extent she is able to express and draw on them, are crucial. Subsequent problems will depend on the diagnosis and other resources that can be marshalled. If there is a permanent impairment the process of identifying problems will be persistent, reflecting changing psychosocial conditions.

The emergency nature of her admission called for quick, timely, focused efforts. If long-range rehabilitation is needed (should she perhaps become paraplegic as a result of the accident), continuing reassessment will be necessary. For example, when admitted to the rehabilitation unit she may seem depressed, reluctant to engage in physiotherapy, and uncommunicative to the point where she no longer asks about her children. How then does the problem search and identification of target problems proceed? Does the depression present a crisis response (for example, Golan, 1978)? If so, how can its components be broken down? Why is she not asking about her children? Is she distancing herself emotionally because she is afraid she will no longer be able to play a mothering role? Are hospital routines contributing to a sense of isolation?

Having used the problem search process, more specific target problems can be identified: (1) finding ways of increasing Mrs. Jones' communication level, (2) ascertaining the motivation for distancing herself from her children, and (3) exploring her particular response to hospital routines. These are the worker's tasks, as may often be the case with traumatic illness and withdrawn, confused, or depressed patients. The family and the other members of the health team are then drawn into the process of trying to understand and specify target problems. Care must be taken not to bypass the identified client. Continuous although brief visits by the social worker may help to break the sense of isolation and despair. Team deliberation may help to identify actions that key staff members can take in drawing people out. For example, bending the rules so that Mrs. Jones' children can visit may help her regain a sense of her mothering role. Perhaps she can give the caretaker some advice on how to help her children with their lessons as she has in the past.

These kinds of actions are considered part of the problem identification and assessment stage because they may clarify the problems as perceived by clients. If asked for advice on lessons or discipline the new patient may for the first time be able to articulate his or her own perceptions.

Particularizing or rank ordering the problem

Shulman, (1979) and Epstein, (1980) converge on an increasingly common theme: breaking problems down into their component parts and focusing on only one or a few parts at a time.

The Hernandez family

The Hernandez family, consisting of Mr. and Mrs. Hernandez, their five children ranging in age from 2 to 17, and Mr. Hernandez's mother, are referred to the community health center by an income maintenance worker from the welfare department.

Mr. Hernandez, partially disabled because of a work-sustained back injury, is unemployed. He also smokes a great deal and has a hacking cough. Mrs. Hernandez is pregnant. Although she talks about having an abortion, she is confused about what to do. Mr. Hernandez is totally opposed to the idea of an abortion.

The school has informed Mr. and Mrs. Hernandez that 10-year-old Maria needs glasses. Juan, the 17-year-old, is involved with a neighborhood group believed to be using a variety of drugs. Mr. Hernandez's mother is becoming increasingly confused and often wanders off.

The family lives in public housing where the heating is inadequate, the elevator breaks down, and the hall lights are often not working. Mr. and Mrs. Hernandez fear for their children's safety and the cold housing exacerbates Mr. Hernandez's cough.

How will the Hernandez family and the social worker approach the combination of health and social problems? As the social worker meets with Mr. and Mrs. Hernandez she asks them to think about what worries them most, suggesting they concentrate on that problem first. Their view of what are the most pressing problems must be considered first. Because their problems are so complex, they have no easy answers. Overwhelmed, they jump from one topic to another. As the worker lists the known problems Mr. Hernandez interrupts, saying, "Everything was OK until she started talking about an abortion." Mrs. Hernandez cryingly agrees, saying she can't win—"How can I do away with a baby, but how can I manage another one?" As the exploration continues the pregnancy clearly surfaces as their major problem. Juan's behavior also worries them.

Together they agree that these are the problems they will consider first. Who can help them make a decision about the pregnancy? Members of the extended family? The physician? Do they feel comfortable talking with the social worker?

They'll talk to a physician about the risks of a pregnancy at Mrs. Hernandez's age. Does Juan know that the youth center has a physical fitness program for adolescents that includes access to a gym and a pool? They say they will mention it to him. Having organized their thinking, Mr. and Mrs. Hernandez seem more relaxed. The worker may feel frustrated because other problems have not yet been addressed, such as Mr. Hernandez's cough, Mr. Hernandez's mother's wandering, and Maria's problems. These need to wait; a beginning has been made.

• • •

The discussion of assessment has pointed to the need for making sensitive efforts to learn about the difficulties clients are experiencing. The rapid pace that prevails in most health settings frequently does not make it possible to engage in extensive exploration before engaging the client. Yet the worker must draw on a variety of sources to compile information so that in early contacts with the client the worker can make an assessment and begin to specify the problems. This process is the first step to intervention.

INTERVENTION

There are many ways of breaking down the components of the interventive process. One relates to the earlier and subsequent stages of intervention. Another is to determine whether contact is to be short or long, time limited or open ended. Crucial are issues of contracting. These issues all relate to the agreement developed between the social worker and the client about how the problem-solving process is to proceed.

I have stated several times that many health care social work clients have limited options about whether or not they will engage with the social worker. When Mrs. Jones, whose situation was discussed earlier, was in the emergency room she had no choice about meeting with the worker. The dialysis social worker is mandated to meet with patients, as are those charged with assessing situations involving child abuse. A hospitalized elderly person's family that no longer has the financial or social resources to care for that person needs to meet with the designated discharge planner.

I am, for the most part, focusing on how to proceed, recognizing that health care clients often do not come seeking the services of a social worker. The emphasis on working with problems in the terms identified by the client and taking into account administrative mandates, constraints, and opportunities aids in developing guidelines. Major among these is the process of contracting.

Contracting

Many definitions of contracting have been offered. I am using the term to refer to the process by which workers and clients engaged in problem-solving activities come to an agreement about the respective work to be done, the objectives sought, the means by which these objectives are to be attained, and others to be involved. These others include not only family, but also a variety of health and welfare agencies and other health care disciplines. A contract in which it is agreed that a cardiac patient will try to begin walking stairs by a certain time involves the physician's judgment of physical status and the family's ability to support the patient's efforts. The decision that the family, social worker and others will support the wishes of the terminally ill patient for hospice care depends on the availability of that care and medical judgment concerning the futility of further therapeutic measures.

Considerations in contracting. The concept of the contract is in many ways a corrective for that mode of practice in which client and worker came together for extensive periods of time, working on goals identified by the worker, but frequently lacked clear purpose for the interaction. In many health care settings workers seldom have the luxury of working in an open-ended way for undefined periods of time. This situation is particularly true in acute care hospitals where decisions about care plans after discharge have to be made within the time constraints imposed by the medical diagnosis and administrative considerations.

Also related to contracting is the assumption that a crisis or other motivation that triggered seeking or receiving help at a particular time activates and speeds up problem-solving capacities. A considerable amount of literature suggests that people in crisis are particularly amenable and responsive to efforts made to help them deal with their difficulties.

Many health care clients are at best semivoluntary. The process of contracting focuses on the clients' options, even when involvement is somewhat coercive. These and other factors suggest that in many facets of health care social work, contracting is a critical component of the initial and subsequent work.

Principles. The foregoing factors suggest a number of principles for contracting in health care:

1. A clear-cut statement about the help and options available despite constraints is essential when clients have little or no choice about being involved. Thus workers may outline the help available as follows:

> *Worker:* Mr. Green, I understand the doctors have told you that you really shouldn't go back to your own home because you live alone, and now after your stroke you'll need someone to look after you. I'd like to know what you think about that. I've been able to help other people think through these kinds of problems.

Mr. Green may be relieved, or he may say,

> "So if I die, I die. I don't want one of those homes."

Since professional responsibility mandates that the worker not stop here, the worker tries to contract by saying,

Worker: It's really difficult. Could we talk about it some more? Let's consider together where you might get the type of care you need.

Hearing this Mr. Green may enter in to a tentative agreement to explore the situation.

Mr. Green: OK, as long as I don't end up in a nursing home.

Without making unrealistic commitments the worker says,

Worker: Perhaps we can begin by talking about what you think you need.

2. The range of services available should be clearly outlined, with an emphasis on the roles the client and worker can play.

Worker: Our senior citizens' center offers lunches, a recreation program, and a counseling program for people feeling lonely or sad.

Client: Well I'd like to get there for those lunches. But you know I don't need one of them psychiatrists.

Worker: You could go a couple of times and see how you like it—see what they do. Then we could talk about it some more and see if you want to continue.

3. The contract should not focus on people changing when system changing is in order.

Worker: Mr. Galeo, I know that when they keep you waiting in that clinic for hours you get awfully angry. Should you and I go to see the administrator together to see if the appointment system can be staggered?

4. When workers seek to contract for psychotherapeutic and concrete services it should be stated explicitly.

Worker: Ms. Jones, when you take your baby home I think you may find it useful to have a nurse come and help you get started learning proper ways to feed the baby. You also might find that you'll get frustrated and angry sometimes being alone with a sick baby. Would you like me to arrange to have someone come in to talk with you about these feelings you may have?

5. Contracting must take into account the cultural and ethnic dispositions of clients. Many people view involvement with social workers or other mental health specialists as shameful. The most they can accept is help with concrete services. For other problems they turn first to the family and community networks. This behavior is not uncharacteristic of many Asians, people of eastern European background, and American Indians (for example, Fandetti and Gelfand, 1978; President's Commission on Mental Health, 1978).

Worker: Mr. Lin, I'm a social worker who talks to most people in this hospital before they go home to be sure they'll get the care they need. Would you like to talk with me? The doctor thinks you might be worried.

Mr. Lin: I'm not worried. I'll be all right.

Worker: It's natural for people to worry when they're all alone and sick.
Mr. Lin: I'll be all right.
Worker: The doctors really think you'll need someone to help you with the housework and getting your meals ready.
Mr. Lin: Maybe my old neighbor could come.
Worker: Have you talked with him?
Mr. Lin: Well, he's pretty sick himself.
Worker: Have you ever heard of homemaker service?
Mr. Lin: No. What's that?

As the worker explains Mr. Lin becomes somewhat more responsive. He tells the worker that most of his neighbors who used to help out are sick themselves. He is willing to consider having a stranger help a little. The worker recognizes quickly, based on knowledge of the Chinese culture, that Mr. Lin is not likely to divulge his worries. The worker tries to contract with him on a concrete service, such as homemaker service. Knowing that it has already been difficult for Mr. Lin to acknowledge that his accustomed caring network has begun to disintegrate, the worker does not push him. However, the worker will continue to search for the best methods of meeting his needs for some supportive care. If these can be found within the Chinese community, Mr. Lin may feel more comfortable about accepting help. Although he may feel lonely and depressed, acknowledging these feelings by contracting to discuss them with the worker could cause him more turmoil than he is already experiencing.

When contracting, the social worker may need to take into account the clients' cultural dispositions with respect to expected gender role behavior.

Mr. Garcia

Mr. Garcia, 34, lost a leg in a car accident. In the rehabilitation hospital the social worker was able to contract with him to share his feelings about the accident as a way of relieving anger and frustration. The worker used an interpreter to talk with Mrs. Garcia (who does not speak English) about all the arrangements that had to be made for Mr. Garcia's return home. These arrangements included discussions with the insurance company to discover if making the house accessible was covered and with Mr. Garcia's employers about disability benefits.

Soon Mr. Garcia became uncommunicative with the worker and increasingly angry with his wife. Another worker pointed out that asking Mrs. Garcia to make specific arrangements without consulting Mr. Garcia further eroded his already damaged male image of himself. When both Mr. and Mrs. Garcia were involved in the planning process Mr. Garcia took on the tasks he could do from the hospital. He made phone calls and wrote letters to identify the benefits to which he was entitled. Once he began to take on the elements of what he considered the male role, in a culturally syntonic fashion, Mr. Garcia resumed his contacts with the worker. The worker gradually was able to contract with him to review his stance on what he would permit his wife to do as he began to recognize that he had certain limitations.

Involving Mrs. Garcia in Mr. Garcia's problems without his consent violated cultural precepts as well as the tenet of client self-direction.

When contracting is not feasible. The concept that worker, client, and other health care providers come to a common agreement on the work to be done represents an important development in social work. Yet there is an implicit assumption that most people share rational conceptions of time and reciprocity and can readily develop the type of trust expected in formal helping institutions. Not all health care social work clients fall into this category. For example, many American Indians view the explicit type of intervention suggested by the contract as interference. Confused, disoriented nursing home residents are often unable to agree on how they will work toward enhanced functioning. Yet they can respond to the regular visits and the empathetic touch of the worker and other health care personnel. Sustained demonstration of interest and concern is important for many people. When this is the only type of service health care clients seem ready to accept, workers need to consider how it can be most appropriately rendered and if the skills of a trained social worker are needed. Volunteers supervised by professional hospital staff may play an important role, as can indigenous community health aides.

When considering the issue of contracting in relation to the wide range of problems presented to health care social workers it is important not to lose sight of some long-standing principles and strategies that are part of social work's tradition. One of these strategies is staying with people in need, in terms defined by professional judgment and the clients' wishes. This is not to suggest returning to the role of "the friendly visitor." A decision about visiting or looking in on a person is based on professional assessment of need and is carried out in the effort to ascertain the client's perception of the difficulty.

Contracting is a process that, when feasible, begins early in the worker/client encounter. How much work can be done and how much recontracting can be carried out after the initial stage of work depends on many factors. In health care, as in other arenas of practice, how the process of problem solving is carried out derives from the needs of the client or client system, the degree to which the agency is committed to facilitate problem-solving needs as they are defined by social workers, and the workers' stance on how the problems identified are best approached.

• • •

In the diverse health settings where social workers practice, the problem-solving process is affected by the health problem at issue and the degree to which administrative constraints of time and function limit the extent to which any one agency or worker can or should take responsibility for problem resolution. For example, the acute care hospital tends to perceive its obligation of attempting to help people deal with psychosocial problems related to illness in more limited terms than do primary care or long-term care facilities. Based on these considerations, in the remainder of the interventive process discussion I will identify a number of issues that arise in the course of intervention and suggest some approaches. These approaches include short-term, long-term, and intermittent contact and the worker's responsibility to help clients take action in accordance with their needs.

Short-term and intermittent contact

The need for parsimonious allocation of resources and organizational mandates in many health settings, especially acute care hospitals, limits the degree to which workers can, on a long-term basis, attend to the problems encountered. For example, in the preceding section on contracting, the situation of Mr. Green, an elderly man needing protected care after discharge from the hospital, was discussed. As the worker reviews alternatives with him he or she may identify many other problems, such as his fear or his feeling of being rejected or abandoned by his grown children. The social worker is tempted to hold on and to help him work through these feelings, as well as to focus on finding resources for him. But, the hospital does not usually see its responsibility in these terms. The worker is obliged to work with the patient only to effect an appropriate discharge plan and is usually not in a position to maintain long-term contact. Nevertheless, the worker's responsibility does not end with developing an individual discharge plan. Workers who have done their homework, as suggested under the general rubric of preparatory work earlier in this chapter, will be able to do much more than this. Quickly establishing relationships based on trust, developing the skills of empathy, focusing on the present reality, and observing patient reactions are crucial skills in health care social work. Equally important are the links the worker has established with community systems because such first-hand knowledge can contribute to a smooth, skillful, and satisfying transfer process.

Many health care social workers are frustrated by what they perceive as constraints on their ability to be effective and view with longing the type of work that can be carried out in other types of agencies. Epstein's recent review (1983) of the "long-term, short-term issue" helps to put this frustration into perspective. She points out that the majority of "casework sequences are in fact brief," and suggests that "casework treatment, when it takes place at all, takes place in spurts, with longer or shorter periods of inactivity interspersed" (p. 78). This is the situation that exists with many health care clients, especially those whose problems call for long-term care. This type of contact with the client may be termed *intermittent.*

The situations of the Hernandez family noted earlier and of patients in dialysis units, rehabilitation centers, and long-term psychiatric settings are cases involving intermittent contact. A different set of issues and needed skills emerges in each of these and similar types of settings in which long-term contact is built into the system. The preceding discussion of the Hernandez family addressed the issue of particularizing and ordering problems with clients. It is unlikely that the Hernandez family or people in other types of settings will sustain long, protracted involvement with the worker. There may indeed be spurts of contact.

This same type of intermittent contact is found in other situations also. Dialysis patients and their families have a long and painful treatment program. When first starting treatment they may be enthusiastic and ready to comply but have a lot of questions. At a later stage they may become weary and not want to go on. By being able to anticipate these kinds of responses workers can gauge the need for varying types of intervention required at different times. In the first stage workers may simply want to make their availability known. Always, as part of an interdisciplinary group, they seek from and share information with others as they keep an eye on the situation. When the dialysis patient becomes weary, stops complying with the medical regimen, and talks about wanting to die, the skills of crisis intervention may be needed. Or the worker may become an advocate for a patient's right to decide if he or she wants to continue receiving treatment. A paraplegic may have similar dispositions, as may many elderly people who are destitute, are isolated, and have limited functioning capacity. When this type of situation arises, workers confront agonizing decisions about the role they feel they must play. This role calls for maximum clinical acumen, collaborative skills, and advocacy skills because it is never easy to distinguish between pathological depression that can lead to apparent suicidal behavior and a conscious, articulate client decision. The wishes of clients and families may clash. It is usually the social worker, along with members of other disciplines, who assumes the difficult task of sorting out and identifying the problem and helping people to make these difficult types of decisions.

Ongoing contact does not always or even usually present workers with these particularly agonizing tasks. Often the worker has an opportunity to use the skills involved in family therapy and group work. Families often have great resilience and capacity to incorporate the new tasks generated by the problems of the ill member and to retain viable family functioning. As social workers incorporate these modalities into health care they will want to pay particular attention to the stressful effects coping with illness has on family members. Whether the work context limits social work involvement to brief interventive efforts or allows for sustained contact, workers must develop the skill of setting priorities.

REFERRAL, TRANSFER, AND TERMINATION

A critical part of the health care social worker's role is the process of referral, transfer, and termination. When I discussed the intervention process I stated repeatedly that much of health care social work involves helping people develop a clear perspective on psychosocial problems related to illness and attempting to ease their struggle of coping with their difficult present realities. During the process of assessment and problem identification health care social workers and their clients come to develop meaningful, emotionally laden relationships. The social worker may have helped someone come to grips with the reality of a life-threatening illness. Women whose husbands are cancer victims may have depended on the worker for comfort and guidance.

It is characteristic of health care social work practice that another facility's services may help fulfill the client's need. *Referral* and *transfer* are major elements of practice in this area.

Compton and Galaway (1979) define referral as a "process that comes into play in a situation that falls outside the parameters of the agency's defined services, or whenever workers define a problem as beyond their expertise or their agency's parameters of service" (p. 433). This definition fits many cases. A patient due to leave the hospital needs the services of the home health agency worker or the nursing home worker. Marital problems beyond the scope of the services offered at the center may surface in a primary health care center suggesting referral to a family counseling agency. Groups of clients angry about limited entitlements under a particular program may, after discussion with the worker, be referred to the public advocate or to any one of numerous health planning and community organization facilities.

Compton and Galaway define transfer as "the process by which the client is referred to another worker, usually in the same agency . . . " (p. 436). Reasons for transfer may be that the worker is leaving or is having difficulty working with a client. This type of situation may arise in health settings where contact is extensive and prolonged, such as dialysis units, neonatal intensive care units, psychiatric facilities, and primary care centers. In health planning facilities a worker may leave in the midst of an intense, prolonged planning process with community residents. In addition, social work students may leave when they have completed their course of study.

Referral

In some types of referral the separation from the social worker may be one in a series of negative, traumatic events. To an elderly person who has counted on the worker's support while in the hospital awaiting a nursing home bed, the worker's absence may add to the person's feeling of isolation and loss. In other instances referral occurs because a positive stage in the illness career has been reached. The patient is truly feeling better and ready to go home. A series of medical treatments has been successfully completed. However, further service, perhaps from the home health agency, may still be needed.

Whatever the reason for referral, workers need to be aware that often such referral is taking place at a critical point in the illness cycle. People may have come to feel comfortable and secure in the hospital. Although some individuals may complain, their complaints may reflect fear of the next stage—the struggle between growing dependence (as with many chronically ill people) and resentment of that increased dependence. Patients who have recovered nevertheless may be fearful of their futures. It is important that workers be aware of these kinds of feelings and help ease the patients' transfer by saying something such as the following:

> I know it's going to be hard to start over with someone else, but you'll be at home finally. And as I've told you, the social worker at the home health agency will visit to see how you manage with that walker alone at home. She'll talk with you about how you're doing and be sure you're getting your Meals On Wheels. Now you know what a social worker does.

or

> You've often said it would be good to talk with other women whose husbands have had a stroke. I think you'll find that group helpful.

Skillful use of the referral process helps people make connections with needed services. Compton and Galaway (1979) identify this type of intervention as a "broker" role for the social worker. They also make the important point that evaluating and drawing on the experience helps people look ahead. An elderly woman being admitted to a nursing home is not likely to be readily comforted although she may appear stoic and accepting. While in the hospital she may have been helpful to others or well liked by staff members and patients. The worker can draw on these positive aspects.

> I know you're scared and sad. But what makes you think there won't be nice folks like us there? Think about how bad you felt when you first had to come here. But even with your pain and loneliness you did OK. Maybe it would help if we talked about how you managed then.

Thus a key element of the referral process is helping people *review* and *evaluate* past efforts so they can look ahead and be able to make good use of the planned service. To play the broker role well workers need thorough familiarity with the services being recommended. If the workers know little about how the home health facility operates or the type of care rendered in nursing homes, they will not be able to give accurate and comforting information.

To best carry out referral workers need to be aware of (1) the fear and sense of loss that accompany any major change, (2) the possibility that the change portends more negative experiences in the future, (3) people's capacity to make positive use of critical life changes to enhance functioning, and (4) the type of service rendered by the other facility. Skill in helping people explore, evaluate, and reflect must be coupled with thorough knowledge of community facilities.

Transfer

Earlier I said that transfer usually takes place when the services of another worker in the same facility are being recommended. Compton and Galaway (1979) review a series of feelings that may be evoked. Both worker and client may experience a sense of loss. Just as the client may feel betrayed, workers may feel they are betraying their clients by turning them over to someone else. Compton and Galaway identify a number of elements to be considered in the termination process that also apply to transfer. These elements include (1) dealing with the loss of a concerned person, such as the worker, (2) reviewing the progress made in the interventive process, and (3) stabilizing those gains that have been made.

For example, in a rehabilitation facility clients may have relied on the worker who helped them prepare for the long treatment process and saw them through stages of anger, denial, and recognition of their disability. It will not be easy for them to adapt to someone else. Nevertheless, progress has been made.

> Yes, I know that you've really struggled hard to realize that you'll never walk again. And you'll get depressed about it again. Ms. Jones understands these matters, too. With your permission I'll go over that with her. I'll tell her that you've really come a long way.

It is important to remember that in most health settings there are other staff members who have a relationship with the client. Workers can draw on their knowledge of the quality of these relationships to help ease the transition.

> You know you've always talked to the doctors and the PTs about your feelings. They'll still be here. And Ms. Jones will also work with them.

There is no question that both referral and transfer can be painful. Yet for both client and worker these processes are inevitable life changes encountered in the problem-solving process.

Termination

Ideally termination is contemplated when the goals set in the early contracting phase have been accomplished, such as when diabetic patients manage their own insulin, adhere to their diets, and feel better about themselves; or when unwed teenage mothers have learned how to care for their babies; or when a community action project designed to work for the opening of a new health center has succeeded.

> My goodness—you've come a long way. When you all started with me you were scared, pregnant kids who didn't know what a baby needs. Now, you've had your kids and you've learned to take care of them.
>
> And some of you are working. You're all nice folks who have learned to take on responsibility. Think about that. You're really ready to be on your own without me. And besides, I'll be you'll be calling each other up all the time.

The worker's last comments are especially important because they point out a major component of the termination process. If termination is occurring because of client progress, the clients usually are ready to proceed on their own, as well as to rely on more informal and natural helping networks. Some of these networks are formed as a result of the social worker's intervention; others occur more naturally in the course of the client's life.

Too often in health care settings termination occurs because the limits of service eligibility have been exhausted. For example, Medicare will not fund more home health care visits and the patient must be discharged from the hospital. While the responsible worker usually seeks to effect a referral rather than terminate, it is not always accomplished. When termination takes place for these reasons workers are obliged to let their clients know that they are distressed also and to share with them plans that may be underway to expand the availability of needed services.

Summary

Transfer, referral, and termination are integral parts of health care practice. These processes can only be smooth and effective if they are preceded by adequate preparatory work, assessment, and intervention. Nothing can totally erase the discomforts experienced by workers and clients during and after a separation, especially if there has been a good relationship.

Having completed my discussion of key elements of the interventive process, I will now continue to review the strategies and skills for health care social work practice. One strategy is to use groups in health settings.

USING GROUPS IN HEALTH CARE SOCIAL WORK

When talking with health students about how services to clients might be enhanced it is not uncommon for many to suggest groups. While groups may be helpful, the view that they are automatically beneficial or cost effective deserves examination. As a social worker is determining when and why groups might be an important component of the interventive process he or she should consider the traditions that guide group work practice, the types of situations that lend themselves to such practice, and the skills required.

I am identifying three traditional approaches to group work practice: (1) the social goals approach, linked to social work's struggle for human rights and social justice (Vinter, 1965); (2) the socialization approach, focused on the development of people who enter a group voluntarily; and (3) the resocialization approach that assumes the existence of dysfunctional behavior (Garvin, 1981). Although these approaches vary in objectives, conceptual underpinning, and style, a number of elements are integral to all of them. These elements include efforts to achieve group objectives through sharing common concerns, developing cohesion, and viewing the group as a mutual aid system. Clearly all three approaches have a place in the problem-solving process of health care social work.

Many of the deficits in the health care system have been and continue to be addressed, often with the aid of a social work professional, by groups of people who work together. The adept community organizer helps groups of people work together to attain shared action goals. For example, not long ago a neighborhood health center in my home community was slated to be closed because of inadequate funding. Community-based groups were joined by health care professionals, including social workers, in the successful struggle to keep the center open. Local, state, and federal officials were contacted and were impressed with the documentation proving the continued need for the center.

The use of socialization or resocialization groups is growing. People experiencing a common loss (for example, husbands or wives of cancer or stroke victims) can be helped to explore their loss and to adapt to the new roles they will have. Grown children of elderly persons who find themselves caring for their parents, who had always cared for them, are experiencing role reversal and trauma. Patients with cancer, end-stage renal disease, or paraplegia all are considered in need of the type of help provided in groups. Objectives of intervention can range from the insight development and behavioral change anticipated in long-term therapeutic groups to limited educational efforts focused on prevention or illness management techniques. The waiting room can be used to provide service to individuals whose relatives are receiving treatment for major problems (for example, Gardner, 1980).

Chapter 6 discussed the importance of having people who are experiencing the same problems help each other. When and how it is useful to form groups in health settings and the problems that frequently surface need to be considered. When determining if groups can and should be used the social worker needs to be aware of (1) the worker's skill, (2) the organization's receptivity and possible source of resistance, and (3) the clients' perception of how groups will help them.

Increasingly schools of social work are including training in group dynamics and group process as an integral part of their curriculum offerings. Many young workers therefore feel comfortable about their capacity to engage groups of individuals. When workers lack this training or experience they need to use consultants and continuing education programs to ensure that they acquire the requisite skill.

The degree of organizational resistance that can surface when efforts are underway to start a group often surprises even workers who have experience with running groups. Such efforts suddenly require administrative approval, or there is no time, or proper place, or administrators suggest that perhaps nursing and social work should run groups together. Therefore considerable organizational skill and savvy is required before clients are even brought together. Sherman (1979) has commented on this problem. Resistance stems from fear of what may go on behind closed doors. Staff members may fear that patients will use the group to complain about the quality of care. Or the professional who runs the group may be seen as developing special relationships with some clients while displacing others. Administrators may fear that groups of people may converge to make demands that are not made in individual sessions. Thus there is a great deal of preparatory work to be done in planning a group. The staff members involved need to be consulted about how they view the needs of the clients to be served. Administrators may want to know if the worker's time will be used as or more efficiently than in individual sessions. Data about past efforts may need to be marshalled to document the advantages of group work.

Social workers also need to be concerned about the clients who are potential group members. Are the individuals comfortable about sharing their concerns with others? What do they hope the group meetings will accomplish? How does the schedule of group meetings conform to their schedules that may already be overloaded because of illness-related activities? Are the group meetings intended to be therapeutic or educational? Are they directed to a personal or community change effort? Some workers have found that work with groups does not always bring the success anticipated. Often people "remain stuck with the surface complaints and demands, coupled with a fear of exposure and avoidance of closeness" (Sherman, p. 24). The idea that groups are cost-effective ways of providing service in health settings has not been fully demonstrated because effective group work often leads to identification of individual problems that cannot be dealt with by the group.

Groups can be an extremely useful mechanism for providing social work services in health care. The worker planning this type of intervention needs to consider group objectives, client need, organizational context, and worker skill.

Before I close this discussion of the strategies and skills for health care practice I will comment on how workers may be involved in institutional change efforts.

INSTITUTIONAL CHANGE EFFORTS

Chapter 6 reviewed a few of the key assumptions of community and organizational change models. The principles for practice presented in that chapter suggested that involvement in such efforts is part of the health care social worker's ongoing responsibility. Sometimes these efforts are large scale and involve working with other concerned professionals and citizens to effect legislative change. Other efforts are part of the "nitty-gritty" daily work and are focused on what Meyer (1979) terms "making organizations work for people." These efforts include redesigning programs to make them more humane and tailored to individual needs. For example, Fisher (1979) carried on a successful effort to redesign routines in an intensive care unit so that dying patients could continue to interact with family members and others close to them. Previous procedures had relegated many patients to an isolated existence.

My own students, assigned field tasks intended to "follow the demands of the client task" (Chapter 6), have engaged in many innovative endeavors. One student assigned to a "geriatric mental health outreach" program based in a hospital was successful in her efforts to change the name of the program. When she went to churches and senior citizens' centers and was identified as a mental health worker people resisted her outreach efforts. These efforts were intended to help with daily living problems such as recreation, shopping, loneliness, and health problems. The senior citizens viewed the "mental health" label as stigmatizing. A "community program for senior citizens" is a more acceptable term for the program and was adopted.

Another student was instrumental in changing policies concerning use of the health services of a congregate living facility. Residents who had their own physician were initially not allowed to use the health center attached to the facility. Their own physician was often not conveniently located and people worried when they developed symptoms. The student successfully advocated with the hospital that was responsible for the health care center and the local medical community. Students placed in nursing homes have engaged clients to voice the concerns generated by small personal care allowances for newspapers and personal items. They have helped articulate leaders emerge and plead their cause to appropriate regulatory agencies.

Gaining open access can be viewed as a major organizational change effort. This effort involved changing the definition of the social work role so that now a "social-health" rather than a medical definition governs social work involvement with many hospitalized patients. Nobel (1972) describes a successful effort made by a hospital social work department to reach out to community residents who were not fully availing themselves of hospital services.

These types of efforts and the public health–oriented approaches considered throughout this book involve a number of perspectives and skills. Understanding the formal structure and goals of the organization as well as the interpersonal processes that hold the organization together is crucial. For example, changing the name of the geriatric mental health program involved a number of steps: (1) identifying the clients' objections to professionals having strong commitments to the mental health concept as initially defined and (2) learning the processes by which such a change is made because funding sources also are tied to certain categorical definitions of their programs. The effort to facilitate clients' access to the health center of the congregate living facility was not easy. Some physicians saw their incomes threatened. Therefore careful negotiation and documentation were required to avoid resistance. These examples illustrate how creative thinking, coupled with skill and commitment to expanding the scope of service, can improve the problem-solving process.

SUMMARY

This chapter focused on the interventive process in health care and related procedures, strategies, and skills. The skills needed for developing familiarity with the community, the organization, and major health problems are an intricate part of intervention in health care. Stages of the interventive process were identified. The distinctions between long- and short-term contact, the importance of developing good referral skills, the use of groups in health settings, and organizational and community change strategies were discussed.

REFERENCES

Campos, D., and Podell, J.: The role of the culture specialist in crisis intervention, Paper presented at the annual meeting of the Society for Applied Anthropology, Philadelphia, 1979.

Compton, B.R., and Galaway, B.: Social work processes, Homewood, Ill., 1979, The Dorsey Press.

Devore, W., and Schlesinger, E.: Ethnic-sensitive social work practice, St. Louis, 1981, The C.V. Mosby Co.

Dockhorn, J.: Essentials of social work programs in hospitals, Chicago, 1982, American Hospital Association.

Drayer, C., and Schlesinger, E.: The informing interview, American Journal of Mental Deficiency **65:**363, November 1960.

Egan, C.: The skilled helper: a mode for systematic helping and interpersonal relating, Monterey, Calif., 1975, Brooks/Cole Publishing Co.

Epstein, L.: Helping people: the task-centered approach, St. Louis, 1980, The C.V. Mosby Co.

Epstein, L.: Short-term treatment in health settings: issues, concepts and dilemmas, Social Work in Health Care **8**(3):77, 1983.

Euster, S.: Rehabilitation after mastectomy: the group process, Social Work in Health Care **4**(3):251, 1979.

Fandetti, D.V., and Gelfand, D.E.: Attitudes towards symptoms and services in the ethnic family neighborhood, American Journal of Orthopsychiatry **48**(3):477, 1978.

Fischer, J.: Effective casework practice: an eclectic approach, New York, 1978, McGraw-Hill Book Co.

Fisher, D.: the hospitalized terminally ill patient: an ecological perspective. In Germain, C.B., editor: Social work practice: people and environments, New York, 1979, Columbia University Press.

Gardner, M.E.: Notes from a waiting room, American Journal of Nursing **80**(1):86, 1980.

Garrison, V.: The Puerto Rican syndrome in psychiatry and *espiritismo.* In Crapanzano, V., and Garrison, V., editors: Case studies in spirit possession, New York, 1977, John Wiley & Sons, Inc.

Garvin, C.D.: Contemporary group work, Englewood Cliffs, N.J., 1981, Prentice-Hall, Inc.

Glass, L., and Hickerson, M.: Dialysis and transplantation: a mother's group, Social Work in Health Care **1**(3):287, 1976.

Golan, N.: Treatment in crisis situations, New York, 1978, The Free Press.
Meyer, C.H.: Making organizations work for people, Washington, D.C., 1979, National Association of Social Workers.
Middleman, R., and Goldberg, G.: Social service delivery: a structural approach to social work practice, New York, 1974, Columbia University Press.
Monk, A.: Social work with the aged: principles of practice, Social Work **26**(1):61, 1981.
Nobel, M.: Community organization in hospital social service, Social Casework October **53**(8):494, 1972.
President's Commission on Mental Health, Task Panel Reports **3:**appendix, 1978.
Public policy and the frail elderly—a staff report, DHEW Pub. No. (OHDS) 79-20959, Washington, D.C., 1978, Federal Council on Aging.
Sherman, E.: Social work with groups in a hospital setting, Paper presented at a conference on Social Work Groups in Maternal and Child Health, New York, 1979, Columbia University School of Social Work and the Department of Social Work, Roosevelt Hospital.
Shulman, L.: The skills of helping individuals and groups, Itasca, Ill., 1979, F. E. Peacock Publishers, Inc.
Vinter, R.D.: Social group work. In Turner, J.B., editor: Encyclopedia of social work, vol. 15, New York, 1965, National Association of Social Workers.
Wolock, I., Nicholas, C., and Russell, N.: A study of hospital social work services: implications for discharge planning, Paper presented at the annual meeting of the American Public Health Association, Montreal, November, 1982.

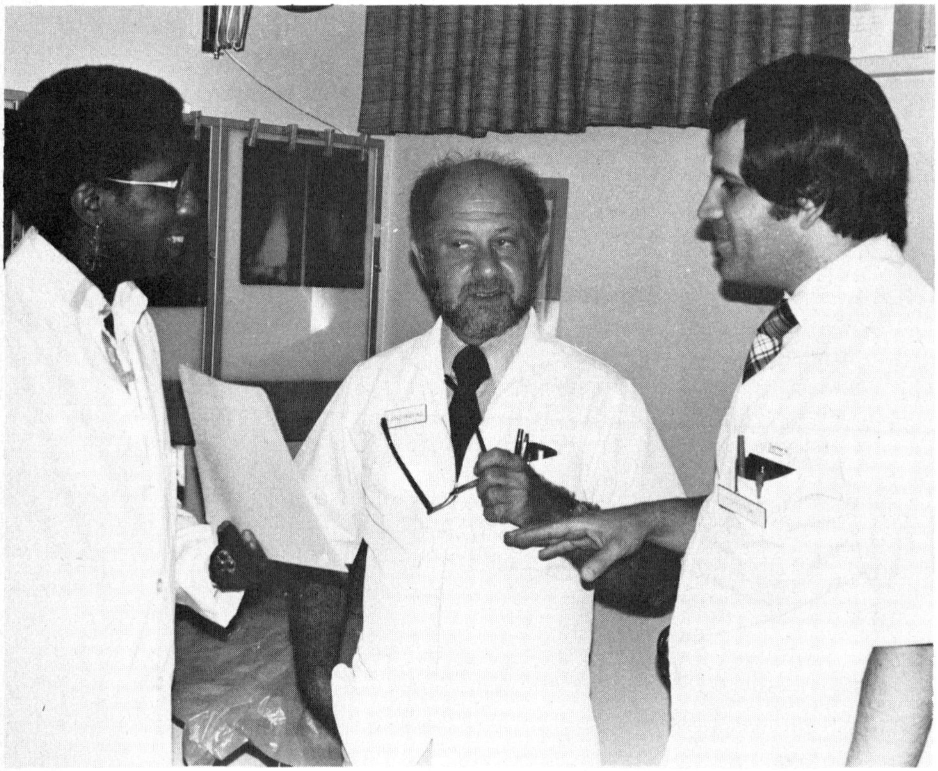

Chapter 8

Interdisciplinary practice

Reflection on the daily, nitty-gritty work of the health care social worker evokes images of a fast-paced, intense, interdisciplinary endeavor. The strategies and skills reviewed in Chapter 7 are almost always carried out in an interdisciplinary context. Thus an impromptu hallway conference between a physician and a social worker is one method of obtaining information needed to facilitate the process of problem identification. A telephone conference between nurse and social worker helps each to keep abreast of the needs of patients for whose care they have different although complementary responsibilities. Planned, regular, highly structured team meetings or rounds, routine in many settings, engage the skills of diverse professionals in the problem-solving process. When epidemiologists, health planners, and social workers join forces with community residents under the auspices of health planning groups, exciting plans for needed restructuring of health care delivery may evolve. These are but a few examples of the interdisciplinary processes typical of health care practice.

Most health professionals cannot, nor are they expected to know and do all that needs to be done about health problems calling for interventive or preventive action. Collaboration, cooperation, and coordination between diverse disciplines are essential components of social work practice in health care. Nevertheless, frustration, tension, and questions about who can or should do what are ever present components of interdisciplinary efforts. Kane (1982) suggests that health care social workers are both fascinated by and preoccupied with these efforts. She characterizes the preoccupation as a "love-hate relationship." A sizeable group of health care social workers cite "the exigencies of multidisciplinary practice and the associated juggling of complex role relationships as the most distinctive feature of social work practice in a health care setting" (p. 2).

Collaborative efforts are usually demanding and often frustrating. Many social workers have the impression that other health care professionals with whom they collaborate are more readily accepted and their roles more clearly defined and understood. Many workers question whether they have sufficient autonomy and whether there are times when collaborative efforts compromise social work values (Dana, 1983; Mailick and Ashley, 1981). These questions and the associated sense of frustration cannot be taken lightly. There is, nevertheless, considerable challenge, excitement, and satisfaction when interdisciplinary efforts are productive and patient care is enhanced.

This chapter draws on a number of formulations that have been used in efforts to understand and facilitate various forms of interdisciplinary collaboration. These formulations serve as the basis for presenting guidelines thought to enhance social work's participation in the collaborative process. Although the inevitable frustrations and tensions cannot be ignored, attention is focused on approaches that may serve to reduce these tensions.

ISSUES IN INTERDISCIPLINARY PRACTICE

A substantial literature has focused on the advantages, dynamics, and problems of interdisciplinary practice. Much of this work has dealt with the interdisciplinary team, defined by Kane (1982) as a "small working group with a commonly espoused purpose, differentiated roles, and ongoing communication processes" (p. 2). Less attention has been paid to other forms of collaboration (Dana, 1983), despite the fact that case-by-case collaboration, case management, and other means by which health care professionals share information and engage in the process of allocating diverse health care tasks are prominent features of daily work in the health setting. For this reason much of the following discussion identifies a number of key issues that are repeatedly noted in discussions of interdisciplinary practice.

Arguments for and against collaboration

Kane (1975), Dingwall (1980), and others have reviewed the rationale that underlies team work. Kane points out the inherent logic of increasing interdependence as knowledge proliferates and tasks become more complex. Dingwall suggests that current professional jurisdictions are arbitrary. However, the problems presented by health care consumers are not neatly arranged in terms of the tasks and functions that have been assigned to various health professions. In the absence of a coordinating structure the burden of integrating, synthesizing, and coordinating services falls on the client. Both Kane and Dingwall point out that incentives for participation in team practice differ for the established and the less prestigious professions. The less prestigious professions like social work—view the team as a "point of entry," as a way of "publicizing their skills," and as a means of "access to clientele." Professionals such as physicians, whose claim to competence is rarely questioned, may be giving up autonomy and some aspects of their function. They also consider the additional time and administrative costs entailed. Kane's discussion helps to clarify why the established professions often resist or ignore the participation and contribution of other professionals. As social workers plan strategies to get a foothold in uncharted areas they might well keep these factors in mind.

When team functions are being planned social workers may introduce new tasks or interventive activities that the established professionals have not considered necessary. In their view these tasks and activities must be justified.

For example, the social worker who wants to introduce group work as a way of enhancing the goals of the rehabilitative team often meets resistance. One reason for that resistance may be physicians' skepticism about how this mode of intervention will further attainment of rehabilitative goals.

The entrenched professions are often persuaded to engage in collaborative efforts if the advantages are clearly perceived. For example, physicians who acknowledge social workers' skill in helping people cope with illness-related anxiety will be ready to collaborate with the social worker. Many may be ready to turn over tasks that they know need doing but prefer not to carry out. For example, convinced that social workers do well with hypochondriacal patients physicians facilitate the referral process. With some exception most health professionals readily identify social workers as the people who link clients to community services.

Thus far I have focused on the incentives and disincentives for participation in collaborative processes, especially the team. These can be summarized both from the perspective of the client and from that of the participating professionals. The client advantages are (1) coordination of skilled services, (2) avoidance of duplication, (3) convenience, (4) relief from the burden of integrating services, and (5) possible introduction of preventive services. Corollary disadvantages are (1) interference with one-to-one relationships, (2) possible miscommunication among team members, and (3) diffused professional responsibility.

The professionals' advantages are (1) simplified access to and communication with other professionals, (2) promotion of learning, (3) access to clients for the less established professions, and (4) awareness that the work of others can facilitate one's own work. Possible disadvantages are (1) the tendency for one profession to dominate; (2) the weakening of any one profession's contribution if roles are blurred, (3) "uninformed" evaluation by professionals outside one's field, and (4) the view of the established professions that the gains are not worth the losses of autonomy or transfer of function (Kane, 1975, p. 12).

When social workers opt for team work the advantages and disadvantages just suggested are worth considerable scrutiny. Although some of the disadvantages also arise in relation to other forms of interdisciplinary practice, they may not be as intense. In considering which type of collaboration is most likely to further patient care goals, and social work's participation in them, it is important to consider the points just presented. The tendency to equate all collaborative efforts with team work may be counterproductive, as is the view that the team is the "epitome of multidisciplinary collaboration, and that all else represents failure" (Kane, 1982, p. 3).

Team processes

Kane (1975, 1978) and Lister (1980, 1982) are two of the many researchers who have analyzed team processes. Kane has analyzed the interprofessional team as a small group. She says the team, like other groups, is composed of individuals encountering diverse norms, making decisions, resolving conflicts, and struggling with leadership. Her classic work is worthy of considerable attention. Only a few of the key concepts, as presented by Kane and elaborated by others, can be touched on here.

These revolve around such issues as the individual's role in the team, team decision making, leadership, size, team communication, and the relationship between personal, team, and professional norms.

The individual in the group. The point that team members are individuals first, professionals second, and interdisciplinary team members third is most important. Kane (1975) and Lister (1982) suggest that success and problems with team approaches can be traced to roles unrelated to the team members' professional status. Referring to personal, formal, and informal roles, Lister suggests that it is both possible and important for team members to identify the respective roles they play. Perhaps as important as learning about their professional roles is attention to the impact of sex roles, ethnocultural roles, and socioeconomic roles.

Kane highlights the fact that some professions tend to be associated with a particular sex or social class (for example, physicians are often middle-class males and social workers and nurses are often women). Analogously, ethnic identification affects perceptions of how pain is expressed or how the sick role is to be played. For these reasons it is often difficult to decide whether professional or personal attributes most explain team members' behavior or intergroup tensions. Lister suggests that health team training programs can serve to identify the sources of judgments. Most interdisciplinary training programs, he suggests, tend to focus on professional roles only, neglecting the impact of interpersonal roles.

Group norms and the team. If teams are to function effectively they must develop team norms and a team culture. These may at times conflict with professional norms or loyalty. Excessive attachment to team norms can have a number of adverse effects. One is the possibility that loyalty to the team will inhibit the application of a distinctive professional viewpoint. Social workers need to guard against the possible violation of client self-determination on such issues as the right to accept or refuse treatment planned by the team.

"Good teams" often seek to reduce conflict to maintain group cohesion. Yet conflict may facilitate the identification of different professional sources of judgment. Social workers, who view themselves largely as team facilitators, run the risk of giving up a distinct social work stance for the sake of reducing conflict. There is also the danger that intense group norms and well-established functioning patterns can lead to inflexibility and resistance to new information that might call for change. For example, for many years I was a member of an "ideal team" at a center for retarded children. Routines and responsibilities were well defined. When appropriate, physicians, social workers, nurses, and speech therapists all participated in counseling parents. The work pace was deliberate, careful, and slow. The clinic's services were highly sought after, and there was usually at least a 6-month waiting list. Because any proposals for reducing the length of the waiting list would disrupt team routines, limited attention was paid to such proposals.

Issues of client advocacy often get lost in team processes. When advocating for a client's right to service or to refuse treatment, social workers may encounter conflict. Mailick and Ashley (1981) have commented on this issue. Social workers, because of their relatively low status and commitment to the team concept, run the risk of abrogating important and distinct contributions if they do not carefully balance these needs and those of the clients served by the team.

Decision making. Closely related to the issues associated with group norms are those involving decision making. The process characterized by Kane as "group think" may deflect attention from articulating the contribution each member can make to decision making concerning patient care. Rubin and Beckhard (1972) suggest that distinct professional contributions will be made if the team consistently asks questions such as the following: Who (or which discipline) has the necessary information? Who must be consulted? Who must be informed? The section of this chapter entitled "The Collaborative Work To Be Done" addresses some of these questions by referring to the types of problems dealt with in interdisciplinary efforts.

The literature on the team has also focused on leadership, team size, and conflict resolution. Large groups tend to need more direction from a designated leader and are more likely to tolerate differences than small, intimate groups.

Clearly teamwork has the potential for conflict as well as cooperation. Mechanisms for tension reduction are essential because tension not acknowledged or resolved can perpetuate mistrust and misunderstanding. Social workers are particularly skilled in facilitating such processes. When using these skills it is important that they do not lose sight of their contribution for the sake of harmony.

• • •

This brief review of the personal and professional issues involved in team processes highlights the potential for effective work and the fact that involvement in such processes is hard work. This work calls for insight, self-discipline, and the ability to compromise when such compromise does not violate basic professional tenets. With these considerations in mind I will now focus on the collaborative work to be done. Some of this collaboration takes place in the context of team work and the remainder is carried out in other ways. With full recognition of the difficulties of collaboration, focus in the following sections is on the work to be done. I hope that the focus on client issues can serve to deflect some of the tensions that consume so much energy.

THE COLLABORATIVE WORK TO BE DONE

In this section attention is focused on a number of health problems and health policy or planning issues. A series of case vignettes illustrates

1. The information needed for efforts of problem identification and resolution
2. The disciplines that are the usual or optimal sources of information
3. The diverse disciplines involved and the tasks they usually carry out in connection with the problem identified
4. The similar or different perspectives and values of various disciplines and the impact these may have on the view of the work called for
5. The impact of the organizational context or auspice on problem definition

Mrs. Mary Jenkins

Mrs. Jenkins, an 85-year-old Black woman, was admitted to the hospital with an ulcerated foot related to diabetes. She is in pain and somewhat confused, although well oriented to time and place. Amputation is ruled out because of her age.

Mrs. Jenkins is widowed and has been living alone across the street from her son, daughter-in-law, and grandchildren. Physicians believe that after discharge from the hospital she should not be left alone because she will not be able to move around unassisted. She would prefer to stay in her own home rather than move into the already crowded family quarters because the family members all work or go to school. The Jenkins are active members of a church that often assists people needing physical, emotional, or financial help.

Kevin Riley

Kevin Riley was born 3 months prematurely to his 17-year-old unmarried mother Joan. Examination revealed low birth weight and meningomyelocele. Because the hospital where he was born was not equipped to deal with seriously ill infants he was immediately transferred to the nearest hospital with a neonatal intensive care unit. That hospital is some distance from Joan's home. Although the prognosis was guarded it was expected that after some months of hospitalization Kevin could be cared for at home with the help of caretakers to tend to his special needs. The long-range outlook for his mental and physical development cannot be predicted at this time.

The Center City Health Planning Council

The social work director of a local health planning group called a meeting of professionals and consumer groups to consider the request of a local hospital to build the additional facilities needed to perform complex cardiac surgery. Three other hospitals in the area already have the capacity to perform such surgery. Previous studies by the council have shown that none of the four hospitals provides comprehensive primary care services.

The Kearny Prenatal Clinic

Kearny Hospital is located in a depressed rural area and serves many low-income women, many of whom are unmarried and in their teens. A review of the records indicates that in the past 5 years a disproportionately high number of these women have given birth to premature infants with birth defects. The rate of repeated out-of-wedlock pregnancies is high, and many of the women do not use any method of contraception.

Mt. Zion Church

Mt. Zion Church serves a Black congregation. The elders are aware that Black men are particularly subject to hypertension and that Black women are particularly at risk for developing diabetes. In an effort to educate their members the elders asked the neighborhood health center for help with providing information and preventive services.

As these types of situations come to the attention of social workers, it becomes clear that the efforts and knowledge of diverse people are needed.

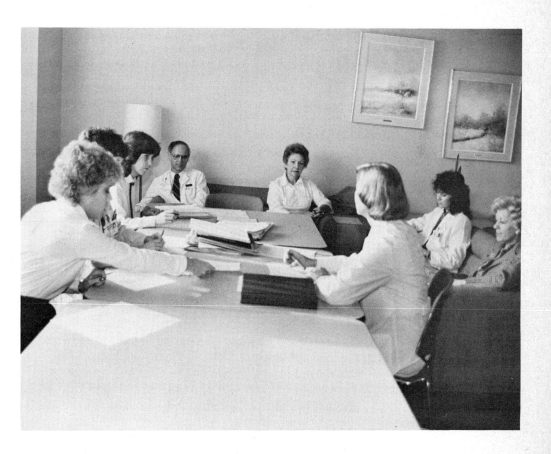

These include health professionals, members of the community, and various welfare resources.

Before any of these problems can be addressed, the issues identified on p. 230 need to be clarified.

Information needed

Although the specific type of information required varies for each situation, some common themes exist. When clear-cut individual medical problems are a major component of the situation, medical information is needed about the disease, its anticipated course, the expected rate of progress or decline, and the type of treatment needed to reverse the course of the disease, slow the decline, or create as much comfort as possible. Also important is information about the physical and psychological impact and the kinds of management routines anticipated (Chapter 5).

The response of patients and those close to them is essential. Do they understand the problem? What are their concerns and questions? What are some of the common consequences when the health problems of populations at risk are involved (such as at the Kearny Prenatal Clinic)? Who would benefit from the allocation of scarce resources (as in the situation of the Center City Health Planning Council)? What would be the likely benefits if money were allocated to build a network of community-based primary health centers?

Likely sources of information

1. Physicians are the logical source of information about individuals' specific medical problems. Their areas of specialty and expertise vary considerably. For example, Mrs. Jenkins' physician might be a family practitioner or a general internist with a subspecialty in vascular disease. A neonatologist is likely to be in charge of Kevin Riley's medical care.
2. Social workers, nurses, and a variety of other health care personnel are all sources of information about the patients' response to the illness. Because of their ongoing contact with patients, nurses often observe if patients and family are despondent or appear to be coping well with the situation. They usually know if there are visitors and how they interact with the patient. A nurse may have a good sense about whether Joan Riley seems comfortable or strained when she comes to visit Kevin in the nursery—and if her parents, as evidenced by how they act on visits, seem ready to help her through the arduous tasks ahead.

   Data on populations at risk are available in written documents from consultation with epidemiologists and others. They need to be combined with information about the community in which work is contemplated and past efforts to involve the population around work on related health problems. Physicians in clinical practice are not likely to be the best source of information because they do not always keep abreast of the information that affects population aggregates.

3. In situations involving judgments concerning the allocation of resources, the preferences of the residents as well as health planners are sources of information. Decisions are less likely to be made on the basis of precise information than on the basis of value judgments concerning a preferred course and influences of the political process.

Resources needed

1. People with defined medical problems clearly have a range of curing and caring needs (Chapter 5). These include medical care, home health care, counseling, financial resources, and many others. Many disciplines, both within and outside the health system, provide such resources.

2. When present problems encompass but move beyond those focused on immediate medical care, perspectives on what resources are needed will vary. Some professionals will perceive the problem in psychological terms and look for psychotherapeutic resources. Others will look to the preventive and ameliorative role of the school, peer group, and family.

3. Resources to aid populations at risk are usually obtained from state or federal funding sources such as the maternal and infant care programs or state health department programs focused on hypertension.

Important in these types of situations is recourse to such resources as churches, benevolent societies, and other community networks. For example, many members of the Mt. Zion Church have undoubtedly been successful in controlling their hypertension. How can their coping skills be used to help others?

Perspectives of various disciplines

Few people are likely to disagree with the basic thrust of the discussion thus far, although they may expand on the formulations or have minor differences. However, more disagreement is likely to be manifest as members of different disciplines draw on their diverse professional and personal values when thinking about the collaborative process. The stress and tension referred to earlier may derive from differences in judgment and values. These differences originate from (1) the incomplete knowledge health professionals often have about the education and expertise of other disciplines; (2) the tendency for most health professionals, especially physicians (Rehr, 1970), to assign most tasks to their own profession rather than to others (Kane, 1975); (3) the difficulties members of different professional groups have communicating with each other; (4) the differences in problem definition that often rise from differences in professional perspectives and education (for example, whether health problems are viewed in narrow medical terms or in social functioning terms); and (5) the fact that in many situations any number of disciplines can provide appropriate service.

One of the more vivid examples of how these differences in perspective affect collaboration is found in the classic work of Banta and Fox (1972). In this study nurses and social workers reflected on overlap and conflicting perspectives on the kind of services required by clients of a neighborhood health center. The nurses viewed themselves as warm, caring, and "intuitively" capable of working with social and psychiatric problems despite their lack of training in this area. Some were reluctant to refer to the social workers who "even though they do service, it isn't sort of rolling up the sleeves . . . I mean touching people" (p. 711). The social workers agreed that the nurses were caring. However, some viewed them as having "rescue-fantasies" and the "inability to set limits," and as being "too ready to get caught up emotionally" and likely to "miss the nuances, because of their absolutist, simplifying view" (p. 712). Other social workers thought the nurses were "inappropriately instrumental" with a tendency to give advice and concrete "things" in an indiscriminate fashion.

The role functioning of the nurses and social workers was in turn affected by physicians with distinct but different views. The social worker's focus on helping people struggle with their own problems contrasted with the views of others who were more likely to provide concrete help and advice is not an uncommon difference in perspective between the two professions. These kinds of differences clearly affect the collaborative process and the variations in perspective.

• • •

These sources of variation may determine whether Mrs. Jenkins is perceived as a patient with a diabetes-related ulceration of the foot or whether she and others like her are viewed as frail, elderly people in need of psychosocial as well as medical care. Social workers will always define the situation in psychosocial terms, but the perspectives of physicians and other professionals usually need to be determined. When physicians define the situation in medical and psychosocial terms they may, and often do, counsel patients and families. Their view of the collaborative work to be done may be limited to asking the social worker to find a home health aide or a nursing home for Mrs. Jenkins. The intricate relationship between Kevin Riley's disability and the family's ability to assume caring functions is likely to be shared by the various professional disciplines involved in neonatal intensive care units.

The effort to reduce the number of low birth weight infants born to low-income women may be defined as a problem calling for environmental modification, resource provision, education, and counseling, or all four. Hypertension control efforts may be defined the same way. Health educators, physicians, nurses, and others may have limited knowledge of the community organization and group process skills that social workers can use in these kinds of efforts.

The organizational context

The organizational context inevitably affects the definition of the collaborative work to be done. Rising hospital costs place increasing limits on extending hospital stays for psychosocial reasons. After all diagnostic and treatment procedures for Mrs. Jenkins' ulcerated foot have been carried out there may be limited time to allow collaborative planning for optimal care to take place. However, in the view of the American Hospital Association (Dockhorn, 1982), the hospital's responsibility does not end when all possible medical procedures related to Mrs. Jenkins' ulcerated foot have been carried out. Part of that responsibility involves engaging in planning for her care after her discharge from the hospital. This includes work with her and others in similar situations on an individual level. It also involves interdisciplinary community outreach efforts.

This discussion of the collaborative work to be done has focused on the complex array of issues confronted by health care social workers. How these issues may be addressed through interdisciplinary functioning is the focus of the balance of the chapter.

INTERDISCIPLINARY BOUNDARIES AND OVERLAP

Given the array of problems presented, it is no wonder that students as well as experienced practitioners are often bewildered. Few situations allow for totally independent decision making by health care social workers. A series of questions about interdisciplinary boundaries and overlap flows logically from the review of the collaborative work to be done. These questions relate to issues of social work autonomy contrasted with dependence on the knowledge and judgment of other health professionals and areas in which there is legitimate and useful overlap between the various disciplines.

1. Which of the identified problems clearly do and do not fall within social work's domain?

For example, linking people with community resources is a long-established social work function. Decisions about whether psychotropic drugs should be used are not social work tasks.

2. Which types of functions may and should be carried out by several disciplines?

For example, many professionals may develop warm, supportive relationships with fearful, anxious people. They may in that process talk with the clients about their fears of their illness, marital problems, and many other concerns. Social workers who view these kinds of interactions as part of their turf are all too likely to feel that their functions are being usurped. This attitude is inappropriate, deprives people of needed support, and can lead to unnecessary turf battles. When social workers are working with someone on explicit problems, they may be able to incorporate the support and advice being given by other professionals into their own work, as follows:

> On the one hand you tell me that people don't care and don't like you. But on the other you keep telling me how helpful the nurse is. Doesn't that tell you something about how people respond to you?

3. How much consultation or "physician sanction" (Dana, 1983) is required when there is no question that social work has expertise in and responsibility for a particular area of work?

For example, does the judgment about what kind of care is required after hospitalization ultimately rest on the medical or psychosocial assessment? In Mrs. Jenkins' situation medical assessment was limited to the judgment that her physical mobility would be seriously impaired. Whether her care could be rendered at home or in a nursing facility depended on a psychosocial assessment of her response and available supports.

4. What circumstances call for independent decision making by the social worker? That is, when does possible resolution of any particular problem essentially relate to psychosocial concerns and social functioning?

For example, if child abuse has been documented, social workers should not need a "doctor's order" concerning appropriate care.

These examples illustrate but do not exhaust the types of issues subsumed under boundary issues. They serve to heighten social workers' sensitivity to and awareness of matters in which they have clear-cut expertise. Energy should be devoted to using that expertise and to demonstrating by action how patient care is facilitated by social work participation. If energy is expended in this way there is less time or need for social workers to fret about being unappreciated.

How does the social worker implement a perspective formed by values, confidence in his or her capability, and understanding of others' contributions? Some of the answers may be found by applying the principles and strategies of the problem-solving process outlined in Chapter 7 to efforts for enhancing interdisciplinary functioning.

INTERDISCIPLINARY EFFORTS AND PROBLEM-SOLVING STAGES

Work before involvement and assessment

Just as workers need familiarity with the community, the recurrent medical problems, and the organizational context, they need a sense of what the prevailing patterns of collaboration have been, especially when first encountering a new setting.

1. When there have been or currently are other social workers in the setting they clearly should be the first consulted to learn how social work is

perceived, sought after, respected, or merely tolerated. Other workers also can provide clues about which disciplines tend to exert considerable control and if this control is exercised through formal or informal channels.

For example, one social worker cites her experience in moving from a psychiatric inpatient unit of a veterans' hospital to a physical rehabilitation center. At the hospital she discovered that nurses made many patient care decisions often through informal means. Therefore she had developed informal relationships with nurses that aided her own work. She assumed the same relationships would be present in the rehabilitation center; however, she quickly learned that the physiotherapists played a major role in the daily management of patients. Consultation with other social workers might have reduced this trial and error stage.*

2. Consultation with other disciplines and administrative personnel can be most useful. Unless there are extreme and untoward tensions, most people will feel flattered when a newcomer seeks their advice on how things ought to be done, how they see social workers fitting in, and what they believe the problems are. Even the most anti–social work chief of surgery may feel pleased when asked and will respond to this kind of approach. When working with community groups such consultation is essential. A stance that conveys the sense of "I need help from you" can set the stage for collaboration.

Launching the interaction process

Most social workers want to be liked and feel needed. They also seek respect for their profession and its contribution. They have strong convictions about the views and needs of human beings that are embodied in social work values. However, because of the frustrations that often accompany interdisciplinary practice, social workers sometimes forget that other professionals have the same need for approval and respect as they do or that they also have major commitments to the norms of their profession. Thus there is some tendency to respond to other disciplines in stereotypical terms. If the social worker is in awe of physicians or perceives nurses as authoritarian and focused on bureaucratic routines, there is a danger that these dispositions will affect the collaborative undertaking. In addition, if social workers seriously doubt that they have an important or unique contribution to make they will readily, albeit unwittingly, convey this message. The techniques of stage setting, tuning in, and attending are important mechanisms for minimizing these and related barriers to collaboration.

Stage setting. In Chapter 7 the discussion of stage setting emphasized the need to be aware of the impact of the physical setting on social work clients. In collaborative work social workers need to think through how the

*Based on conversation with Pat Costante, a former student and current social worker in a rehabilitation institute.

characteristics of the physical setting affect the work. Considerations include attention to the purpose of the exchange, the available space, and how that space can be used to convey a sense of social work autonomy when it is essential. A mental review of possible meeting places includes the hallway, the lounge, the nurses' station, and the workers' or other people's offices.

A creative mix of flexibility and structure can go a long way to facilitating collaboration. Much of the work in many health settings requires continuous, on the spot sharing by health professionals of information needed to carry on daily work. For example, the social worker needs to know from the physician whether a firm diagnosis has been made. The physician may want to know if there will be someone at home to care for Mrs. Jones. A flexible approach to exchanging information suggests that much of this type of work is most productive if carried out on the spot. Despite other more formal collaborative structures, this type of exchange is important and attests to flexibility and readiness to respond to the situation at hand.

Social workers who have established good working relationships with their non-social work colleagues are easily spotted. When they enter a hospital floor or clinic waiting room nurses, patients, physicians, and secretaries stop them to ask questions about resources or progress on plans previously made. The workers also ask questions of the others.

When a formal team structure or rounds are an integral part of the process they need to be planned in advance and a designated space used. Advance planning is needed when the purpose of interdisciplinary encounters is to develop plans, share detailed and sensitive information, or resolve conflicting perspectives. A telephone call or message suggesting a brief meeting in the worker's office or the floor conference room usually brings a positive response. When considering these and other settings for collaboration social workers will not accomplish their objectives if they are oblivious to routines, other people's schedules, or the relative priorities others place on the exchange with the social worker as compared to other elements of their work.

> Doctor, I know you're due in surgery in an hour. I think it will take only a few minutes of your time to tell me what specific types of care Mrs. Polansky needs at home.

There are strategies that convey the message of "I'm in charge." Examples are getting to a meeting early to ensure a place at the head of the table (Middleman and Goldberg, 1974) or holding a meeting on one's own turf.

Chapter 7 briefly referred to high-risk screening. High-risk screening procedures are predicated on the assumption that social work plays a unique and autonomous role in planning for patient care. Implementing that stance can be facilitated if social workers play a key role in planning and organizing how they share the information obtained from screening processes. A daily 30-minute meeting organized by the social worker can translate that stance into action.

The worker's office, if conveniently located, is an ideal spot for such a meeting, but other sites will do. The major point is that in setting the stage social workers not only make a point about their autonomy but also demonstrate their contribution by how they seek and share information and present proposals for action. The worker may review the situation with the physician as follows:

> Six patients were admitted to coronary care this week. Mr. Wu, Mr. Adams, and Mr. Jacob have wives at home who are already asking how they can take care of their husbands when they get better. Mr. Campbell is a bachelor. He apparently has no relatives or close friends near by. Mrs. Smith is a widow; her children live fairly near to her. Mr. Johnson is an alcoholic. We need to worry about Mr. Campbell, Mrs. Smith, and Mr. Johnson. I'll meet with them when you think they're medically ready. Have any of you learned more about their social situations? So far I haven't seen anyone visit Mr. Campbell.

Tuning in and attending. Tuning in and attending are crucial parts of the initial as well as the ongoing work. Although workers may have a good sense of the flow of work and how social workers are perceived, they need to continuously tune in to daily reactions. Is the surgery about to be performed particularly trying or risky? If so, perhaps the request for information can wait. Have the floor nurses developed an especially protective attitude toward an abused child, making them particularly fearful about returning this child to a mother who has battered her in the past? Does this particular group of staff members understand the social worker's role in making judgments about child abuse and in planning for the care of abused children?

Although the hospital has a firmly established open access policy, which of the physicians is skeptical? Which of them consider talking to seriously ill cardiac patients exclusively their function? How do they convey this? By not coming to meetings? By brusque responses to the social worker's questions? When social workers sense these kinds of concerns how might they deal with them?

> Doctor Gray, I know this procedure of meeting daily with me is new. Do you have any questions or suggestions for a different way of sharing information?

or

> Dr. Collins, Mrs. Smith tells me she's very grateful for the conversation you had with her daughter about her condition. She's asked me to ask you how you would feel about me talking to Mary about how it would work out if Mrs. Smith went to stay with her for a few weeks when she's ready to leave the hospital. I could give her information about how a home health aide might help with daily care. Or perhaps you'd rather tell her about it. She can call me if she wants to go ahead with the plans.

PROBLEMS AND ISSUES IN INTERDISCIPLINARY COLLABORATION

Although the issues are clearly varied and complex, for the present purposes I will identify two major types.

1. What are, from the social worker's perspective, the most appropriate and fruitful types of collaboration, given the major problems and tasks and the organizational context?
2. What are the difficulties encountered, regardless of the collaborative process being used?

What type of collaboration

The following questions and others similar to them, if systematically thought through, can facilitate social workers' attempts to affect decisions about the part they can and should play in the collaborative process:

1. What kind of problems lend themselves to "situation-by-situation" collaboration (Dana, 1983)?
2. Do the problems that are typically presented call for sustained, formally planned interaction characteristic of team functioning? If so, what kind of evidence can the social worker present to support the view that a team structure contributes to better care than other forms of collaboration? If a team structure is suggested, which disciplines should logically participate and what are the probable distinct contributions of each? What types of problems can be anticipated in relation to who or which discipline seeks to control team function? In relation to the ways in which members of different disciplines tend to define client problems and their own roles? What are the costs of a team structure compared to those of other types of collaboration?
3. Which forms of collaboration are most likely to allow social workers to function autonomously?
4. Which forms of collaboration are likely to encourage the achievement of health care goals derived from a social work perspective?

The case for situation-by-situation collaboration

Dana (1983) points out that situation-by-situation collaboration is the oldest and remains the most characteristic mode of collaboration. Information and ideas are shared and plans are made as the need arises. Despite the other types of collaboration in use, situation-by-situation interaction should and will remain an integral part of the collaborative process. Examples of this type of collaboration are impromptu hallway conferences about a newly referred patient, information about resources given to a non–social work colleague, and a one-time lecture to a parents' group on problems of drug abuse at the local school.

Research findings on the outcome of team efforts

In her review of the literature on the interprofessional team Kane (1975) found few examples of systematic efforts to evaluate teams on their effectiveness in achieving stated goals, efficiency compared to other types of collaboration, and appeal to clients and professional staff. Halstead (1976) found three categories of studies: (1) statements of belief or faith in the team, (2) descriptions of programs and team concepts, and (3) efforts to investigate the effectiveness of team care in various settings. The last category contained the least amount of work. Some of the literature answered the question "What is the effect of coordinated team care on patients with chronic illness?"

Team care was the treatment variable applied to one population of patients but not to another. Ten studies were involved. In five studies treatment was provided at home or in a clinic by nurses and allied health personnel. In five other studies treatment consisted of comprehensive care provided by a rehabilitation team. The findings are equivocal. In five groups of patients, functional status improved to a greater extent in the experimental group than in the control group. In two no major differences were observed. In the rest there was less physical deterioration in groups treated by the team than in the control group. Although these are limited findings, Halstead does provide some encouraging support for the team concept. He suggests that (1) coordinated team care appears more effective than customary, fragmented care received by people with long-term illness, (2) functional status is more likely to be improved through team care, (3) there seems to be less deterioration and more disease control with team care, and (4) team care is usually associated with increased use of health services.

Blatterbauer, Kupst, and Schulman (1976) focused on another area—the physician-patient relationship. They studied social workers' participation as observers of physician-patient contact and as interpreters of medical information. The social workers' involvement appeared to help parents of children with serious illness incorporate and understand the difficulties more than when the information was transmitted only by the physician.

Beloff and Korper (1972) studied the use patterns of families with multiple social and health problems in relation to a family-oriented health team that included physicians, nurses, health aides, and social workers. The model appeared to increase use of services and decrease amount of physician time involved. The objective was to demonstrate the efficacy of an integrated approach as contrasted with the fragmented and specialized community resources usually used. The results are encouraging for those committed to using teams to improve health care delivery for the poor.

Some conceptual formulations on collaborative models

Mailick and Jordan (1977) identify three types of interdisciplinary models: (1) the authoritative model, (2) the consensus model, and (3) the matrix model. The *authoritative model* is appropriate when the degree of technology inherent in the team task is high and the work clearly requires the direction of one individual. Each member of the group has a high level of expertise and responds to direction of the leader without challenging his or her authority.

This is often true with surgery and medical crisis situations in emergency rooms and with admission to intensive care units. Authoritative team members need clear-cut knowledge of and respect for each other's functions.

If the social worker is a member of this kind of team, agreements about the social worker's role need to be made in advance. For example, there may be an agreement that no new patient in intensive or coronary care will be interviewed by a social worker unless the physician indicates that the medical condition will not be jeopardized by discussion of psychosocial problems. Social workers should be available in the emergency room and know the resources that can and cannot be marshalled in a crisis, such as child protective workers or a list of shelters for the homeless. The social worker should also be skilled in crisis intervention.

The *consensus model* is applicable when task and time constraints are less urgent and there is no single occupational group whose competence is essential for survival. Many teams fall into this category. In rehabilitation centers physicians may determine the thrust of physical rehabilitative efforts. However, physiotherapists are also active, usually on a long-term basis, in efforts to help patients regain mobility. Social workers should focus on the long-range process of identifying responses to the illness and helping coordinate resources for return to the home. This process involves making needed physical alterations and accepting the functional limitations imposed by the illness.

This kind of long-range planning involves intense team deliberations. There may be disagreement about how the patient's physical and psychosocial status is affecting progress. Patient care may be enhanced or constrained by the degree to which the team successfully solves its own role strains and jealousies about who is in charge of the patient. Certain components of dialysis care fall in this category. The technical job of dialysis is clearly a medical one with nurses performing most of the work involved in treatment. However, patient response is monitored by both nurse and social worker, whose roles may overlap in the degree to which they become involved in emotional issues.

In the *matrix model* communication patterns are informal, and roles are highly interchangeable. The psychiatric ward, where milieu therapy is operative, or the medical ward are characteristic situations in which the unique quality of each profession's expertise is likely to be submerged in daily activities. Because occupational boundaries can easily overlap there is potential for both conflict and ideal collaboration responsive to patients' needs. In this type of collaborative model the social worker's role involves resource delineation and linkage with community systems.

In their discussion Mailick and Jordan (1977) underscore the point made by Kane (1982) that team work, in its formal sense, is only one type of collaboration. The previous illustrations suggest that the team is most useful when the problems addressed are protracted, prolonged, and shifting. The work of Halstead (1976) and of Beloff and Korper (1972) suggests that use of health services by those who have difficulty dealing with traditional delivery systems is enhanced by well-planned team approaches.

Other collaborative models such as case-by-case or on-the-spot collaboration are viable ways of bringing diverse skills to bear on patient care, as are the coordinating functions carried out by the case manager.

A number of people have raised questions about whether confidentiality is violated in the collaborative process. There is no ready-made answer to this question. Professional judgment and ethics determine when it is appropriate to withhold information for fear that the team will use the information in a destructive manner. If that fear arises frequently the social worker needs to reexamine the relationships that have been established and the values that are operative.

Similar concerns are raised about advocacy. Mailick and Ashley's point (1981) on this issue is well taken.

> Social workers cannot lay special claim to having a higher level of knowledge or devotion to the welfare of the client than other professions. Each professional group has a formal or informal code of ethics that espouses the primacy of client need (p. 135).

Nevertheless, the definition of primacy varies. Advocating in opposition to team culture may generate tension between team members. Persistent accusations that other professionals' stances are anti-client will negate the social worker's contribution. As stated in respect to withholding information, reevaluation is indicated if other collaborators constantly appear to be violating patient rights or defining problems in ways antithetical to social work.

The social worker should develop guidelines that determine what practices of other professionals require a social work advocacy stance. Implicit reference was made to this in the discussion of values in Chapter 6. These guidelines include violation of the right to self-determination (such as efforts to impose treatment modalities or other forms of care) and judgments based on stereotypes of race, class, or gender that may lead to attributing pathology when little exists.

No one mode of collaboration is ideally suited to enhancing social work autonomy. Independent case finding facilitates control over quality and quantity of work. Mailick and Ashley (1981) suggest an answer to the question of autonomy.

> The collaborative process is useful to social workers because it encourages a structure for cooperation, a culture for consultation, and development of consensus among professionals. It promotes the inclusion of social workers in planning and execution of services . . . regularizes . . . social workers' contacts with other professionals and secures their inclusion in the interprofessional group (p. 133).

SUMMARY

This chapter has focused on various components of interdisciplinary practice. Key dynamics of such practice were summarized. A series of case vignettes was used to identify the diverse problems that call for collaborative efforts and the contributions that can be expected from diverse professionals. Some components of the problem-solving process were used to illustrate the procedures and strategies that can facilitate interdisciplinary work. Three models of collaboration were reviewed to highlight how differences in technology and task urgency affect formal and informal role definition.

REFERENCES

Banta, H.D., and Fox, R.C.: Role strains of a health care team in a poverty community, Social Science and Medicine **6**:697, 1972.

Beloff, J.S., and Korper, M.: The health team model and medical care utilization, Journal of the American Medical Association **219**(3):359, 1972.

Blatterbauer, S., Kupst, M.J., and Schulman, J.L.: Enhancing the relationship between physician and patient, Health and Social Work **1**(1):45, 1976.

Dana, B.: The collaborative process in social work. In Miller, R.S., and Rehr, H., editors: Social work issues in health care, Englewood Cliffs, 1983, Prentice-Hall, Inc.

Dingwall, R.: Problems of teamwork in primary care. In Lonsdale, S., Webb, A., and Briggs, T.L., editors: Teamwork in the personal social services and health care, Syracuse, N.Y., 1980, Syracuse University School of Social Work.

Dockhorn, J.: Essentials of social work practice in hospitals, Chicago, 1982, American Hospital Association.

Halstead, L.S.: Team care in chronic illness: a critical review of the literature of the past 25 years, Archives of Physical and Medical Rehabilitation **57**(2):507, 1976.

Kane, R.A.: Interprofessional teamwork, Manpower Monograph No. 8, Syracuse, N.Y., 1975, Syracuse University School of Social Work.

Kane, R.A.: The interprofessional team as a small group. In Bracht, N.F., editor: Social work in health care, New York, 1978, The Haworth Press.

Kane, R.A.: Teams: thoughts from the bleachers (editorial), Health and Social Work **7**(1):2, 1982.

Lister, L.: Role expectations of social workers and other health professionals, Health and Social Work **5**:41, 1980.

Lister, L.: Role training for interdisciplinary health teams, Health and Social Work **7**(1):19, 1982.

Mailick, M.D., and Ashley, A.: Politics of interprofessional collaboration: challenge to advocacy, Social Casework **62**:131, 1981.

Mailick, M., and Jordan, P.: A multimodel approach to collaborative practice in health settings, Social Work in Health Care **2**(4):445, 1977.

Middleman, R., and Goldberg, G.: Social service delivery: a structural approach to practice, New York, 1974, Columbia University Press.

Rehr, H.: Comparison of health care professionals in predicted outlook of patient compliance and in general attitudes regarding collaboration in health care, doctoral dissertation, New York, 1970, Columbia University.

Rubin, I., and Beckhard, R.: Factors influencing the effectiveness of health teams, Milbank Memorial Fund Quarterly; Health and Society, **50**:317, July-Oct. 1972.

COLLEGE of
MEDICINE and DENTISTRY
of NEW JERSEY

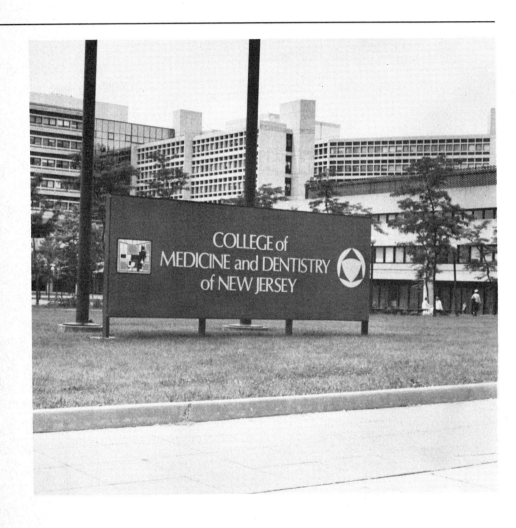

Chapter 9

Social work in hospitals

Social work's involvement in health care is as old as the profession itself. The subspecialty formerly known as "medical social work" originated in 1905 when Dr. Richard Cabot of Massachusetts General Hospital in Boston invited social worker Ida B. Cannon to join the staff of the hospital for the purpose of "(opening) our eyes to the *backgrounds of medical work*" (Cabot, 1915, p. 32)—social, educational, and preventive activities. Cabot and Cannon are viewed as pioneers in the development of this new form of social service. Commenting on Cannon's work, Bartlett (1975) states:

> She always kept the individual patient's needs in the central focus, continually interpreted the social aspects of illness as a basic concept, and emphasized the teamwork of the professions—medicine, nursing, social work, and others. Thus she built an enduring model which spread throughout this country and beyond (p. 208).

From these early beginnings has grown a recognized and expanding sphere of social work practice. Phillips (1977) points out that despite the expansion of medical social services into a variety of settings, they are still predominantly offered under the aegis of hospital social service departments.

The hospital social worker's role is complex and includes many functions. Some of these are commonly carried out in all hospitals; others are either stressed or deemphasized, depending on the focus of the medical services rendered. A number of issues concern all hospital social workers—the degree of autonomy concerning decisions about their work, the extent to which their work is understood and appreciated, the part they can or should play in determining policies of hospital-wide care, and the hospital's relationship to the community.

Most health care social work is carried out in hospitals. The hospital, as already noted, plays a key role in contemporary health care. Together these factors suggest that it is important to continue to clarify the role of the hospital social worker. That is the aim of this chapter. First I will focus on the hospital and the various types of services rendered. I will discuss some theoretical formulations that help clarify the nature of hospital decision making and the social worker's role in the hospital hierarchy. I refer in particular to the dual authority system (Smith, 1958) and to the compelling demands for cure and care that face most hospitals. I will also consider the organization of hospital social work departments, their relationship to the hospital's administrative structure, and their responsibility for a socially oriented approach to care.

In the past decade there has been considerable refinement of research in hospital social work practice. The results of these efforts have quickly been translated into guidelines for practice, especially in such areas as identifying hospitalized patients most in need of social work intervention. Discharge planning, or effective planning for hospital care after discharge, has always been one of the major functions carried out by hospital social workers. For some time social workers tended to downgrade this function, viewing it as concrete "scut" work not worthy of trained professionals. Rising hospital costs, the role of third-party payers, and the thrust toward accountability have once again put the issue of discharge planning at the forefront of hospital social work concerns. Considerable attention is paid to discharge planning, which may be viewed as work with people who are often facing the most frightening, threatening, and life-altering situations they have ever had to confront. Relationships with other disciplines also are discussed as appropriate.

THE HOSPITAL IN AMERICAN SOCIETY

Hospitals can be characterized along a number of dimensions. One revolves around the degree to which they are organized to provide acute, chronic, or specialized care. Each of these types of hospitals provides both in patient and outpatient care.

Many people have the general hospital in mind when they think of THE HOSPITAL. It is often glorified, as in many current television programs, or vilified, as in periodic exposés. Whichever description is presented, neither conveys the total complexity. The general hospital has been termed "the fastest growing component of health care since the turn of the century, particularly since the '30's [and] has increasingly replaced the home and the doctor's office as the focus of physician's treatment and nursing care" (Anderson and Anderson, 1979, p. 373). More recent analysis (Anderson and Gevitz, 1983) suggests that

> Despite all the rhetoric to deemphasize it relative to other elements in the health services spectrum, the general hospital will remain a pivotal component. This is inherent in the technological imperative of medicine and society in general (p. 315).

Various factors are responsible for the increase in hospital care and the central role it has come to play in health care delivery. These include the provision of health insurance to cover the cost of care, federal financing of hospital facilities (particularly the Hill Burton Act of 1946), and the rapid escalation of medical care technology. As suggested by Anderson and Gevitz, much technology-intensive care can only be rendered in hospitals.

The term *hospital* conjures up many images in contemporary society. Some equate it with the large, awesome, new medical center complex, the "house of hope" (Fuchs, 1974), and the place where medical miracles occur. Eager, well-trained staff members are viewed as ministering to a variety of needs. Others view the hospital with fear and as a place to die, as many people did years ago when only paupers went to hospitals. Still others think of the small community hospital where a homelike atmosphere prevails. Hospitals also include large state psychiatric hospitals, veterans' hospitals, and other hospitals serving special population groups. Clearly the term *hospital* encompasses many meanings.

Fuchs' description (1974) is apt:

> The American hospital is large, impersonal, and dominated by elaborate technology. The American hospital is small, inefficient, underequipped, and understaffed. The American hospital exists primarily to further the professional and economic interests of physicians. The American hospital exists to serve the community. The American hospital is crowded to the point of inefficiency and even danger, and serious delays are encountered in obtaining admission. The American hospital is often half-empty, and many of its patients should be at home or in extended-care facilities. The American hospital is the noblest expression of the philanthropic impulse. The American hospital is a business run to show a profit for its owners. Will the "real" American hospital please stand up? (p. 79).

Fuch's tongue-in-cheek description captures many truths about the contemporary American hospital. It is not uncommon to characterize hospitals as the "physicians' workshop in which physicians practice their skills in line with available scientific knowledge and technology" (Boaz, 1977, p. 551). In university-based hospitals, teaching and research goals are often paramount as patient care is organized to serve these goals.

Hospitals are clearly multifaceted institutions that employ a wide variety of personnel and serve diverse costly health care needs. Hospital costs account for about 40% of total American health care expenditures. The growth in hospital costs has been of major concern to many. Half of the increased costs are accounted for by inflationary labor, food, and supply costs; increases in use are responsible for another 10%; the remaining 40% results from increases in service intensity. Service intensity is in large measure related to the technological advances variously noted. Much attention is paid to increasing hospital costs and ways to reduce these costs. Discharge planning is dramatically affected. Efforts to control cost, including the new reimbursement mechanisms (such as the prospective payment plans discussed in Chapter 2), all affect the hospital social worker's daily activity. Who owns hospitals and for whose benefit hospitals are operated are questions that become more and more difficult to answer.

Hospital ownership: increase in public/private mix

It was customary for many years to identify three basic types of ownership: (1) government, including federal, state, and local; (2) nonprofit, private, or voluntary; and (3) proprietary. Traditionally there was a clear-cut distinction between proprietary hospitals, which, like businesses, are run to make a profit for their owners, and the nonprofit voluntary hospitals. These distinctions are becoming increasingly blurred in hospitals, as in other sectors of health and social services (Kane, 1982; Reichert, 1982). Reichert points out that the health care system, especially the hospital, is now thought of as an industry. Stock is purchased by major investment firms and "economic concentration in chain enterprises, franchise operations, conglomerates, and large hospital complexes has taken place" (p. 173). The "impelling dynamic toward competitive growth" and the "focus of profit" are the same for voluntary and profit enterprises (p. 174). Writing in the *Journal of the American Medical Association,* Wright and Allen (1983) echo a similar theme. Large investor-owned *mediglomerates* "own, manage, and/or operate hundreds of hospitals . . . " (p. 48).

A number of factors have contributed to this trend. They include the high costs of running hospitals, the influx of funds via third-party payers, and the increasing managerial skill needed to run complex organizations such as hospitals. "Indeed, hospital administrators have already become financial managers. . . . To survive in an ongoing struggle for resources, the hospital will have to take on more corporate characteristics . . . (Anderson and Gevitz, 1983, p. 315). This trend is of major concern to some social workers. Reichert (1982) has made a comprehensive analysis of the existing and potential impact of what he terms "market system penetration" into the health and social services. He suggests that an emphasis on marketing and profit has a negative effect on efforts to ensure access to care, "service comprehensiveness and continuity," and public health–oriented efforts to identify and reach out to populations at risk. He contends that services enhancing the hospital's competitive position will receive emphasis. Wright and Allen's comments (1983) suggest there is validity to Reichert's contention. Referring to the mediglomerates, they state

> These organizations have discovered marketing, know the relationship between marketing and advertising, and consequently do extensive marketing research and analysis on customers within their geographical target market areas. . . . They advertise and promote their hospitals in an attempt to create appealing images of their facilities, thus engendering "customer loyalty" and repeated visitation behavior (p. 48).*

Services for the most needy populations are not always profitable. Social workers are asked to engage in efforts to effect "cost savings through stringent discharge programs . . ." (Reichert, 1982, p. 177). Social workers will want to watch these developments carefully. As they function in hospitals they need to be acutely aware of these facts about hospital costs, ownership, and the increasing business orientation of the hospital. However social workers view this development, it surely has an impact on the nature of services rendered.

Services provided

Regardless of ownership, complex and multiple services are rendered. Anyone who has ever sought to find a loved one in one of the hospital's many wings will notice the profusion of signs, signals, and arrows that indicate the diverse work carried out. One set of colored arrows may point to the "blue wing" where one finds patients being treated for general medical or surgical problems. Signs indicating that only members of the immediate family may visit in small groups of two for brief periods are often posted in intensive and coronary care units where those most seriously ill may be attached to cardiac monitors, respirators, and intravenous bottles. In dialysis units people spend many hours several times weekly undergoing this intensive form of treatment. In the emergency room are those with minor fractures or suspected heart attacks, and accident victims. There are also lonely, destitute, disoriented people and those who, lacking a home, hope the hospital will offer food and shelter for a night or two. An inconspicuous sign on which is inscribed "Project Haven"* tells the initiated that the hospital has a "hospice program" designed to provide special care for the terminally ill—either in their own homes or in the hospital. That type of care usually involves the cessation of active life-saving efforts and seeks to help those who can no longer benefit from active treatment to die in comfort and dignity.

A more cheerful atmosphere pervades the "yellow areas" that may include the obstetrics wing where happy families bring toys and clothing for welcome newborns. Tension and distress may surface in the nearby neonatal intensive care unit where premature infants or those with multiple physical problems are kept under close observation. A busy ambulatory care division also is found in many hospitals. There people come with a variety of illnesses. The social work department may be located near the main entrance or scattered through a variety of floors.

Hospitals, now often called medical centers, may have more than one dimension. For example, a mental health institute and an institute for physical rehabilitation may be relatively autonomous units within the larger complex. If the center or hospital carries out major teaching functions, students of various health professions may be seen eagerly watching their mentors, waiting for the opportunity to carry out important procedures. Some hospitals have developed extended care facilities for those no longer needing acute care. These facilities

*Noted on a recent visit to a hospital developing a hospice program by that name.

may be located on the grounds or nearby. Primary care units—such as family practice residency programs—may be located on the hospital grounds—as they train various providers to provide comprehensive care in settings simulating the conditions of private medical practice.

The modern hospital can indeed be awesome, exciting, and confusing.

Who works in hospitals?

Chapter 2 referred to diverse types of health professionals. Emphasis was on physicians, nurses, and social workers. Other people working in a hospital are administrative personnel, office staff, aides, orderlies, clergy, physiotherapists, occupational therapists, and psychologists.

Amidst this array of services, needs, personnel, and technology social workers seek to delivery social services and to make an impact on how the services of the hospital are rendered. Social workers working with these individuals require an understanding of the major ways in which hospitals are organized and administered and the prevailing sources of power and decision making.

Organizational goals and administrative structure

A number of conceptual formulations are useful in efforts to identify primary hospital goals, their administrative structure, the basis on which decisions are made, the source of power, expertise, and the delegation of function. The literature on human service organizations, on the source of physician dominance, and on the increasing importance of caring functions aids in clarifying both the tension and the satisfaction experienced by many hospital social workers.

One important work (Hasenfeld, 1983) makes a distinction between organizations that aim to change, process, and sustain people. The first type of institution, including schools, prisons, and hospitals, hopes to effect dramatic alterations in the way people think, believe, and behave. Most treatment organizations fall into this category. The second type of institution is less concerned with shaping people's lives than with assigning a label that evokes reactions from other people. An example is the label *cancer patient,* which is expected to make others behave to those labeled in an appropriate manner. Sustaining organizations seek to prevent, maintain, or retard deterioration of their clients' condition. In this classificatory scheme they do not attempt to change their personal attributes.

Clearly these goals overlap. Hasenfeld points out that hospitals have both "people-processing" and "people-changing" goals. The physician who performs successful coronary bypass surgery is fulfilling a people-changing goal. Others may give palliative treatment and suggest that functioning has diminished to the point that lifelong skilled nursing care (such as that provided in a nursing home) is required. These physicians are fulfilling a people-processing function.

In terms of the themes developed in this book, a curing stance can roughly be equated with people-changing; a caring stance involves many activities, some of which are people-processing and others are people-sustaining. For the social worker these translate into efforts to locate the proper nursing home, home health facility, or school for a disabled child or helping patients and others accept their newly defined states of disability.

When hospital social workers attempt to alter the feelings and behavior of the mentally and physically ill they assume a curing stance. Many view themselves as allies with physicians or as independent participants in the therapeutic or curing process. However, many health professionals view the social worker as carrying out a people-processing role because that term is appropriately applied to efforts to move patients who can no longer benefit from medical intervention out of the hospital.

Based on her study of several Canadian hospitals Watt (1977) concludes that others view the function of the medical social worker as intervening in some way with patients who do not fulfill physicians' expectations of appropriate attitudes and behaviors related to illness or hospitalization. This category includes those whose illness does not have an organic base, those with chronic illness requiring alternate forms of care, and those who "in one way or another, disrupt the highly routinized functioning of the acute treatment hospital" (p. 14).

As social workers compare their goals to those of the hospital and the dominant professionals within it (physicians), their own people-changing goals may be at variance with the people-processing goals and functions with which others identify them. The view of cure and care presented earlier suggests that hospital social workers can usefully carry out both functions. However, their claim to a clearly defined technology, one that is associated with curing, is tenuous. Social work's claim to expertise about the social response and antecedents of illness is more solidly based, as is its knowledge of community resources and its ability to use and link hospital patients with those resources.

The distinctions between people-processing and people-changing help categorize and define the hospital social worker's diverse roles. Both are legitimate, useful functions. However, many social workers have traditionally identified with and preferred to play a therapeutic or people-changing role. Many resent the view that social workers primarily provide support services and are instrumental in obtaining concrete resources. This resentment is one of the sources of tension between hospital social workers and other hospital personnel. Closely related to this is the fact that increasing numbers of people need the type of care provided by sustaining institutions. Often more of these institutions are needed than are available. Many individuals explicitly or implicitly blame social workers for being unable to move people out of the hospital quickly. Tension also occurs because efforts to carry out these activities in a caring way are not as highly valued as are the functions performed by physicians.

Dual authority system and decision making

The value placed on physicians' services derives from the hospital's major goal of curing and the physicians' presumed technological expertise. The value of the physicians' services and the resultant power to affect all areas of hospital functions relate to the physicians' command of technology. Technology is based on "a body of knowledge that ensures, within certain limits, the success of the transformation process, enabling the training of personnel to perform necessary tasks" (Hasenfeld and English, 1974, p. 13). It is characterized by the degree to which desired outcomes are clearly defined and the knowledge assuring that, given a certain state, application of the technology will yield predictible outcomes. Clearly social work is far from achieving this level of technology. However, physicians presumably possess this level of technology. In a seminal article Smith (1958) relates this belief in the physicians' command of technical expertise to two lines of authority in the hospital—lay and professional.

> There is almost no administrative routine established in hospitals which cannot be (and frequently is) abrogated or countermanded by a physician claiming medical emergency or by anyone acting for the physicians claiming medical necessity. . . . Although the conventional organization chart portrays the position of the medical staff as outside the line of authority, we observed physicians to be exerting power throughout the hospital structure at all levels. . . (p. 469).*

Bracht (1978) expands on this line of reasoning, suggesting that hospitals are characterized by a dual authority system, a division of labor, and an authoritarian nature. He suggests that while the physicians' authority and power rest primarily on medical knowledge and skill, social workers expand this base of authority and power by participating in planning and policy groups in the hospital. Such participation places more emphasis on expertise than on the caring components of treatment.

Schlesinger and Wolock (1982) support the validity of this proposal in their 1975 and 1981 comparisons of selected New Jersey hospital social work departments. The study revealed that in the intervening period the departments increased their participation in hospital-wide planning activities and in diverse hospital groups that plan various aspects of patient care. The data showed increasing social work integration in hospital decision making. This finding is in keeping with the position of the American Hospital Association (Dockhorn, 1982) that social workers must participate in planning and developing programs involving the social components of care. Numerous investigators have identified the importance of such activity as one way of increasing the

* Noting that these observations were made more than 25 years ago, I asked an astute social worker who is now a hospital administrator whether this conception had perhaps become outmoded. His vehement response was "You must be kidding!"

scope of social work influence (Hirsch and Lurie, 1969; Wattenberg, Orr, and O'Rourke, 1977; Wax, 1968). Much of this work suggests that "as the structure and mission of hospitals has changed and expanded, the social components of health care has had increased acceptance" (Wattenberg, Orr and O'Rourke, 1977, p. 286).

These are promising developments for expanding and enhancing social work's long-standing participation in hospital-based care. They indicate a greater recognition of the need for care as well as cure, social work's accelerating efforts to refine its knowledge and skills base, and the functions carried out by social workers.

> Concomitant with the excitement and challenge experienced by social workers in a hospital setting is the long standing sense that their role is misunderstood, undervalued and secondary to that played by other more dominant and prestigious members of the hospital staff. Blackey's 1956 analysis of social work in the hospital . . . remains pertinent as a synthesis of the source of strain, challenge and professional goals. She identifies the struggle of the profession seeking recognition in a host setting where the authority and prestige of medicine—the dominant profession—are closely linked to the hospital's major focus on illness and its treatment. Social work's emphasis on health and social strength is contrasted with the focus on pathology inherent in the medical model.
>
> The recent but accelerating emphasis on hospital cost control and earlier patient discharge has focused extensive attention on the social work role.
>
> [This] emphasis can be perceived as a "double edged" sword. Direct and indirect positive effects of cost consciousness can be see in the proliferation of work focused on the development of peer review mechanisms, identification of problem taxonomies, specification of outcome criteria and patient information systems. . . .
>
> Clearly, hospital social work is in a period of ferment . . . (Schlesinger and Wolock, 1982, pp. 59-61).

That ferment is reflected in numerous ways. The remainder of this chapter focuses on various aspects of hospital social work organization and function that help social workers further identify those components of hospital practice that promise productive response to challenge, excitement, and ferment.

THE HOSPITAL SOCIAL WORK DEPARTMENT

In an official publication of the American Hospital Association, Dockhorn (1982) delineates the role of the hospital and social work's responsibilities in the hospital.

> Today the hospital has responsibilities that not only include preventive, rehabilitative, and follow up services, but also extend beyond these services to leadership in making comprehensive care a reality for persons in the community it serves (p. 1).

When meeting these responsibilities the hospital is obliged to draw on social work expertise in (1) counseling patients and families about the internal and external stresses that may interfere with the effectiveness of medical treatment; (2) establishing relationships with community groups and developing community resources, including developing new programs for people whose needs are not met by established programs; (3) and helping people with diverse ethnic and cultural backgrounds whose needs for care may not be met by prevailing programs.

Several broad service categories are identified by Dockhorn (1982), including services to patients, their families, and the community. Participation in key hospital committees is expected of social workers, and service to the community is encouraged. Social work participation on health and welfare councils and in community action groups joins the hospital and the community in efforts to achieve common goals. Participation in professional organizations such as the Society for Hospital Social Work Directors and the National Association of Social Workers enables social workers to share knowledge with other concerned, informed professionals and community leaders. They can initiate and support activities aimed at providing facilities and services needed by various patient groups, as well as promote coalitions to develop the power necessary to influence policy and regulatory and legislative changes. Social workers' management skills "combined with their abilities to collect and analyze data and document needs, can be forceful spiers to action" (Dockhorn, 1982, p. 14). Consultation, advocacy, collaboration, education, and research to document current needs are thus viewed as proper and necessary activities of hospital social work departments.

Organization

Although the sizes of departments and hospitals vary considerably a number of guidelines apply to all. Social workers may be assigned to a number of different units but are expected to be professionally accountable to the social work department. In large hospitals assignment to various departments or program units (for example, medicine, surgery, pediatrics, or psychiatry) is desirable. Such assignment facilitates joint planning and ongoing participation with other personnel in that unit. It also improves the collaborative processes discussed in the preceding chapter because it allows ongoing relationships to develop.

Personnel

Social work directors should have a master's degree in social work, administrative experience, and preferably experience in another health setting. Such experiences will help them cope with the complex and delicate administrative tasks that arise when social work functions in a host setting. There are also other levels of social work personnel. They are those with master's degrees in social work who, by virtue of such education, are held accountable to act in accord with professional ethics and have command of prevailing knowledge and skill. BSW or other undergraduate level workers should have consistent supervision from a person with graduate training.

Departments may and do employ social service technicians and community or family health aides who live in the community and can be helpful in interpreting local mores and customs. Volunteers and clerical specialists also perform important functions. Additionally, it is not uncommon for members of other disciplines to function as part of the social work program. These may be researchers or nurses with expertise in determining nursing needs for those about to be discharged from the hospital.

Although the specific lines of responsibility and authority vary, the hospital social work director is ultimately accountable to the hospital administration and must function within mandates operative in the hospital.

Financing

Usually hospital social services are not directly reimbursed, either by direct patient fees or by third-party payment mechanisms. The costs are considered overhead costs in the hospital's budget. The emphasis on hospital cost control was noted earlier. Consequently, hospital social work departments are under increasing pressure to demonstrate that they are efficient and that their services can save the hospital money. An increasing amount of literature has been devoted to finding ways of documenting such cost savings and to the revenue-producing components of hospital social work services (for example, Nason and Delbanco, 1976; Rosenberg, 1980; Rosenberg and Weissman, 1981; Simmons, 1978). This thrust and the implied emphasis on cost compared to care is distressing to some. However, it is a trend that is not likely to diminish. Social workers who understand financing mechanisms and can contribute to hospital income without violating the tenets of good patient care will make a major contribution.

Management

It is not the intention of this section to review the diverse management and supervisory skills called for in managing a social work department in a large, complex organization like a hospital. Rather, this discussion is focused on a number of strategies that are useful in enhancing the quality of care. Hallowitz (1971) describes one way of conveying the message that the department is understaffed—reduce coverage. Although this was difficult for the social workers in his department, he obtained an increase in his social work staff. Services were selected for reduced coverage on the basis of social work assessment of need, receptivity of other staff to social work, and the social worker's interest in following through with the decision to reduce coverage. Redefining priorities via such mechanisms as high-risk screening highlights areas of need.

Fisher (1982) presents examples of reimbursement for hospital social work services using data on the revenue-producing components of service. She calculates the fiscal impact of providing social work services in an outpatient clinic and in the emergency room. She shows that without social work evening coverage in emergency rooms the number of admissions for protective services (for people without medical need) is increased at substantial cost to the hospital. The same is true for many frail elderly individuals who need community support services and not medical care when they come to the clinic or emergency room.

These and other reports (for example, Coulton and Butler, 1981; Rosenberg, 1980) suggest contrasting the costs of paying for social work services with the costs generated when such services are not available has increasingly become an important management function. This fruitful approach requires a "hard nosed" look at what we do, and a willingness to take risks such as those identified by Hallowitz.

THE HOSPITAL SOCIAL WORKER IN ACTION

There are a number of ways to describe and categorize the hospital social worker's activities. One way is to categorize by activities commonly performed, such as discharge planning and screening. Another method of categorization is by tasks commonly generated by attachment to a particular hospital service or program. Although these two methods overlap considerably (for example, almost all hospital social workers carry out discharge planning functions), this effort to present an image of the hospital social worker in action focuses first on those actions that apply to all areas of hospital social work and second on some of the unique and distinct elements that characterize various programs.

Discharge planning

The traditional function of discharge planning has not always received the thought or attention it deserves. Kane (1980) cites comments made by a student that are familiar to those involved in education for social work health care practice. The student believed that social work in hospitals does not require a high level of psychosocial skill because it consists largely of discharge planning. Kane's efforts to refute this "fallacy wrapped in a fallacy" demand detailed examination. One belief revolves around the identification of discharge planning as a "low-skill" activity, "alleged to be concrete, routine, and apart from the world of high emotion and troubled relationships" (p. 2). The present discussion takes as a given Kane's assertion that

> Nothing could be further from the truth! In fact, discharge planning is one of the most intellectually demanding, skill-dependent activities in the social worker's repertoire. Few time-limited social work interventions have such significance for better or worse, particularly when the discharge plan may be life long institutional care (p. 2).

Kane's comments point out that much planning for care after hospitalization is laden with fear and uncertainty.

The perfunctory emphasis that is too often placed on discharge planning and the low esteem attached to this work result in negating the basic social work tenet of actively involving clients in decisions affecting their own future. Instead, faced by hospital pressures to "get the patient out" and their own need to leave time for "more therapeutic work," social workers "rush to a decision prompted by helplessness; or conversely, rush to a decision prompted by panic and a sense of time running out. In either case, thoughtful consideration of the practical and emotional consequences of the various alternatives have been short-circuited" (p. 3).

To counteract these negative perceptions Kane identifies the situation confronting both client and worker, pointing out that "every iota of clinical acumen" is needed in such efforts. Discharge planning, especially from acute care facilities, often takes place in a context where utilization review procedures "count each excess hospital day as a cardinal sin" (p.3), where alternative sources of care are often not readily available, and where institutional placement is viewed as a ready answer since reimbursement mechanisms encourage such care. These pressures minimize the likelihood that people will have sufficient time to express despair and anger and play a part in crucial decisions affecting them. Viewed as an important clinical process, discharge planning can enhance understanding of how people cope with difficult decisions and can lead to the discovery of creative options.

There are no panaceas that can readily alter the negative evaluation and dilemmas involved in the discharge planning process. These problems are compounded by current cost control thrusts and emphasis on short-term stays. These problems and the increased number of elderly and others with chronic problems compel concerted, creative attention to this activity. Some of the newer modalities such as early screening and aggressive case finding will be considered later in this chapter. These approaches can individualize patient care and give the social worker more time to carry out discharge planning in a professional manner.

Although responsibilities for discharge planning are mostly, and appropriately, lodged in the social work department, interdisciplinary approaches are increasingly being developed. In Morristown Memorial Hospital's discharge planning manual (1982) such planning is defined as "a multidisciplinary program developed to ensure that each patient admitted to the hospital has a planned program for needed continuing care and/or follow up upon discharge" (p. 1). In this hospital the involved personnel are usually physicians, nurses, social workers, home health care personnel, and the utilization review committee. The social work department has primary responsibility for planning and implementing the program.

The Discharge Planning Update (1980) points to the discharge planning conference as the mechanism for sharing information about the patients' perceptions of their problems, their own plans for discharge, and significant others' views of the patients' plans. The update presents a number of models that identify individualization, coordination, and screening criteria for patients most likely to need help with planning. Any such model must take into account and balance "the central purpose of discharge planning, namely the patient's continuing care needs, and administrative and regulatory requirements" (p. 27).

The mounting pressures for rapid discharge and cost control have generated legislative thrusts to systematize and regulate the process, especially when continuing expenditure of federal funds is involved. These thrusts have led, for example, to nursing home preadmission screening programs and to other projects that examine the efficient use of community supports required after discharge. Social work must examine these projects to ensure that fundamental social work tenets are not buried under the miasma of regulations and protocols. This objective is difficult to achieve, especially with high case loads and resource deficits. A number of studies have highlighted this point, including the following.

Coulton and Vielhaber (1977) surveyed a group of hospital social work directors in Ohio to obtain information on several components of planning services. In the hospitals surveyed 42% of all patients were discharged to their homes, 38% to nursing homes, and 11% to other hospitals. Between 27% and 65% of the time workers spent with patients was devoted to discussion of feelings. Social workers spent significantly more time considering the patients' feelings than did nurses involved in discharge planning. The average age of patients was high; some departments served geriatric patients almost exclusively. These departments were likely to be heavily involved in sending patients to nursing homes.

Lindenberg and Coulton (1980) presented findings of a follow-up study of patients who received social work assistance after discharge. The most common diagnoses were cardiovascular disease, cancer, orthopedic problems, and cerebrovascular disease. The degree of impairment was high (23% were severely impaired and thus unable to carry out basic tasks of daily living and 45% were moderately impaired). Although social workers were active in planning for needs after discharge, many of those needs were not met adequately. Among these were needs for financial assistance, social activities, and environmental modification. More adequate follow-up is proposed.

Wolock, Nicholas, and Russell (1982) interviewed patients following discharge and found that in one hospital the majority of patients and families seen by a social worker expressed satisfaction with social work services, which they perceived as having been focused on concrete services. This despite the fact that half of the respondents had little or no choice about discharge plans. Many said this did not matter. Despite patient satisfaction the workers fear that limited time (one or two contacts with the worker) precludes the possibility of providing adequate psychosocial care. Although these authors did not try to determine if planned services were actually received, it is probable that resource deficits like those identified by Lindenberg and Coulton might be found.

Although the workers surveyed by Lindenberg and Coulton spent considerable time on emotional matters, their follow-up data suggest that this time did not substitute for a lack of community-based services. The fact that half of the clients questioned by Wolock and her colleagues thought "it did not matter" that they had limited choice about decision making is disturbing. It raises questions about the quality of service rendered as well as the self-image of those with the most serious medical problems. If so many people no longer care how much discretion they have about what happens to them, what does that tell us about how society views the elderly, the disabled, and their families? If they are beginning to give up, hospital social workers need to find means to reverse this process. Therefore social workers' application of their particular perspectives to discharge planning becomes especially important. These perspectives derive from social work values and a number of the practice approaches that were considered in Chapter 6. These perspectives include the view of social work as a problem-solving endeavor, the importance of focus on the immediate and pressing reality and on the primary role clients need to have in making decisions and identifying problems, and the importance of seeking to make environmental changes. These considerations make it possible to suggest some guidelines for discharge planning. Although the following guidelines are not exhaustive they convey important elements of the social worker's style and the values from which they derive.

1. The situation of the person to be discharged is conceptualized as a problem stemming from disability, resource deficit, or both.

Despite the severity of the situation, the problem, when viewed from a social work perspective, suggests that the involved people should be treated as having problem-solving capacities. This suggests that in approaching people there should always be a stance that helps to activate these problem-solving capacities. Regardless of the difficulty, people must be engaged in the discharge planning process in terms that they can identify.

2. Unless patients are completely unable to communicate or there are no significant others who can be located, efforts to involve patients and their families in care plans must always be made.

3. Patients and their families must always be engaged to determine their views of what is necessary or probable.

Too often because of the hectic, last-minute nature of discharge planning the worker assumes that people will need to go to a nursing home or need formally organized home health care. However, discussion often reveals resources that are more comfortable and consonant with people's life-styles. For example, discussion with an apparently destitute elderly man living alone may reveal that a neighbor has for years been making sure that he gets his meals regularly. Discussion focused on his view may reveal that he has already made arrangements for his neighbor to take care of him.

Time must be devoted to activating the problem-solving process and to discovering people's views of the problem. This does not mean that everyone need be or can be seen for long periods. While time is an asset in the effort to help people struggle through some of the most difficult decisions they have ever had to make, some matters can be attended to in brief encounters.

> 4. Take time not only to talk and listen but also to observe people's physical stance; their degree of tension, relaxation, or anxiety; and signs that indicate a crisis state.

Some of these types of observations are facilitated by good relationships with other staff members because they can give important information that may help the worker make observations and judgments. Knowing the person and degree of tension or comfort present makes it easier to consider available alternatives, even those of a most limited nature. When alternatives are limited because of resource gaps workers are obliged to acknowledge this, and to share the pain and anguish. They may, and need, to help identify the positive aspects of a grim situation, but they should never suggest that "it's for the best." For example, if people are to be discharged to their home instead of to a nursing home because the latter is not available, workers can share their anger with clients and family. Most important, the client or family must not be blamed for the situation.

> 5. Do not assume a "person-blaming stance" when a "systems-blaming stance" is in order.

Sensitive discharge planning will be facilitated if efforts are made to identify and generate resources. The time taken to explore new resources, document unmet needs, and work with existing agencies can pay off in the long run in less harried discharge planning. All this is easier said that done when utilization review procedures terminate payment for patients no longer needing acute care and the social work department is held accountable for implementing discharge plans. This role can be played on a case by case basis by mentioning the need for a few additional days to plan. This task can be simplified when the social worker's credibility as a member of the team has been established and his or her judgments are known to be sound. And it can be played by careful documentation of resource deficits that prevent early discharge. Dockhorn (1982) suggests that the American Hospital Association not only sanctions but encourages such activities. For one really doubts that physicians (whose authority is so pervasive) really support discharging patients who will not receive adequate care. Have we social workers sought to enlist their support of coalitions developed to enhance care? In 1981 the Medical Society of New Jersey was engaged in a statewide effort to increase services available to the elderly. A social work intern worked with the group in that effort. Such efforts are feasible and need to be increased.

Effective discharge planning requires thorough knowledge of policies; the capacity to relate these in an individualized manner to the situation at hand; quick and systematic ability to engage the patient and others, regardless of their physical or psychological state; and, most importantly, the ability to identify the problem. Often the problem is considered in terms of the hospital's need for the bed or the cost of extra hospital days. Real as these considerations are, they are not the terms on which the social worker initiates interaction. The following illustrates the manner in which interaction may be initiated:

Worker: Mrs. Green, they tell me that you're getting a bit better. There's not much more the hospital can do for you. Have you thought about how you might manage when you're discharged?

Mrs. Green (crying): But I've got nobody home. I still don't feel good. I can hardly get around.

Worker: I know. I can see that you feel awful. Sometimes it helps to cry.

Mrs. Green: I do feel a bit better now. I really don't want to go to one of those nursing homes. On the other hand, they do take care of you there. Are the people there all crazy, or could I find folks to talk to?

Worker: There are lots of folks like you there. Remember Mrs. Smith who was in the next bed the last time you were here?

Mrs. Green: Yeah. But she was sicker than me. Maybe I could get one of them nurses to come every day again. But then, what do I do at night?

Worker: Let's think about it. You'd be alone. You would have to have your phone by the bed. I would keep in touch with the nurse and she could probably find a social worker to come and talk to you at home. We'll need to decide in a couple of days. You know, pretty soon they'll start sending you a bill if you stay here past the time they think you're ready to go. Think about it. I know it's tough. I'll be back tomorrow.

And so, despite most limited options, the worker helps the patient to express her worries, cry, and think about alternatives. In this process the regulations are not forgotten; both worker and client are aware of them and work within that framework. The American Hospital Association guidelines previously referred to (Dockhorn, 1982) suggest that follow-up and coordination are social work department responsibilities. If Mrs. Green chooses (or must) go home with minimal support services, follow-up is essential, as is a well-developed relationship with the home health service. In such a relationship the hospital social worker and those in the community-based service will regularly track the progress of Mrs. Green and others like her.

High-risk screening

Considerable attention has been given to how hospital social workers come to serve those thought to need social work intervention. The dysfunctional aspects of a system in which other health professionals determine who is in need of services has been noted in a number of works for example, (Berkman, Rehr, and Rosenberg, 1980). In characteristic referral systems where physicians, nurses, and others refer patients, referrals are often made late, thus limiting the time available for planning. In addition, many who could use help with illness-related psychosocial problems are not referred.

As early as 1973 Berkman and Rehr identified early social work intervention with reduced hospital stays. Schrager and others (1978) also found that early referral reduced the length of stay by an average of 3 days, at considerable cost savings to the hospital.

Also important is social workers' dependency on other disciplines for defining the terms of their work and the resultant lack of autonomy. Recognizing the limitations of the traditional approach, the social work department at the Mount Sinai Medical Center in New York City undertook a series of studies designed to (1) identify those patients at risk for illness-related psychosocial problems, (2) test mechanisms by which social workers screen all admissions where the length of stay is expected to be 7 or more days, and (3) determine if screening uncovered high-risk situations. The findings, presented in a series of papers (Berkman, Rehr, and Rosenberg, 1980; Rehr, Berkman, and Rosenberg, 1980) show great promise. The departments determined, based on professional judgment, those categories of patients thought to need social work intervention. Following this a series of steps, variously detailed in these and other works for example, (Paneth and Lipsky, 1979), were carried out.

Early screening can be done by a clerk who checks the slips of newly admitted patients meeting high-risk criteria. Volunteers and others can help in this effort. Once patients are screened into the social work system workers become involved with them. Ideally patients are seen within 24 to 48 hours of admission. The screening procedure is intended to select cases of psychosocial need that the traditional referral system misses (Rehr, Berkman and Rosenberg, 1980). Appendix C discusses in more depth the criteria used in high-risk screening. Population characteristics (for example, the elderly living alone) and health problem areas (for example, abused children) serve as an organizing framework. The reader is encouraged to examine these lists and adapt and expand them based on practice experience, literature review, and research.

If the screening procedure increases work load without a simultaneous increase in staff size, reordering priorities in the service delivery pattern is essential. Needs for additional staff may be documented. When screening identifies those in need of service who are not ordinarily referred, social workers can be more confident that limited personnel provide care for those most in need, in the terms identified by the profession. This mechanism has potential for enhancing social work autonomy. Social work then assumes major responsibility for hospital patients particularly at psychosocial risk.

Schlesinger and Wolock (1982) found that between 1975 and 1981 procedures for identifying high-risk patients increased substantially in New Jersey hospitals. (Dockhorn 1982) states that each social work program should have a clearly defined screening mechanism to identify populations at risk and is obliged to develop a way of carrying out the procedures in a timely fashion.

Discussions with New Jersey hospital social work directors reveal various difficulties in implementation. One is acceptance by medical and administrative staff of the social worker's right to meet with patients without medical clearance. One director* gives a vivid account of a 1-year effort to obtain consent for an open access system from the involved medical groups. On successive occasions her well-documented reports were met with suggestions for further study. As each request for more study was met, additional suggestions were made until the plan finally met with approval.

Not surprisingly, some social workers are reluctant to shift from engaging patients on the basis of referrals made by other caretakers to engaging patients whose needs for social work service have not been previously identified by others. Rehr, Berkman, and Rosenberg (1980) and Paneth and Lipsky (1979) point out that workers feel awkward in this latter type of encounter.

Epstein's work (1980) on strategies that facilitate intervention with those who do not seek service further elaborates the skills required for engagement. She consistently points to the importance of working on problems in the terms identified by the client, regardless of the basis of intervention. When social workers arrive on the scene without prior preparation by the physician or others, the likelihood of eliciting the patient's concerns may be enhanced. The following examples will clarify this point.

Mr. Smith has been told by his physician that a social worker will come to see him about arranging for transportation to the clinic after discharge.

> *Worker:* Mr. Smith, I understand that Dr. Jones has told you I'd be coming to talk with you about how you'll manage after you leave here.
>
> *Mr. Smith:* Well yeah, he told me you'd arrange for a van to get me to the clinic.
>
> *Worker:* Yes, that's one of the ways I can try to help. Perhaps you're worrying about other matters also.
>
> *Mr. Smith:* Nah, doc just said you'd get me a van.

Now consider the same Mr. Smith, a 75-year-old man who lives alone and has cancer. He needs to come to the hospital regularly following discharge for chemotherapy. He's been picked up by screening procedures.

> *Worker:* Hello Mr. Smith. I'm Miss Jones, a social worker. One of us always

* Mrs. Jo Marshall, Director, Department of Social Service, Morristown Memorial Hospital, Morristown, N.J.

comes to talk with people having a pretty rough time with painful treatments that will continue after discharge from the hospital. Would you like to talk to me?

Mr. Smith: Well, I've always taken care of myself—never needed welfare before. But from what the doc tells me, it's going to be pretty hard for me to get on a bus to come down here twice a week. My son works and he can't afford to take time off from work.

Worker: Sounds like you have a lot to think about about how you'll manage at home.

Mr. Smith (sighing): Yeah. It's rough. The doc says I really shouldn't stay alone. My son says I should come to stay with him, but I don't want to bother him.

In the first example Mr. Smith feels compelled to maintain the definition of the social worker's service presented by the physician. In the second, approached by the worker in an open-ended way, he uses the opportunity to explore the other facets of his situation. A less skillful worker responding to the physician's referral may simply have said:

> Dr. Jones has asked me to help arrange for your transportation to the hospital for your treatments after you leave.

Thus put it is unlikely that Mr. Smith would begin to reveal his other concerns.

An unskilled worker involved in screening may say:

> Mr. Smith, I'm a social worker. I'd like to help you with other problems you have.

Mr. Smith, who tends to identify social work with welfare, may well turn away and say,

> Oh no, I'll be OK. My doctor's taking care of me.

At least one further problem arises in addition to issues of reversing ingrained medical staff resistance to open access systems and worker's reluctance to alter practice habits. The fact that an open access/high-risk screening system is in operation does not mean that the usual referral procedures are totally replaced. The process does not always pick up all of those who want service. Often well-established routines continue to operate. Given a choice between meeting screening deadlines and responding to requests from traditional referral sources, many workers tend to *carry on as usual.* Some directors point to powerful physicians and administrators who want their patients or the problems they identify cared for, despite other compelling demands on the worker's time.

The studies by Coulton and Vielhaber (1977) and by Wolock, Nicholas, and Russell (1982) both implicitly touch on this issue. Coulton and Vielhaber's social work respondents doubted whether earlier intervention would have affected the outcome. Of the patients interviewed by Wolock, Nicholas, and Russell, 69% thought that nothing would have been gained if they would have been contacted by the social worker earlier in their hospital stay. Clearly much more research is needed before it can be stated with certainty that high-risk screening procedures have clear-cut, positive effects on length of stay, social quality of hospital care, and progress following hospitalization.

There is little doubt that high-risk screening presents an important development in hospital social work's long-standing attempt to define the conditions of work and render care in a manner governed by a social work perspective and autonomous decision making.

The preceding discussion has centered on the range of activities that tend to be carried out by hospital social workers, no matter what their assignment. The balance of this chapter focuses on how assignment to particular services or programs shapes the social worker's activity and how the social worker in turn affects the service rendered. There are many types of services and units in hospitals. Space considerations make it impossible to deal with all of these. Three have been selected for discussion: (1) the medical/surgical service—a very common and important assignment and (2) specialized units. In the latter category two examples are presented—work in dialysis units and in neonatal intensive care units.

THE MEDICAL/SURGICAL WORKER

Social workers assigned to the medical/surgical services of an acute care general hospital work at a hectic pace with patients who suffer from a variety of conditions and who stay in the hospital for relatively short periods of time. Like other health care social workers they interact with many health professionals, among them many medical specialists, nurses who have different levels of training, and the usual array of orderlies, attendants, and aides.

A wide variety of health problems are encountered: heart disease, malignant neoplasm, pneumonia, and emphysema. Many are hospitalized for such problems as heart attacks and strokes and have major surgery such as a mastectomy. Those who need highly monitored specialized care, like that provided in intensive and coronary care units, are also often cared for on medical and surgical services. A disproportionate number of those hospitalized on medical/surgical floors are elderly. Almost all of the five types of illness careers identified in Chapter 5 are represented in this service. Berkman and Henley's point (1981) about the wide variety of pathology that confronts practitioners in medical/surgical services is well taken. During several hours on the ward the social worker may encounter a young mother hospitalized briefly for pneumonia, a woman awaiting the results of a biopsy that will determine if she needs a mastectomy, someone who has had a stroke, and someone recovering from major surgery for cancer.

How does the social worker cope with this diversity in situations where time is short and pressures are great? Berkman and Henley (1981) point out that short-term casework services are the primary modality used. Workers need to develop skills in making quick, accurate assessments and in contracting for limited service. Berkman and Henley cite the 1977 New England Regional Study of Social Work Practice in which it was found that workers tend to be mostly involved in working with families experiencing difficult life changes related to illness and locating home care services or long-term institutional care. Emotional support and advocacy were the most frequent interventions used. Advocacy was related to delayed discharge because of inadequate community facilities.

The chapter on interdisciplinary practice made implicit reference to a number of additional interventions that are and need to be used by social workers in medical/surgical services. Sharing information with other personnel, especially nurses, can complement the worker's efforts to help people struggle with difficult life changes. Sometimes sharing information involves interpreting for other personnel and sometimes it means using their insight to facilitate the social worker's assessment. For example, the worker can learn from other staff members whether or not there are visitors and what is the patients' level of tension.

Important components of practice in the medical/surgical service are (1) how workers organize their time and work load; (2) their availability to patients, families, and other staff members; and (3) the leadership role they play. If assigned regularly to a unit, workers need to be aware of routines, visiting hours, and the best time for formal or informal communication. The time of day when various medical procedures tend to be carried out is not usually the best time for workers to be on the floor regularly. Desk work, telephoning, or in-office interviews might be scheduled then. However, workers may want to formally inform staff members and patients of the hours they will usually be on the floor. Arrangements for evening and weekend coverage should be made explicit, and if at all possible, social work departments should be physically open during key weekend and evening hours. Think for a moment about the impression created concerning the importance of the social work department when, unlike most other departments, its doors are tightly shut on evenings and weekends.*

Making arrangements to keep a department accessible at key hours and developing routine relationships with other staff members involves developing a leadership stance vis à vis the department and other staff. The advocacy and planning roles must be carried out not only on a case by case basis but also in relation to policy and organizational decisions. For example, the medical surgical worker will have special insight into the need for an extended care facility the hospital may be contemplating.

*I have often had that experience when visiting a friend or relative during "off hours." As a working woman who wanted the social worker's help with a relative, I found this to be most disconcerting.

These and similar functions are often disregarded because of time pressures and the need to effect discharge planning. However, in the long run sufficient attention to these kinds of issues can enhance patient care and reduce worker pressures. Berkman and Henley (1981) identify a number of related issues as "future agendas" for this arena of hospital practice. One relates to efforts to influence insurance companies and those who regulate Medicare and Medicaid to regard social work services as direct-cost items. This would generate income from social work services for the hospital and probably increase staff size. Another relates to the need to more clearly differentiate the tasks carried out by workers with various levels of training. Such efforts can give highly trained staff more time for direct service and planning roles. Lower level staff can carry out important but more routine tasks such as checking on the availability of resources. Most important is Berkman and Henley's suggestion (1981) that the departments must be instrumental in developing the "aftercare network of social services to provide a sufficient variety of posthospital options to prevent unneeded bed-days and improve the quality of life of patients" (p. 275). This involves the kind of linkage and systems change activities that have been stressed throughout this book.

THE WORKER IN SPECIALIZED UNITS OF HOSPITALS OR SPECIALIZED HOSPITALS

An issue not yet resolved by health care social workers is whether various subspecialties of health practice areas require specialized knowledge and skills (for example, *Health and Social Work* supplement to volume 6, 1981). This question arises in relation to practice both inside and outside the hospital. Although I do not claim that the issue is resolved, it is useful to attempt to identify the particular types of knowledge needed and practice roles enacted by workers in those segments of the hospital that tend to focus on one particular set of problems. The examples I have selected are dialysis units and neonatal intensive care. These examples mainly focus on describing the types of psychosocial problems and reactions triggered by the medical problem. Before discussing work with dialysis patients and in neonatal intensive care units I will call attention to several issues that confront workers in a variety of specialized settings.

Practice issues. The worker needs to be particularly knowledgeable of the specific medical problems and the typical associated psychosocial problems involved in the case. Team members will expect such knowledge from the social worker. Only the worker with such familiarity can make an accurate psychosocial assessment. The stroke worker needs to know how different types of strokes affect speech, mobility, and memory. The worker in a cancer center needs to understand specialized treatment protocols. Team work is likely to be intense. The authoritarian model of team practice (Chapter 8) may prevail in critical care decisions. In addition, many professionals are usually involved with the patients' emotional and physical well-being. Roles may greatly overlap as issues of counseling and helping people cope with management regimes arise.

Contact is more protracted in neonatal unit service than in acute medical/surgical service. Discharge planning, although important, may not have to be carried out under the same kinds of pressures as exist in acute care. Assessment procedures also can sometimes proceed at a slower pace. Social workers in these as well as other segments of the hospital use all types of social work intervention. Simultaneous attention to micro and macro issues (Chapter 6) is as important in these as in other settings. For example, there may be subtle or overt pressures placed on dialysis patients to continue treatment at all cost. Advocating for the patient's right to make decisions on these and similar issues is a crucial function of the social worker. Stroke victims and newborn infants and their families usually require more resources than are currently available. Thus resource and network building based on knowledge acquired in the course of specialized work is a major social work responsibility.

The dialysis worker

Fortner-Frazier (1981) and Frazier (1981) discusses the medical facts associated with kidney malfunction, the hemodialysis process, the types of diets

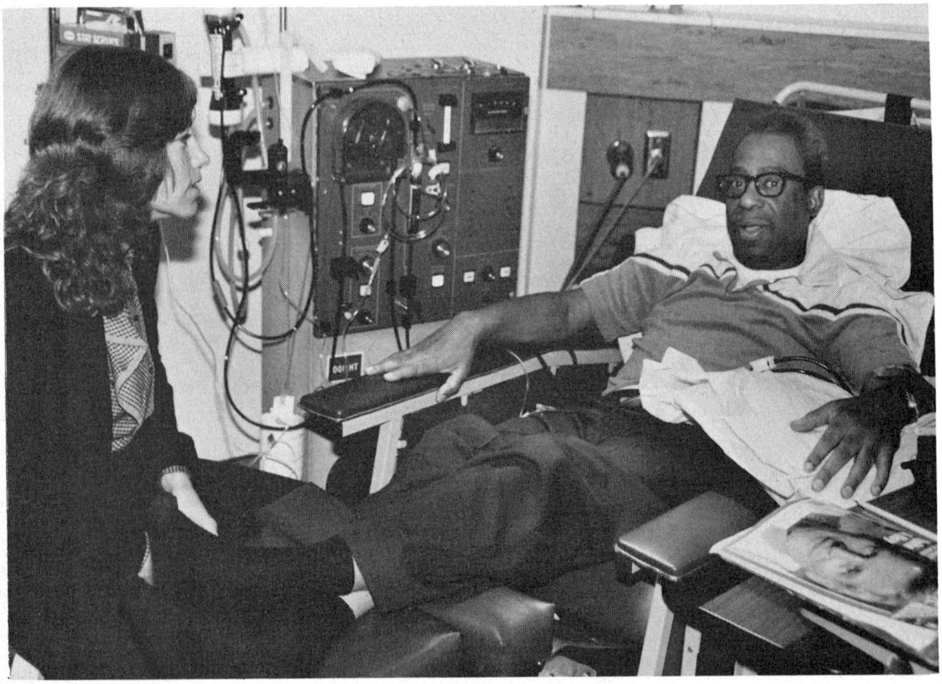

and medication regimens to which dialysis patients must adhere, and the recurring psychological problems faced by many people receiving dialysis treatments or kidney transplants. For each area Frazier identifies the particular contribution social work can make in helping people cope with the various adaptations entailed. It is not possible or appropriate to review each of these contributions in detail here. However, several key points deserve mention.

The dialysis process "involves the use of machines to rid the body of poisons that accumulate because of the lack of adequate kidney functioning" (Fortner-Frazier, p. 755). People with end-stage renal disease will die if they do not undergo one of three types of treatment or receive a successful transplant. Dialysis may be carried out at home or at the hospital. Another form of treatment, peritoneal dialysis, involves inserting a permanent catheter into the abdominal wall, instilling "dialysate" into the abdominal cavity, leaving it in for a specific amount of time, draining it, and replacing it. Each of these forms of dialysis involves complex medical procedures and has the potential for generating frightening complications.

Hospital dialysis requires patients to spend many hours several times weekly attached to the machine, entrusting their lives to the staff. Home dialysis requires both patient and home caretaker to be fully cognizant of all needed procedures and be thoroughly trained. Peritoneal dialysis does not involve attachment to the machine. However, the catheter may be visible or people may develop a "pot-bellied" appearance because large amounts of fluid are carried around all day.

Each of these types of treatments markedly affects every aspect of the patient's and the family's lives. Whether or not family members are willing and able to take on home dialysis, which is the least expensive and most convenient method, is often a tortuous decision. Leff (1975), Palmer (1978), and others comment on the problems of adapting routines and of the fears generated by treatment. Fortner-Frazier (1981) suggests that in many dialysis settings the social worker's psychosocial evaluation is important in helping to determine which mode of treatment is most suited for particular patients and their families. The dialysis and transplantation worker must develop a working knowledge of the disease, the related procedures, and the range of common effects. Without such knowledge he or she will not be able to make an accurate psychosocial assessment or be alert to physical danger signals.

Fortner-Frazier's comments on offering in-depth therapy are instructive.

> As a rule of thumb, it is best to determine if patient's coping skills are interfering with the basic requirements of dialytic treatment such as coming in for treatment on a regular basis, making responsible compliance with diet and activity restrictions, and taking medication properly before assuming that in-depth psychotherapy is needed (p. 148).

The following are matters to which social workers in dialysis units must pay particular attention.

1. In respect to diet and medication a number of issues arise for the social worker's consideration. One is understanding the effect of both on levels of fatigue and psychological distress. Thus in assessing patients' psychological states, the effects of medication and diet must be separated from other psychological indicators. Fortner-Frazier (1981) suggests that eating binges can often be correlated with a change in emotional state. Collaboration with dietitians becomes most important. Social workers can alert dietitians to the possibility of binging by noting the patient's psychological state. Conversely, they can get clues about how the patient is coping by asking about his or her dietary habits (Fortner-Frazier, 1981).
2. Just as people with other chronic conditions, many dialysis patients go through varying stages of adaptation. The fear of death is always present, although denial may be great. Therefore the fear may not be articulated.
3. The dialysis social worker has an opportunity for a relationship that is relatively unique in a hospital setting; the long-term involvement with people with complex psychological, medical, and family problems seems ready made for the kind of intervention in which social workers are particularly skilled and enjoy carrying out. In addition, successful group approaches have been described (for example, Leff, 1975). Yet often students are disappointed when they get their "much longed for" assignment with a dialysis patient. Many patients are reluctant to engage in conversations about their emotional states, and groups often do not respond well. Fortner-Frazier (1981) points out that most dialysis patients do not view themselves as having emotional problems.
4. Although federal policy now makes costly treatment available to all, there are many concrete financial problems.
5. Obtaining transportation to the hospital is a problem shared by many patients.

A case study will highlight some of the issues just identified.

Mrs. Smith

Mrs. Smith, a 45-year-old Black mother of three, was advised of her need for dialysis following unsuccessful efforts to keep her kidneys functioning. For some years, Mrs. Smith had been diabetic and hypertensive. Although she took medication regularly she found it difficult to control her salt and sugar intake. She was considerably overweight.

Discussion with her revealed that she was a cheerful person who coped well with the fact that she has two children with developmental disabilities. John, now 18, is mildly retarded; William, 16, is also retarded. In addition, William exhibits some schizophrenic-like behavior.

Mr. and Mrs. Smith have a good relationship. They always tended to the children's special needs together.

The family and the dialysis team agreed that Mrs. Smith would come for hospital based dialysis three times weekly following a brief period of hospitalization. Because Mr. Smith's job as a carpenter did not allow him to take time off from work, arrangements for transportation were made through the local ambulance service. Mr. and Mrs. Smith could manage the small cost.

Mrs. Smith's initial adaptation seemed good. She was cheerful, came regularly, and did better in adhering to her diet than she had before the onset of kidney failure. In a routine outreach interview while Mrs. Smith was being dialyzed the worker tried to engage Mrs. Smith to learn how she was doing. The worker indicated she was aware that Mrs. Smith had additional problems (the two retarded children) and suggested that dialysis might be just another blow. Mrs. Smith was quite matter-of-fact, saying "The Lord takes care." She clearly did not want to talk with the worker about such emotionally-laden issues as her dialysis and her children. The worker simply let Mrs. Smith know that she was available if needed.

One day in a routine team meeting the dietitian said she was quite dismayed because she was sure Mrs. Smith had been binging. She had gained weight and the laboratory findings were not good. The nurse remembered that on her last two visits Mrs. Smith seemed quite agitated and had made a passing remark about needing to find another school for William. The worker decided to seek out Mrs. Smith. Although she said things were fine, she made it conditional "as long as that rotten school leaves me alone." The worker was successful in helping her discuss why the administrators of the school William attended wanted him to stay home for awhile (he was destructive) until they found another school more suited for him. Mrs. Smith seemed agitated and depressed. "It gets rough. What's the use of living? First the kids, now this. My husband needs a real woman."

Slowly over the next few days she revealed her despair over her children, her fear that she would die, and her complete loss of sexual interest. She also admitted she had not been watching her diet. The worker acknowledged the need to express these feelings and she said it did seem that Mrs. Smith had more than her share of problems. This recognition of her feelings enabled her to decide with the worker that they would work together on helping her think through her binging, and discovering if any help with the school situation could be arranged.

Mrs. Smith recognized the implications of her binging. Without prompting she said "I'm not ready to go yet." Mr. Smith assured her that he could wait until she felt better and regained her sexual interest.

The worker contacted the school, where a difficult situation existed. The administrators were willing to keep William temporarily now that they knew of his mother's illness. The possibility of a residential school will be considered when Mrs. Smith's bout of depression diminishes.

This case illustrates certain components of work with dialysis patients. The worker was able to establish contact early in Mrs. Smith's treatment. Not uncharacteristically, Mrs. Smith was not ready then for the worker's intervention. She was managing and did not want to put herself in another client role.

However, the ongoing experience and pressure of the illness combined with external pressures generated a problem that Mrs. Smith was willing to discuss. Mrs. Smith had many difficulties that were exacerbated by her dialysis. Perhaps William was more agitated because his mother was ill. Contact may be minimal after problems with William decrease and it may increase as new problems arise. The worker will continue to be available.

Mrs. Smith's problems other than her kidney disease may have been more extreme than those of others. However, most dialysis patients will have some difficulties related to other areas of life. These problems, combined with those generated by the dialysis, require the worker to be available as needed. Mrs. Smith may become more seriously depressed. As the treatment continues she may say again "What's the use?" The worker will need to be available to discuss that question with her.

The dialysis worker, like other health care social workers, has the responsibility to be aware of coping styles and resource needs. When these are kept in mind there is considerable opportunity for the worker to make a major contribution to an interdisciplinary endeavor.

The neonatal worker

A network of regionally organized neonatal care centers provides highly specialized care to infants with difficulties or believed to be at risk for developing problems. Infants are frequently transported to such centers within hours after birth. Often the mother remains in the original hospital while recuperating from the delivery. Often there is much drama and physical, psychological, and social tragedy in neonatal intensive care units. Infants sometimes weighing as little as 1 pound are intensively cared for by highly trained nurses, neonatologists, and others. The infants may be attached to a wide variety of equipment. The chance for life or normal development is often not known. Many infants die. These children's parents confront a range of problems. For many a welcome, joyfully anticipated event is instead an unexpected tragedy.

In a review of research and clinical practice in this area Trout (1983) suggests that the parents of severely disabled children often experience grief analogous to that following a child's death. They are grieving for the normal child they expected and about which they continue to fantasize. Anger, fear, and guilt are common feelings that must be handled simultaneously with the arduous problems of daily care. The parents ask what they did wrong or blame their partners as they struggle with this turn of events. Bonding with the child may be delayed because of physical separation or the risks involved in handling the child. Those families whose children live often confront difficult lifelong tasks of caring for a disabled child.

The severity of the situation confronting these children and their families is exemplified by a series of studies concerning the relationship between child abuse, prematurity, and other disabling illnesses during the first year of life.

Hunter and others (1978) point out that infants discharged from neonatal intensive care units are eight times more likely to be abused than those not requiring such care. Trout (1983) cites data showing that 60% of a group of abused children had histories of recurrent illness in the first year of life. This 60% is in contrast to the nonabused siblings of such children, 10% of whom had comparable difficulties.

A discussion of the tasks faced by parents of these children is needed if this distressing finding is to be put in perspective. Many children discharged from neonatal intensive care units still require its elaborate equipment. Some need to wear cardiac monitors that could possibly malfunction. This possibility causes tension and necessitates constant surveillance. Other children constantly need to be administered oxygen. Some have to use orthopedic appliances; others are disfigured. Many do not go through the usual developmental stages at the expected time. Life is never the same for many families and the most routine aspects of living can become major sources of difficulty.

David Lacona

David Lacona, born 2 months prematurely, was discharged to home at age 3 months with a diagnosis of bronchopulmonary dysplasia. He required a constant supply of oxygen delivered through his nose. This complication related to his premature birth began 2 days after birth. When David went home it was not possible to predict how long he would need the oxygen—perhaps as long as 6 months. In addition, his long-range developmental prognosis could not be determined. He might be subject to recurrent viral pulmonary infections.

Although his 22-year-old mother and father had visited regularly, they felt David was like a stranger who had been cared for by others. Both recent college graduates, the parents had planned to have David cared for by a sitter. Both Mary and David Sr. had expected to go to graduate school. Grandparents planned to help with finances and child care. Mary and David discovered that the sitters they can afford were afraid to care for David. Even Mary's mother, a capable woman, did not want to remain alone with him for a long time. Mary decided to drop out of school for awhile.

The worker learned of these problems during a follow-up telephone call. She also discovered that Mary was quite agitated. Mary acknowledged that sometimes she had to restrain herself from throwing David when using the equipment. David Sr. was spending a lot of time at the library, and having to always stay inside agitated her.

Mary was very angry about having to drop school for now. The worker let Mary express her feelings and asked David Sr. to join them. He admitted he was forcing Mary to accept great responsibilities. Together they agreed to find a sitter who could manage David and give both parents some free time. The worker told them about other young couples who had children with similar problems. They agreed to contact some of them. Two months later, although the oxygen was still in use, both Mary and David Sr. were more able to cope with David's problems.

Problems will continue to surface until David recovers. The worker needs to be aware of this potential and of the possibility that this young couple could abuse this child. The strain of the birth of a disabled child added to Mary and David's struggle to reorganize their own lives and long-range life goals greatly increases the potential for child abuse.

Where functioning is limited other problems need to be considered. For example, ethical issues often surface sharply as staff members and parents must make decisions about prolonging or maintaining the life of infants whose functioning is likely to be minimal (for example, Cohen, 1976 President's Commission, 1983).

Interdisciplinary practice can be very gratifying because all disciplines involved usually have a high commitment to comprehensive care and feel very close to the families. However, this level of commitment can generate role conflicts and different definitions of the problem (for example, Donohue and Mack, 1982).

Neonatal workers also need medical information as they seek to help parents cope. They are likely to work with parents whose children have many different problems. Some will be confronting the fact that the problems are genetic and may influence their decisions about having more children. Neonatal workers are constantly confronting new diagnoses with which they need familiarity. Some children may remain hospitalized for many months and others may leave quickly. Many cases provide the opportunity for intense, ongoing work to continue for weeks or months. When children go home they may need various services not offered by the neonatal unit. Often families live considerable distances from the hospital. It is essential that the social worker develop relationships with the network of health and social services that are both close and far away.

SUMMARY

In this chapter I focused on key elements of hospital social work practice. The diverse types of hospitals and their structure, financing, and major role in American health care delivery were discussed. I introduced some theoretical formulations to examine the possible source of distinctions between hospital social workers' view of their role and the way others perceive them. I identified discharge planning as a key social work function and I made an effort to indicate the high level of skill required for effective practice. I also discussed high-risk screening mechanisms and their potential for enhancing social work autonomy and the quality of care. The medical/surgical worker was characterized as confronting many and varied problems. Short-term contact is characteristic of this service and workers need to acquire skill in rapid assessment and contracting for brief, limited services.

I reviewed the particular medical and psychosocial problems encountered in dialysis and neonatal intensive care units to suggest the differences and similarities in practice between work in acute medical/surgical services and in more specialized services such as stroke units, psychiatric units, cancer care centers, and others. All social work interventions are applied to each specialized setting. A working knowledge of the particular medical problems and related psychosocial issues is essential.

REFERENCES

American Hospital Association: Discharge Planning update—an interdisciplinary perspective for health professionals, **1**(1):entire issue, Fall 1980, National Health Standards and Quality Information Clearinghouse.

Anderson, O.W., and Gevitz, N.: The general hospital: a social and historical perspective. In Mechanic, D., editor: Handbook of health, health care and the health professions, New York, 1983, The Free Press.

Anderson, R., and Anderson, O.W.: Trends in the use of health services. In Freeman, H.E., Levine, S., and Reeder, L.G., editors: Handbook of medical sociology, ed. 3, Englewood Cliffs, NJ, 1979, Prentice-Hall, Inc.

Bartlett, H.M., and Ida, M. Cannon: Pioneer in medical social work, Social Service Review **49:**208, 1975.

Berkman, B.: New England regional study of social work practice, (unpublished). Cited in Berkman, B., and Henley, B.: Medical and surgical services in acute care hospitals, Health and Social Work (suppl.) **6**(4):22S, 1981.

Berkman, B., and Henley, B.: Medical and surgical services in acute care hospitals, Health and Social Work (suppl.) **6**(4):22S, November, 1981.

Berkman, B., and Rehr, H.: Early social service case finding for hospitalized patients: an experiment, The Social Service Review **47**(2):256, 1973.

Berkman, B., Rehr, H., and Rosenberg, G.: A social work department develops and tests a screening mechanism to identify high social risk situations, Social Work in Health Care **5**(4):373, 1980.

Boaz, R.F.: Health care system. In Turner, J.B., editor: Encyclopedia of social work, Washington, D.C., 1977, National Association of Social Workers, vol. 1, p. 550.

Bracht, N.: Social work practice in hospitals: changing directions and new opportunities. In Bracht, N.F., editor: Social work in health care, New York, 1978, The Haworth Press.

Cabot, R.C.: Social service and the art of healing, New York, 1915, Moffat, Yard, & Co.

Cohen, M.: Ethical issues in neonatal intensive care: familial concerns. In Jonsen, A., and Garland, M., editors: Ethics of newborn intensive care, Berkeley, Calif., 1976, Health Policy Program, Institute of Governmental Studies University of California Press.

Committee on Discharge Planning of the Society for Hospital Social Work Directors: Discharge planning, reference article, Kensington, Md., September 1980, National Health Standards and Quality Information Clearinghouse.

Coulton, C.J.: Social work quality assurance programs: a comparative analysis, Washington, D.C., 1979, National Association of Social Workers.

Coulton, C.J., and Butler, N.: Measuring social work productivity in health care, Health and Social Work **6**(3):4, 1981.

Coulton, C.J.; and Vielhaber, D.: Patterns of social work practice in post hospital planning, Cleveland, 1977, Northeast Ohio Society for Social Work Directors.

Davidson, K.W.: Evolving social work roles in health care: the case of discharge planning, Social Work in Health Care **4**(1):43, 1978.

Discharge planning manual, Morristown, N.J., 1982, Morristown Memorial Hospital.

Dockhorn, J.: Essentials of social work programs in hospitals, Chicago, 1982, American Hospital Association.

Donohue, E., and Mack, S.P.: Interdisciplinary problems in a neonatal intensive care unit: an approach to enhancing social worker-nurse understanding and effectiveness, paper presented at the Sixth National Conference on Perinatal Social Work, Houston, May 1982.

Epstein, L.: Helping people: the task-centered approach, St. Louis, 1980, The C.V. Mosby Co.

Fisher, D.: Reimbursement for hospital social work services in the ambulatory care setting, Paper presented at the annual meeting of the American Public Health Association, Montreal, November 1982.

Fortner-Frazier, C.L.: Social work and dialysis, Berkeley, 1981, University of California Press.

Frazier, C.L.: Renal disease, Health and Social Work (Suppl.) **6**(4):755, 1981.

Fuchs, V.R.: Who shall live? health economics and social choice, New York, 1974, Basic Books, Inc., Publishers.

Hallowitz, E.: Redefining the role of hospital social work, Paper presented at the National Conference of Social Welfare, May 1971.

Hasenfeld, Y.: Human service organizations, Englewood Cliffs, N.J., 1983, Prentice-Hall, Inc.

Hasenfeld, Y., and English R.A., editors: Human service organizations, Ann Arbor, 1974, The University of Michigan Press.

Health and Social Work (Suppl.) **6**(4):entire issue, 1981.

Health, United States, DHEW Pub. No. (PHS) 80-1232, Washington, D.C., 1979, U.S. Government Printing Office.

Health, United States, DHHS Pub. No. (PHS) 83-1232, Washington, D.C., 1982, U.S. Government Printing Office.

Hirsch, S., and Lurie, A.: Social work dimensions in shaping medical care philosophy and practice, Social Work **14**(2):75, 1969.

Hunter, R.S., Kilstrom, N., Kraybill, E.N., and Loda, F.: Antecedents of child abuse and neglect in premature infants: a prospective study in a newborn intensive care unit, Pediatrics **61**(4):629, 1978.

Kane, R.A.: Discharge planning: an undischarged responsibility?, Health and Social Work **5**(1):2, 1980.

Kane, R.A.: Entrepreneurs, Health and Social Work **7**(3):170, 1982.

Leff, B.: A club approach to social work treatment within a home dialysis program, Social Work in Health Care **1**(1):33, 1975.

Lindenberg, R.E., and Coulton, C.: Planning for posthospital care: a follow up study, Health and Social Work **5**(1):45, 1980.

Nason, F., and Delbanco, T.L.: Soft services: a major cost effective component of primary care, Social Work in Health Care **1**(3):297, 1976.

Palmer, S.E.: Social work in home dialysis: responding to trends in health care, Social Work in Health Care **3**(4):363, 1978.

Paneth, J., and Lipsky, H.: Utilization review and social work's role. In Rehr, H., editor: Professional accountability for social work practice, New York, 1979, Prodist.

Phillips, B.: Health services: social workers. In Encyclopedia of social work, ed. 17, Washington, D.C., 1977, National Association of Social Workers, p. 615.

President's Commission for the Study of Ethical Problems in Medicine and Biomedical and Behavioral Research: Deciding to forego life-sustaining treatment: a report on the ethical, medical, and legal issues in treatment decisions, Washington, D.C., 1983, U.S. Government Printing Office, p. 197.

Rehr, H., Berkman, B., and Rosenberg, G.: Screening for high risk social work: principles and problems, Social Work **25**(5):403, 1980.

Reichert, K.: Human services and the market system, Health and Social Work **7**(3):173, 1982.

Rosenberg, G.: Concepts in the financial management of hospital social work departments, Social Work in Health Care **5**(3):287, 1980.

Rosenberg, G., and Weissman, A.: Marketing social services in health care facilities, Health and Social Work **6**(3):13, 1981.

Schlesinger, E.G., and Wolock, I.: Hospital social work roles and decision making, Social Work in Health Care **8**(1):59, 1982.

Schrager, J., Halman, M., Myers, D., Nicholas, R., and Rosenblum, L.: Impediments to the course and effectiveness of discharge planning, Social Work in Health Care, **4**(1):65, Fall 1978.

Simmons, J.C.: A reporting system for hospital social services departments, Health and Social Work **3**(4):100, 1978.

Smith, H.L.: Two lines of authority: the hospital's dilemma. In Jaco, E.G., editor: Patients, physicians and illness, Glencoe, Ill., 1958, The Free Press.

Trout, M.D.: Birth of a sick or handicapped infant: impact on the family, Child Welfare **62**(4):337, 1983.

Watt, M.S.: Therapeutic facilitator: the role of the social worker in acute treatment hospitals in Ontario, doctoral dissertation, 1977, University of California.

Wattenberg, S.H., Orr, M.M., and O'Rourke, T.W.: Comparisons of opinions of social work administrators toward leadership tasks, Social Work in Health Care **2**(3):285, 1977.

Wax, J.: Developing social work power in a medical organization, Social Work **13**(4):62, 1968.

Wolock, I., Nicholas, C., and Russell, H.: A study of hospital social work services: implications for discharge planning, Paper presented at the annual meeting of the American Public Health Association, Montreal, November 1982.

Wright, R.A., and Allen, P.H.: Marketing and medicine, Journal of the American Medical Association **250**(1):47, 1983.

HIGHLAND PARK SENIOR CITIZEN

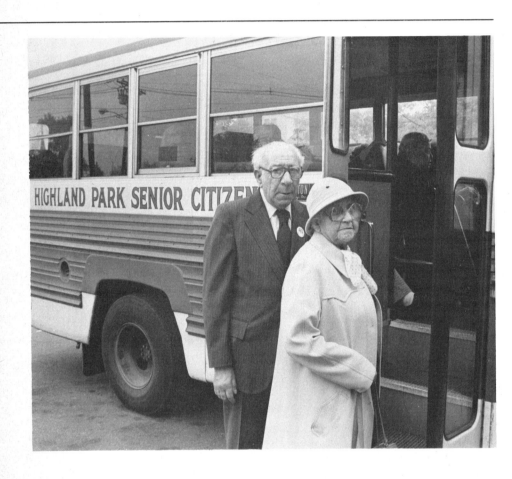

Chapter 10

Social work practice in long-term care

In the introductory chapters considerable attention was paid to the health problems that confront us. Data were presented on the growing numbers of people who have one or more chronic health problems that require lifelong attention. These include those severely disabled as a result of strokes, accidents, lifelong disabling emotional disturbance, or mental illness; the developmentally disabled, who may be impaired physically, mentally, or both; and many of the elderly. This chapter focuses on the various modalities for long-term care, the issues that confront those who provide and who receive such care, and social work's participation in service provision and planning.

Considerable effort has been devoted to finding the most effective ways of providing care for those with minimal capacity to sustain themselves. Major efforts have been focused on reducing the number of people confined to large institutions, on responding to the needs of those in nursing homes and other small, community-based facilities, and on serving the many people who, with assistance from families, community networks, and formal care arrangements, remain in their own homes.

Human service professionals have studied and described various forms of long-term care. An extensive literature has focused on theoretical, philosophical, policy, and practice issues. Some of the major themes that emerge are reviewed. These themes, and the conceptual formulations for health care social work earlier presented (Chapters 5 and 6), highlight the issues that confront health care social workers in long-term care. Together these form the basis for the guidelines for social work practice in long-term care that are presented.

ISSUES IN LONG-TERM CARE

Care for those who cannot care for themselves

Taber (1980) begins his incisive analysis of the literature on alternative care for the physically and mentally handicapped by asking "Who will care for those who cannot care for themselves?" (p. iii). Along with others (for example, Brody, 1974; Lerman, 1982), he focuses on the movement toward deinstitutionalization. This movement has emphasized "normalization" and the ideals of providing "appropriate care" in "least restrictive settings" with "maximum possible independence" (Lerman, 1982, p. 156).

Normalization. Nirje defines normalization as:

> Making available to the mentally subnormal, patterns and conditions of everyday life which are as close as possible to the norms and patterns of the mainstream of society (cited in Lerman, 1982, p. 156).

This view corresponds to that presented by the President's Commission on Mental Health (1978):

> A responsive mental health system should provide the most appropriate care in the least restrictive setting. Whenever possible, people should live at home and receive outpatient treatment in the community. When they cannot, the facility in which they are cared for should offer the maximum possible independence (p. 16).

These ideas are viewed as the basis for formulating standards of care (Lerman, 1982). Mercer and Kane (1979) stress the role of client choice and a sense of control of important elements of the environment as associated with increased hope and participation in the daily activities of living. They suggest that,

> The research base for understanding helplessness, hopelessness, control and choice should be incorporated into the social work curriculum . . . [for] Such concepts provide an empirical base for the profession's cherished values of client self-determination and individualization (p. 112).

These are important components for all population groups needing care over a protracted period or a lifetime.

Deinstitutionalization or alternative care? Whether the deinstitutionalization movement has in fact reduced the number of people who live in institutions is open to question and depends on how one defines the term *institution*. Lerman (1982) proposes that an institution is an establishment that provides food and shelter to four or more persons unrelated to the proprietor and one or more of the following types of services: (1) medical, personal, or social care; (2) treatment or training for skills and habilitation; (3) supervision and/or custodial control; (4) protection and/or social shelter; and (5) diagnostic assessment and/or background investigation. When an institution is defined in this manner it appears that more, rather than fewer, people are now cared for in protective environments (Lerman, 1982). However, in place of the large state hospitals and schools, which have dramatically reduced their populations, care is rendered in a variety of alternative facilities. These include nursing homes, shelter care homes for the mentally ill and mentally retarded, and group homes.

As social workers and other health professionals have sought to develop alternative modes of care, considerable resources, ingenuity, and imagination have been brought to bear. Focusing her comments on review of work with the elderly, Brody (1974) proposes that one central theme has been identification of strengths and assets, as contrasted with an emphasis on losses and deficits. The comments have relevance for diverse population groups. She suggests that "existing and latent strengths constitute the foundation on which constructive treatment programs can be built" (p. 67). In keeping with this view, there has been increasing emphasis on identifying and helping people to make use of those capacities that enhance functioning. Major attention is on developing, retaining, or restoring the skills associated with the needs of daily living. These range from efforts to foster basic self-care skills to helping people move around the community to shop, socialize, or engage in limited work.

Types of long-term care for those with extensive need

There are a number of ways of categorizing types of care. One category is triggered by the care needs generated by the degree of functional disability. For example, people who are not mobile have markedly different needs than the severely mentally disturbed who can get about physically but are actively hallucinating or disoriented as to time and place. Those with diverse types and degrees of functional impairment can be and are cared for in a variety of situations, including their own homes and large, traditional institutional facilities.

Long-term care can also be defined by the particular population groups for which programs are targeted, for example, the mentally ill, the mentally retarded, or the elderly. Such care may also be categorized in terms of *where* it is offered, at home or in small, community-based residential facilities.

Taber (1980) made a systematic review of the literature on "alternative contexts of helping" for a variety of populations. His findings led him to identify three major types of program innovations that have evolved from the movement toward deinstitutionalization. He terms these "new wine in old bottles," "old wine in new bottles," and "new wine in new bottles." These essentially revolve around the fact that much innovation has occurred in traditional settings, in newer settings, and in the type of care rendered. This holds true both for the mentally and physically impaired and for the elderly. These intriguing characterizations provide interesting imagery in respect to the thrusts that have taken place and are therefore used here.*

New wine in old bottles. Reference is to a number of innovative program efforts in such traditional settings as large state hospitals and training schools. Many of these programs have attempted to counteract the characteristic inactivity, boredom, and depersonalization of an earlier day by providing opportunity for verbal interaction, scheduled recreation, and focused attention on the activities of daily living. As might be expected, developmental goals replace custodial goals for those for whom discharge is considered a feasible alternative. These goals are usually geared to the activities needed to live in the community. Efforts to increase the functional capacities of patients with little prospect for discharge are also noted. For example, social clubs are formed and

*The bulk of what follows is abstracted from Taber (1980). Where additional materials are used, they are cited separately.

weekly discussions that provide the opportunity to reminisce and discuss current events are common. The elderly find the opportunity to reminisce especially helpful. The programs described claim benefits "in terms of better relations to current reality, higher morale and somewhat better self care" (p. 13).

Reports of programs in traditional types of community agencies and clinics show, with few exceptions, limited innovation or effort to meet the needs of the particularly disabled. There are reports of successful aggressive team treatment efforts to keep psychiatric patients out of the hospital and programs that "delivered counseling, advocacy or training in whatever setting was most convenient" (p. 17). These tend, however *not* to be based in an agency; settings are as diverse as a factory or a model city project. Most of these projects have not generated new programs. Rather, workers are put into the community to meet people in need at whatever point they express their need. Most of the programs attempt to pick up alcoholics or ex-mental patients at a difficult transition point and then arrange a sequence of services to achieve more normal functioning. A multiple model outreach program is reported wherein a community organization approach organizes self-help and social activity groups for ex-mental patients. Families and discharged ex-mental patients are helped with relocation, group activities, employment, and recreation. In some cases the rate of rehospitalization has been much lower than with more traditional efforts.

The report by Mercer and Kane (1979) of experimental efforts to increase the degree of control that nursing home residents have of their environments is instructive. Experimental variables include the nursing home administration giving clear messages about the residents' opportunities for decision making and to have their ideas or complaints heard by participating in a resident's council. Comparison between residents of the experimental and control nursing homes shows significant decreases in the degree of hopelessness and increase in activity level of the experimental group.

One review of these innovations focuses on moving those in need of long-term care from larger to smaller facilities, such as community homes, halfway houses, family residential centers, and "crisis hostels." Many of these programs aim to prevent admission to large institutions, to ease discharge from such institutions, and to create long-term living situations. Where clear-cut research evidence is available, it appears that concerted programs are successful in helping residents move toward employment and self-reliance and avoid rehospitalization.

Old wine in new bottles. Much work has focused on the effects of moving people from larger to smaller facilities. Where clear-cut research evidence is available, here too it appears that concerted programs are successful in increasing self-reliance, facilitating engagement in paid work, and avoiding rehospitalization.

Day-care center programs designed to maximize family or community living have been described. However, little research has been carried out to assess the extent to which these centers achieve their goals.

New wine in new bottles. The category of alternative care programs that Taber terms "new wine in new bottles" he characterizes as "absorbing." Reports of efforts to place retarded adults in group homes and ex-mental patients in a community work situation and other deliberately designed "contexts" for severely handicapped populations are instructive:

> Practice experiments where effective help was delivered to very needy and handicapped populations were characterized by an environment that was at once highly structured but also supportive. The person being helped, for a period from 4 months to several years, lived within a regime of activity where classes, duties, recreational activities, and social interaction were all directed toward specified goals (p. 27).

These goals include such activities of daily living as grooming, carrying out household chores, engaging in recreational activities, and where possible, working within or outside the facility. Scheduling is tight and days fully planned by a supportive staff that assumes supervisory roles. Resident-staff ratios are high. For the most part, supervision of the day-to-day activities of living is not carried out by professionals.

Implications and questions

This review of the newer approaches to long-term care suggests that some common themes emerge for all of the population groups considered. Whether the need for care is lifelong—as with the developmentally disabled—or comes at the last stage of the life cycle—as with the elderly—structured activity, the opportunity to participate in decision making, and help at crisis points are crucial.

The review also raises a number of important questions. One relates to the effectiveness of standard techniques of therapy and the level at which professionals are needed to make a service effective. A second relates to the permanence or long-term nature of intervention. A third focuses on the advantages and disadvantages of integrating the handicapped with "normal persons" or segregating them with others like themselves.

Clearly, these questions—and the answers—differ to some extent for the varying population groups subsumed under the rubric of long-term care and for the level of care at issue. Those who need day-to-day physical supervision and care, which includes the frail elderly and the severely disabled, can clearly use the services of nonprofessionals. Many of the population groups considered need lifelong care, though much of that care may not be termed explicitly therapeutic, in the traditional sense of that term. A theme of deinstitutionalization is normalization. Whether that means people will be most comfortable in a mixed situation is yet to be determined. And of course, the degree of mixing is an issue.

• • •

Turning again to Taber's review for preliminary answers to the questions just posed aids in organizing the material in terms of the effectiveness of standard therapy techniques, by population groups, by the role of practical help in training in everyday skills, and by the effect of segregation versus integration.

Standard therapy in long-term care

Relatively few substantial research efforts to evaluate the effect of prevailing and accepted therapeutic modalities have been located. Among those located are the effects of drug therapy, group and individual psychotherapy, street work, and social casework. Sadly, most reports that focus on schizophrenic ex-mental patients show no significant difference between kinds of treatment. Drug therapy for schizophrenics outside the hospital more often yields positive results. One study claims reduction in pathology where aftercare treatment involved the combined use of drugs, psychotherapy, and social services.

Work with the "vulnerable" aged, including individualized social work services in the home, shows higher rates of mortality among people receiving those services than among the control group. This classic study by Blenkner et al. (1971) has received considerable attention. It has been suggested that the protective services offered lead to higher rates of institutionalization as social workers become increasingly concerned about the plight of the elderly alone. Wood (1978) wonders how much choice the elderly involved have about their care. Thus posed, the relationship between control over the decisions about one's life—no matter how disabled—and the quality of that life surfaces repeatedly as an issue for long-term care.

By and large, "conventional modes of treatment made a very poor showing among the studies" (p. 36) covered by Taber's review. Those few studies that were multimodal community programs (including standard health and social services) and showed positive findings involved people at crisis points related to their handicaps. These included schizophrenics at the point of admission to treatment facilities.

Practical help and training in everyday skills

A much more encouraging picture emerges from review of service where training in self-care, development of interpersonal skills, or practical services are provided. Criteria used to assess outcome are skill performance or "conforming behaviors" rather than clinical status. Many of these programs include those for the aged handicapped and psychogeriatric patients.

> These practical services were aimed at the most immediate and practical deficits in the behavior repertoires of handicapped persons. Desired role behaviors—conversational skill, attendance at meetings, grooming of self, verbal disagreement without violence . . . were encouraged by social or other reinforcement, by modeling, or in one study by payment of salary (p. 37).

These successful programs were mostly targeted to those said to be underserved by mental health services—among them the aged, the seriously retarded, and alcoholics. Also of importance is the fact that the authoritative, cure-oriented components ascribed to the medical model, with the professional assuming a dominant decision-making role, were largely absent. Another closely related feature was the "deprofessionalization" of service. Aides, members of the target group trained to give care, and other nonprofessionals "recreated the parenting, protecting and guiding functions of a family" (p. 40).

Length of long-term care

The issues of how long people need care and whether treatment fosters further treatment and dependence have long been of concern. Practical questions about readmission to various facilities predominate. Though the data vary, there is some suggestion that previous care fosters the search for subsequent care. Perhaps the most distressing component of the effort to limit care has been the depopulation of many state hospitals without making adequate provision for alternatives—thus the many homeless and street people. A caring perspective suggests that limits on care for vulnerable groups must be most carefully weighed.

These findings may reflect the fact that many of the people considered under the rubric of long-term care simply need continued care. It is also possible that persistently being placed in the sick role or client role minimizes the capacity for independent living; caretakers may reinforce the negative self-images initially generated by the disability. However, the groups considered here have limited potential for living without some help, formal or informal.

Integration or segregation

The current deinstitutionalization movement takes as a given that the handicapped should not be segregated. Nevertheless, whether the handicapped require the protection of segregated settings remains an issue. Taber's review, limited to work on the effects of separate versus integrated education for handicapped children, yields equivocal findings. For some variables, separation is associated with better achievement, while the opposite is noted for others.

This question needs considerable systematic scrutiny. There is comfort in living or being with like-placed others. The growth of self-help and mutual support groups attests to that. Nevertheless in pondering this issue, care must be taken not to find a rationale for segregation that is not based on the needs of people with disability. The subjective response to some segments of the deinstitutionalization movement suggests that life can be enriched for all by mixing. The handicapped and nonhandicapped alike enlarge the scope of their experience.

Public Law 94-142 (the Education of All Handicapped Children Act, 1975) and subsequent amendments mandate the provision of educational services for young handicapped children. Experiences with implementation of this legislation suggest that both specialized and mixed educational opportunities need to be provided.

Conclusions

The preceding review of alternative approaches to long-term care has highlighted the following trends:

1. Significant numbers of people continue to need, and receive, supervised care in situations where their rights or ability to control their own lives is diminished.
2. There has been substantial effort to reduce the degree of external control and to create situations that make it more likely the handicapped, elderly, and disabled will have some say in determining the direction of their lives and nature of activity. Much of this care is provided in homes and in small institutions.
3. Conventional modes of psychotherapeutic intervention appear to be less successful in increasing levels of functioning than programmatic efforts focused on practical help in enhancing training for everyday skills and efforts that aim to facilitate decision making and control.
4. Interventive modalities of a highly protective, supervised, and supportive nature—usually involving high client/staff ratios—show much promise.
5. Much of the daily work of caretaking can be carried out by paraprofessionals and others with limited training, as well as members of the target population. Professionals usually play a significant role in planning and coordinating the wide variety of efforts.

SOCIAL WORK'S ROLE

When health care social workers turn their attention to the needs of those requiring long-term care, a number of concerns common to all of social work health practice emerge. The conceptual formulations developed in Chapter 5 can serve to order and specify our thinking about long-term care tasks. The public health perspective helps to focus on the conditions of life that generate long-term care needs, while at the same time heightening sensitivity to those components of prevention that are at play in long-term care needs. These include secondary prevention—as in efforts to prevent further decline of the elderly, or habilitation of the mentally retarded. The perspective of person-environment fit can help to clarify thinking about whether the needs for long-term care can best be met by environmental modification, efforts to help people alter their behavior, or both. Those new modes of care characterized by Taber as "absorbing" are compelling examples of successful efforts to alter or create caring environments. At the same time they focus on helping people acquire skills that serve them in the daily business of living. The discussions of the continuum from cure to care and the typology of caring presented help to call attention to the range of care needs of those who need long-term or permanent care. The elderly in their own homes or in residential facilities need medical attention and counseling designed to help with depression, anxiety, or other disabling emotional states. The same holds true for many other physically and mentally handicapped people. Efforts to increase the amount of control the elderly have over their environments can yield a profitable shift from custodial or maintenance tasks to those designed to "promote," "enhance," or restore functioning. Kane et al. (1976) have demonstrated that nursing home residents show improvement in memory, thinking, mood, and participation in activities when they receive social services.

Nevertheless, there remains a core of people—in nursing homes, in facilities for the retarded, or in their own homes—whose ability to participate consciously and deliberately in the activities of daily living is most limited. In their exciting experiment designed to reduce helplessness and hopelessness among nursing home residents, Mercer and Kane (1979) included in their study sample only those who were receiving intermediate levels of care, were ambulatory, and could communicate. Those who have virtually no potential for improved functioning nevertheless require "tender maintenance." Their families, or others, need much help.

The concept of *careers of illness* aids in thinking about care needs at different stages of illness or disability. Those whose deficits are identified early in life and expected to last a lifetime, face different tasks than adolescents who, following an accident, become quadriplegic. These differ in turn from the issues confronting the elderly who face increasing decline and role loss following a full, productive life.

Social work tasks

To each of these types of problems social workers bring a fundamental orientation to the social components of care. Brody (1974) has delineated the responsibilities of those whose attention is focused on the elderly. The relevance for all social work practice in long-term care with diverse population groups is clear. She cites the following as particular areas of social work responsibility: individualization, integration of different aspects of the treatment plan, avoidance of fragmentation, capitalizing on individual strengths, mobilization of resources, help for individuals in adapting to their changed situations and in using available programs, development of new resources and programs, and modification of the environment (p. 68). This listing encompasses the range of social work repertoires that require use of the skills reviewed earlier (Chapter 7) and is clearly consonant with the model of health care social work practice developed in Chapter 6.

Though these tasks refer to the gamut of social work practice in long-term care, some illustrations of their specific application are useful. Individualization is most crucial. It is not uncommon to think of *the elderly* or *the handicapped* and to forget that each individual has a unique experience that has brought him or her to the present state of affairs. Thus some elderly like to continue to "parent" while others have long been happy to give up that role. The latter will not readily respond to efforts to involve them in becoming "foster" grandparents to a disabled child. Avoidance of fragmentation and help in using available programs are especially significant for people needing long-term care. Case management strategies are particularly important here. For it is a characteristic of the life of this population group that they require the help of the patchwork system of services so typical of service delivery systems in this country. Coordination becomes a major task.

In carrying out these tasks, social workers are often confronted with barriers that relate to the current pattern of organization of health and welfare services. In long-term care, as in other areas of service delivery, no one profession or discipline currently has responsibility for planning and coordination. Morris and Anderson (1975) review the consequent difficulties and make suggestions that are worthy of serious consideration.

Long-term care—a core social work responsibility?

In "Personal Care Services: an Identity for Social Work," Morris and Anderson (1975) propose that social work could be the profession identified by society as responsible for planning, developing, managing, and administering a variety of programs. Such a programmatic thrust, they suggest, can match psychosocial insights with responsibility for care. A number of models are identified. The first, the *coordinating model,* is most prevalent today. The model assumes that a variety of service organizations will continue to exist, but that more efficient coordination is possible and desirable. Information and referral centers are key components of the proposals for better coordination. Another model is the *cashing out of services.* This approach assumes that given enough money, people will be able to command the resources needed.

In contrast to these prevailing models, Morris and Anderson (1975) propose that the variety of agencies dealing with long-term care issues assign responsibility for managing various tangible and concrete services to the profession of social work.

> Thus assembled could be day centers, halfway houses, foster homes, residential arrangements, home help, home-delivered chore services, home nursing, and many similar services. Skilled assessment or evaluation and personal counseling needs to be provided, but this function is not severed from the concrete services which the assessed and at-risk population also require. Various classes of staff would be employed, with several levels of training but held together coherently by the leadership of one profession which accepts the obligation for seeing to it that this significant segment of modern society is cared for—namely, social work (p. 167).

A health system version is proposed. In this version a social service or a community department of a health agency would be staffed by social workers and social work administrators. This department would employ home health aides and attendants and would have authority to purchase services.

Though consideration of the viability and feasibility of such a model is beyond the purview of this book, its essential elements nevertheless provide a useful way of thinking about the social worker's role in long-term care. The emphasis on planning, control, and integration of services that rely on an amalgam of professional and nonprofessional care services is congruent with the finding that those services focused on skillful efforts to provide practical services were the most promising of the long-term care approaches tried so far. Taber (1980) comments on this. He suggests that successful programs involve program design and planning by professionals (that is, psychiatrists, psychologists, or social workers).

> Actual direct service was performed by aides or non professionals who were trained on the job. Possibly the scope of small-scale programs to provide care for several hundred thousand persons unable to care for themselves can only be provided when scarce professional manpower is amplified in that way.
>
> With the attempts to create new settings for help or to insert chronically handicapped persons into existing community institutions problems of coordination have become acute. [This literature review] supports the general impression that there is indeed a problem of coordinating helping programs in different agencies under different auspices (pp. 99-100).

The need for a "broker" function to facilitate access to multiple services is mentioned by many who have looked at issues of long-term care.

Social workers need to engage actively in policy analysis, formulation, and political activities that would enable the profession to play the role envisioned by Morris and Anderson. Whatever the outcome of such efforts, the profession of social work must, nevertheless, play a leadership role in efforts to assure that coordinated, integrated care takes place.

Official statements by the American Hospital Association (Dockhorn, 1982) recognize such a role for social workers who are involved in planning care for persons to be discharged. When social workers function in statewide mental health associations or branches of the Association for Retarded Citizens, they are often in a position to take a role akin to that proposed by Morris and Anderson. That role needs to be explicitly developed.

For example, in many areas of the country social workers are employed in county Associations for Retarded Citizens. They have responsibility for contracting with state agencies to plan and coordinate a variety of services. These include (1) working with retarded citizens and their families around decisions concerning discharge from large institutions; (2) helping those involved to determine whether a community-based group home or the retarded citizen's own home will meet needs; (3) hiring and supervising those paraprofessionals who manage and work in community-based facilities such as group homes; and (4) planning with and for the residents the types of programs that are most likely to foster normalization. In turn, they are responsible for liaison and linkage with the families, medical facilities, and sheltered workshops.

Many hospitals are beginning to expand their services to include intermediate care nursing facilities for those no longer in need of acute hospital care. Some also develop liaison with congregate housing facilities for senior citizens in their communities. Social work has major responsibility for coordinating these efforts, as well as providing a direct service component.

These types of programs are illustrations of how social work can assume a key coordinating, planning, and service delivery function. That function derives from a social work perspective on social functioning and the emphasis on the person-situation interface. To this function social work brings a knowledge of person-in-situation, sensitivity to the unique dispositions of varying ethnic and cultural groups, and intimate acquaintance with the community and its available resource systems as well as analysis of additional resources. In addition, special attention must be paid to the assault on self-image of those affected and their families when confronted with severe disability. Given the expanding need for long-term care, for innovation, and for continued development of new models of delivery, an approach that focuses simultaneous attention on individual and systemic change needs (Chapter 6) is particularly crucial in long-term care.

With these considerations as a backdrop, the rest of this chapter is devoted to identifying some guidelines for social work participation in long-term care delivery and planning.

GUIDELINES FOR PRACTICE

To illustrate how experience with varying approaches to long-term care can help social workers in further sharpening and delineating their role, the concept *careers of illness* is used to suggest how the tasks of direct service provision are integrated with efforts at planning and coordination.

As suggested earlier, the stage of life at which the need for long-term care arises and the point in time of the illness career have major impact on the type of care needed, as well as on how social work responds to diverse needs. The first type of population in need involves people whose lifelong handicaps are identified at birth or early in life. The second is composed of those who develop disabilities, as a result of illness, injury, or previously undetected genetic defect, while leading a productive, satisfying life. The third type includes those elderly who are facing physical or mental handicaps and who find themselves to be frail and declining, following a long, fruitful life. As these careers are discussed, effort is made to identify direct service tasks and those calling for coordination, planning, and interdisciplinary endeavors.

Needs of those with lifelong disabilities

Many handicapping conditions are identified early in life. Too numerous to be listed here, they variously involve physical and/or mental impairment of sufficient severity to preclude the possibility of independent functioning at any point in their lives. For these children, and their families, a number of stages of the illness career and the accompanying needs and tasks can be identified.

Stage 1—suspicion, recognition. Stage 1, or early recognition or suspicion of defect, can entail the utmost trauma for the family. My work with the parents of children diagnosed as having Down's syndrome, cerebral palsy, hydrocephaly, and other disorders points to a mixture of desperate hope and denial, coupled with gradual and reluctant emotional and intellectual acknowledgment that "something is not right" (Drayer and Schlesinger, 1969).

The social worker, as one of a number of professionals working with such families, plays many roles at this stage. Individualizing and understanding any particular family's response and concerns are major social work responsibilities. Knowledge of the usual and typical reactions to this type of problem must be used as a way of developing an image of the unique and particular set of concerns generated. Some families will focus on what needs to be done now—medical examinations, special type of care required, cost, and the problem of bringing the child for a variety of services when there are other young children needing care. Many families are not ready to share their grief or to raise questions about long-range implications. Others may become immobilized or said to be in a crisis state. Anxiety and tension may reflect guilt, anger, and a blow to self-esteem. All of the skills involved in crisis intervention may need to be marshalled (see particularly Golan, 1978, Chapter 5). Efforts to help people to articulate their reaction, coupled with a focus on action, are particularly helpful.

If people are able to respond by crying or by beginning to express their disappointment, loss, and fears, it is usually helpful to begin to identify what needs to be done. In a neonatal intensive care unit the worker may begin by telling parents about the regular visiting times and giving them the opportunity to participate in some aspects of the child's care. With a somewhat older child, a visit to a day-care center to see how children are treated may be suggested.

Whatever the parental reaction, there is little question that the family will be in contact with a variety of care-takers—hospitals, schools, and other organizations that can contribute to maximum development. Social workers can and must assume responsibility for integrating services. Many families will want to—and should—seek the opinions of a number of specialists to make certain that they have done all that is possible to learn what is wrong with their child and what can be done. However, the long, arduous path of going from clinic, to physician, to one school after another often adds to the family's difficulties. The social worker who is readily available and knowledgeable about resources, links people to those resources, and is ready to provide concrete help or emotional support as indicated can help people through this early stage.

Efforts to project the long-term picture, to help parents and others to acknowledge lifelong disability, may be premature and dysfunctional at this stage. For most, focus is appropriately on their present situation.

Stage 2—the long haul. In stage 2, denial or doubt may persist. Nevertheless, a process of settling in often takes place. Parents learn to cope with the daily tasks of managing a handicapped child. They become accustomed to lifting or diapering a child long past the point when that is ordinarily expected. Nevertheless, crises are not uncommon. Fatigue sets in at the same time that the true implications of the disability are reinforced by the daily experience of living with a child whose growth is slow and faltering at best.

Though scarce social work services may not make it possible for the social worker to be available continuously, a case management stance is considered essential.* Social workers make themselves available for periodic discussion to review the situation. At the same time they call on nurses, child development specialists, and others who can help in training for self-care. Day-care centers, cerebral palsy treatment centers, preschools, and special schools for speech and hearing are but a few examples (Evans, 1983). The social worker may be located in a specialized hospital setting, in a home health agency, or elsewhere. Whatever the case, the basic principle is the same: that is, to use or develop programs that facilitate individualized, coordinated care.

Stage 3—moving beyond the confines of the home. For those children and their parents where physical or mental development has been slow but steady, there is a point when the child moves about, interacts with peers, and begins to communicate. At this point most families are eager to get their child into an educational program, but this often precipitates anger or fear of rejection. Unrealistic hopes may again surface: "Perhaps he can go right into the first grade so he can catch up."

At this point, the family and the child—now in a different way—confront the reality of the disability as decisions must be made about how the child will interact with the larger world. Here as before, there are no panaceas or clear-cut answers. Workers, recognizing this to be a crucial phase, individualize as they bring their knowledge of resources to bear. Where the community schools have developed good programs for "mainstreaming," the situation is different from where segregation has been the rule. Workers can share the fact that knowledge about which is better is incomplete (see earlier discussion). Evans (1983) points out that information as to whether special schools are good and essential for moderately retarded individuals is not yet clear.

Stage 4—adolescence and adulthood. Like other people, the mentally

*Recent developments suggest a core role for social workers as case managers in coordinating services for this population (National Conference on Social Welfare, 1981).

and physically handicapped and their families face especially important developmental tasks in adolescence and adulthood. Sexuality in one deemed unable to handle it may evoke many fears. Neighbors who in the past were friendly and ready to have their children "play with Johnny" may begin to withdraw. At this stage, both the handicapped and their families need information, counseling, and help in locating recreational groups, sheltered workshops, or counseling facilities.

A major issue that begins to surface at this point focuses on "What will happen to Johnny when I'm gone?" Or, "Shouldn't he be living with others like him?" Workers need to help families anticipate and articulate these concerns. Most importantly, handicapped persons—within the limits of their capacity—must be involved in decision making.

The discussion earlier in this chapter identified a number of programs that have been developed for the permanently mentally or physically impaired. Small group homes or supervised apartments may be suitable for those whose families are no longer available or for those who see this type of living as a step toward independence. Sheltered workshops provide skills training and a sense of accomplishment. Counseling may help cope with despair or a sense of worthlessness.

This effort to sketch out the career of mentally and physically impaired persons from birth to adulthood has sought to identify some major themes: (1) the tasks and crises often associated with several crucial stages; (2) the different types of concerns that tend to arise at infancy, childhood, adolescence, and adulthood; and (3) the mix of services required at each stage. The social worker's effort at each stage must always be focused on how unique responses and needed or available resources interact to facilitate or hamper functioning.

Social workers have a particular obligation to be alert to the emotional needs of the developmentally disabled and other handicapped people. Evans (1983) vividly describes the degree to which "normal" people will distance themselves from the mentally retarded. Intellectual deficit does not imply emotional numbness. Thus counseling the retarded themselves and others about such feelings must not be overlooked.

The needs of those dealing with unanticipated disability

Quadriplegia following an automobile accident, dramatic and rapid decline of functioning following the onset of multiple sclerosis, and disabling stroke in midlife are but a few examples of major health problems that trigger long-term care needs. Emphasis is on those needs that confront people who develop these problems somewhere between late childhood or adolescence and the fifties and early sixties. For the most part they have led and planned their lives in accord with routine expectations. They hope to raise families or are already parents. They are making vocational plans or are actively involved in their life's work. Most function as sexual beings.

Their needs for care, medical, emotional, and physical, are extensive. They, too, go through stages of response to their illness; in turn, each of these stages generates a common pattern of needs.

Stage 1—recognition. Not unlike the parents of young children whose deficits are noted early on, response to the onset is coupled with denial and anger. Few people come to grips all at once with the enormity of their difficulties. Paraplegics and quadriplegics may often respond well to intervention while in the rehabilitation center and may eagerly plan a weekend home to test out the skills learned in the hospital. On returning to the hospital, they may reveal to the social worker that in anticipating the home visit, they had retained an image of their former selves. Somehow, magically, the disability would disappear, and they would be able to navigate stairs, bathe, and otherwise do things as they had before.*

Anger may be projected on the spouse or children, while the model patient role is sustained. During the period of hospitalization, life itself is perceived as being in the hands of the medical staff. Some patients fear that overt criticism and refusal to cooperate with treatment may alienate those on whom they are now dependent.

When social workers can help people to develop trust, they may be able to help them to verbalize these fears. This is important because it can serve to release energy and emotion for realistic coping. Coping takes the form of developing a new set of skills, of maintaining a viable self-image, and of beginning to modify or change cherished life plans.

The social worker's role usually begins early in this stage. Too often, social workers attempt to force acceptance and early recognition at the expense of focusing on the incremental steps needed to enhance functioning, not recognizing that the psyche needs time and concrete evidence to incorporate the enormity of what is going on.

Stage 2—return to the community. In Chapter 5 the types of management problems that confront those with permanent residual disability were reviewed. Homes need to be adapted or modified to enable those in wheelchairs to get around. Others need to be on hand to help with anticipated or unanticipated medical emergencies. Career goals need modification, or new ones need to be developed.

The social worker need to be knowledgeable and skillful in identifying or creating concrete resources for help with these problems. Group experiences, such as "stroke clubs," have been shown to effect maximal use of limited capacities. The broker role becomes critical as social workers link people with needed services. Advocating for the client's right to terminate treatment, even when eager rehabilitation staffs seek "just a little more progress" from those who are tired of playing the eager patient role, is often crucial. Where social

*Based on conversation with Pat Costante, rehabilitation social worker.

work is successful in contracting and monitoring diverse services this can be extremely helpful. It can avoid the arduous task of determining eligibility for a variety of categorical programs where so many people inevitably fall between the cracks.

Although the current pattern of fragmented service delivery does not facilitate this type of coordination, any effort in that direction can enhance life for those who face protracted dependency. Some will remain with their families. Others will require the combination of medical and social care available in group homes or nursing homes. All need a say in how they will live, as well as concrete and emotional help in minimizing the negative impact of dependency.

The needs and wishes of the elderly

The elderly are not a monolithic group, all of whom present a common set of needs. Decline is sometimes gradual and imperceptible. For others, medical, biological, and psychological events converge to generate rapid and dramatic shifts.

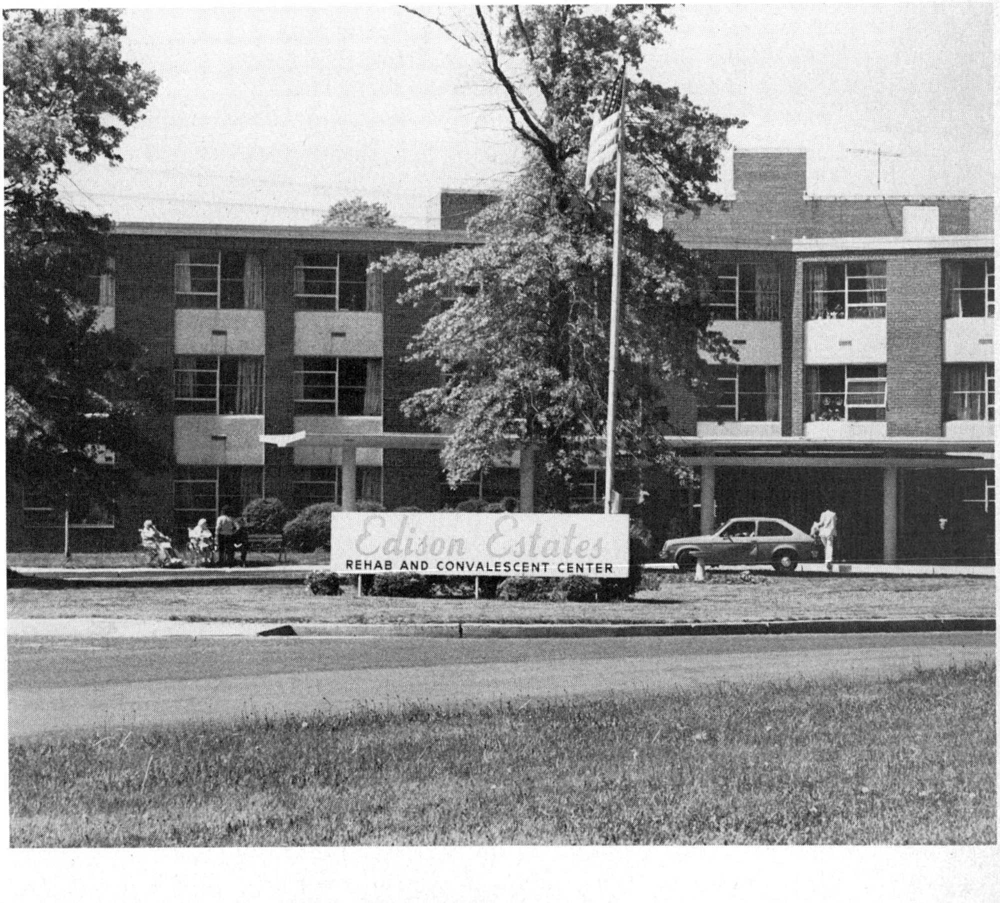

Levels of functioning rather than chronological age determine the care needs of the elderly. Though recognition of one's own mortality and the imminence of death surface more sharply with advancing age, it is difficult to classify a progression or stages of aging, as was done with the situation of disabled newborns and young children and those who acquire disabilities between adolescence and midlife. For this reason, this discussion of the elderly focuses on a number of issues that are repeatedly noted in the literature.

In "Social Work with the Aged: Principles of Practice," Monk (1981) suggests that:

> The professional interventions of social workers are exceptional because they ultimately take into account the totality of clients' lives, even when they are designed to search for the last threads of clients' remaining strength amidst tangles of chronic impediments and the overwhelming bombardments of successive losses (p. 61).

In exploring the question "Does social work have a distinctive purpose in regard to the aged?" Monk identifies three perspectives. One relates to the fact that this is a distinct stage of life when life experiences are integrated, and death is never far. The second focuses on past devaluation of practice with this age group derived from "a deeply ingrained therapeutic nihilism that views the aging as rigid and impervious to change" (p. 62). The third focuses on a view of aging that does *not* involve a cyclical reenactment of prior life events, but instead has its own characteristics. This view points to the need for special supports. These include those from family, the community, and the health and welfare system.

Recognizing that this chapter cannot begin to capture the full complexity of knowledge, resources, and social work tasks required for this group, this section seeks to identify some major findings that point to the needs of the elderly and social work tasks in relation to these.

In Chapter 1 some basic data on the number of elderly in the population, the degrees of disability, and their need for medical and social care were reviewed. The *frail elderly,* those over 75, have been the subject of particular concern and inquiry.

The preferences of those elderly persons who need some form of protective care are firmly established by a number of investigations. Bell (1973) found that 85% preferred to remain in their own homes. Many of those who need help in caring for themselves request homemaker service (Gold, 1972). A survey focused on what services were considered the most desirable ranked transportation and home maintenance services as the most important, and counseling and casework services as the least important.

A number of workers have commented on the fact that the family is the major provider of social support for the elderly.

> The stereotype of the lonely or abandoned older person has not been confirmed by research. . . . Families do more for their elderly relatives than they

> are given credit for. The family, rather than formal service systems, provides most of the home health services for incapacitated or homebound relatives (Monk and Dobrof, 1980, p. 146).

By the same token, the elderly prefer to live in their own homes rather than with relatives. Class and ethnic differences affect the degree to which primary support networks are available. Among nonwhite minorities* Hispanic elderly were most likely to be involved in close-knit family networks. In one study Cantor (1973) found that Blacks were experiencing declining support from their offspring. Wolf (1978) found that the number of elderly Blacks in nursing homes is low in proportion to their number in the population. Lowy (1979) suggests that discrimination continues to play a role, as does the tendency for Blacks to "care for their own." Role loss, coupled with greater reluctance to accept services to which they are entitled, results in particular trauma for many of the white elderly.

Though the family assumes substantial responsibility, this form of care is not adequate for all. Further, such attention takes its toll on adult offspring, many of whom are beginning to approach senior citizen status. Those who care for elderly parents while they are still busy in efforts to launch their own children into adulthood face dual pressures. The difficulties experienced by the adult offspring of the frail elderly are being increasingly recognized. Senior citizens' outreach centers are developing outreach programs to work with such families, in groups or as individuals, to help them cope with the daily pressures of trying to meet diverse sets of demands, to cope with guilt around "not doing enough," and to help locate proper services.

The increase in reported cases of abuse of the elderly by their adult children is symptomatic of the types of pressures being experienced by this population group.

Types of care. Using the approach to categorize care by type or nature of facility, a number can be identified. They include the home, foster care, adult day-care centers, nursing homes, and homes for the aged.

Home care includes home health care, homemaker services, the services of home health aides, and visits from the social worker. Meals on Wheels and other senior citizen nutrition programs whereby the elderly are transported daily to centers that provide meals and the opportunity to socialize are crucial elements of service facilitated by recent legislation. Monk and Dobrof (1980) point to the recommendations of the 1978 President's Commission on Mental Health that "home care must become an essential component of mental and physical care of the elderly" (p. 150). Research on such programs points to the need for more case management and quality control. In creating the Area Agencies on Aging under Title III, it was hoped that these agencies would monitor

*This group includes Blacks, Puerto Ricans, Chicanos (the term *Hispanic* is often used for the latter two groups), American Indians, and Asian Americans.

existing services and develop those needed. These agencies experience the same dilemma as do others seeking to provide and coordinate long-term care services. Guidelines for an appropriate mix of planning and coordinating services and direct service delivery are not clear; the power to sanction and make major policy and administrative decisions is not clearly assigned.

Legislation has long required social work consultation to nursing homes (which care for some 5% of the elderly). A number of studies (for example, Mercer and Garner, 1981) suggest that these consultants have had a limited view of their function. Considerable time and effort were spent in teaching clinical skills to social work designees.* "Their stated purposes did not include the bringing about of systems change, and their most preferred and time consuming functions had little to do with such change" (Mercer and Garner, 1981, p. 12). Gehrke and Wattenberg (1981) found that social work nursing home consultants and designees considered the work of planning for residents' care as most important. Advocacy, though considered important, was seldom done. The use of groups was limited, as was involvement of residents in formulating their own care plans, despite the important findings of workers like Mercer and Kane (1979), who showed that participation in daily decision making by nursing home residents considerably enhances functioning.

This emphasis on increasing the advocacy and system change role does not imply a negation of the importance of direct work with the elderly on a one-to-one basis. Surely, whether at home or in an institutional facility, the elderly need the opportunity to complain, to reflect on their life, and to anticipate impending death.

Increasing attention is paid to groups in which the elderly reminisce about past experiences as a way of bringing closure on past successes or on the basis of failures. In our rapidly changing society, there is still room to draw on the wisdom and experience accumulated in a long life that will have, for the most part, been marked by some achievement. Where decline has set in to the point that this kind of reflection is not possible, family members need help in coping with the facts of such decline.

• • •

This review has touched briefly on the wishes and needs of those elderly and their families who require one or more social and health supports, the types of settings where these supports are provided, and the difficulties encountered in providing and planning for services. The challenge for enhancing practice with this group is a continuing one. The objectives of practice with the elderly enunciated by Monk (1981) are consistent with the themes for health care social work practice presented in this book and congruent with the guidelines for practice with various groups needing long-term care. These are (1)

*These are persons, often without professional training, who perform social work tasks.

helping people to enlarge their competence and increase their problem-solving capacities, (2) helping the elderly to obtain resources, (3) facilitating interaction between individuals and others in their environment, (4) influencing interactions between organizations and institutions, and (5) influencing social and environmental policy.

As is true with other groups of the disabled, the principles of appropriate service delivered in the least restrictive environment that fosters maximum possible independence is crucial. A focus on social functioning, on service geared to the given level of capacity (including available supports), can serve to individualize need. As is the case with other groups of those with long-term care needs, careful attention is needed to differentiate between the services required from professionals, nonprofessional caretakers, family, and community networks, and above all, to what the elderly can continue to do for themselves.

As social workers grapple with these issues, they need to sharpen their assessment and counseling skills, as well as those coordinating and political skills that may facilitate their ability to develop and manage caring programs for the elderly.

SUMMARY

This chapter has reviewed some major themes in the literature on long-term care, among them the current thrust toward deinstitutionalization and normalization.

The emphasis on normalization and providing care in least restrictive, supportive environments extends to a variety of populations in long-term care. In this chapter it was pointed out that these populations include those whose disabilities are lifelong, as exemplified by the developmentally disabled; those who develop difficulties during adolescence or adulthood, as exemplified by paraplegics or those with multiple sclerosis; and the elderly.

A review of the literature on long-term care pointed to three major types of care: (1) new interventive modalities offered in traditional institutions; (2) traditional modalities used in new types of facilities; and (3) new modalities in new settings. All point to the importance of enhancing the skills of daily living and enlarging the decision-making role of the disabled and elderly.

Review of current service delivery patterns showed them to be highly fragmented. Several models for developing more integrated service structures were reviewed. One model that would assign a major role to social work in managing, coordinating, and planning such services bears particular scrutiny by the profession. Policy analysis and political activity are essential if social work is to obtain a mandate to play this role. Social work has a long, historical tradition in watching out for the needs of those afflicted by lifelong problems.

How social work can attend to those difficulties, at both individual and systemic levels, was illustrated by reference to the illness careers concept, which was used to develop suggested guidelines for practice in this area.

REFERENCES

Bell, W.G.: Community care for the elderly: an alternative to institutionalization, The Gerontologist **13:**349, Autumn 1973.

Blenkner, M., Bloom, M., and Nielson, M.: A research and demonstration project of protective services, Social Casework **52:**489, October 1971.

Brody, E.M.: A social work guide for long term care facilities, Pub. No. (ADM) 76-177, Rockville, Md., 1974, Department of Health, Education and Welfare.

Cantor, M.: The elderly in the inner city: some implications of the effect of culture on life styles, Paper presented at the Institute on Gerontology and Graduate Education for Social Work, New York, March 1973, Fordham University.

Dockhorn, J.: Essentials of social work programs in hospitals, Chicago, 1982, American Hospital Association.

Drayer, C., and Schlesinger, E.: The informing interview. In Wolfensberger, W., and Kurtz, R., editors: Management of the family of the mentally retarded, 1969, Follett Educational Corp.

Evans, D.P.: The lives of mentally retarded people, Boulder, Colo., 1983, Westview Press, Inc.

Gehrke, J.P., and Wattenberg, S.H.: Assessing social services in nursing homes, Health and Social Work **6**(2):14, 1981.

Golan, M.: Treatment in crisis situations, New York, 1978, The Free Press.

Gold, J.: Comparison of protective service projects, The Gerontologist, vol. 12, Autumn 1972.

Kane, R.L., Jorgensen, L.A., Teteberg, B., and Kuwahara, J.: Is good nursing-home care feasible? Journal of the American Medical Association **235**(5):516, 1976.

Lerman, P.: Deinstitutionalization and the welfare state, New Brunswick, N.J., 1982, Rutgers University Press.

Lowy, L.: Social work with the aging, New York, 1979, Harper & Row, Publishers, Inc.

Mercer, S.O., and Garner, J.D.: Social work consultation in long-term care facilities, Health and Social Work **6**(2):5, 1981.

Mercer, S.O., and Kane, R.: Helplessness and hopelessness among the institutionalized aged: an experiment, Health and Social Work **4**(1):90, 1979.

Monk, A.: Social work with the aged: principles of practice, Social Work **26**(1):61, 1981.

Monk, A., and Dobrof, R.: Social services for older persons: a review of research. In Fanshel, D., editor: Future of social work research, Washington, D.C., 1980, National Association of Social Workers, Inc., pp. 139-161.

Morris, R., and Anderson, D.: Personal care services: an identity for social work, Social Service Review **49**(2):157, 1975.

National Conference on Social Welfare: Case management: state of the art, HEW Grant No. 54-p-71542/3-01, Administration on Developmental Disabilities, Department of Health, Education, and Welfare.

President's Commission on Mental Health: Report and recommendations to the President, Washington, D.C., 1978, U.S. Government Printing Office, vol. 1.

Taber, M.A.: The social context of helping: a review of the literature on alternative care for the physically and mentally handicapped, DHHS Pub. No. (ADM) 80-42, Washington, D.C., 1980, U.S. Department of Health and Human Services.

Wolf, R.S.: A social systems model of nursing home use, Hospital Research and Educational Trust, p. 111, Summer 1978.

Wood, K.M.: Casework effectiveness: a new look at the research evidence, Social Work **23**(6):437, 1978.

LYONS
FAMILY HEALTH CENTER
entrance
LYONS
FAMILY HEALTH CENTER

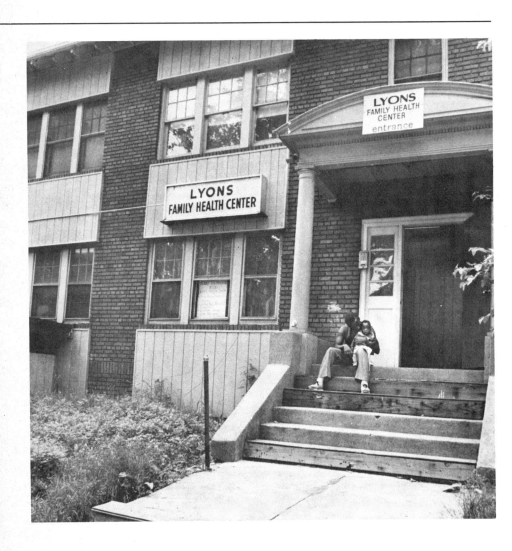

Chapter 11

Social work practice in primary care

In the introductory chapter to a recent volume entitled *Primary Health Care: More Than Medicine,* Miller (1983) points to the complex issues that have led to increasing attention to this most exciting, yet elusive component of contemporary health care. She points to humanistic yearnings for the ready accessibility of continuous, comprehensive care for all implied by increasing emphasis on primary care. She suggests, however, that "it would be simplistic to think of primary care as a throwback to the erstwhile family doctor" (p. 1). Much of the material reviewed in this book suggests that Miller's point is well taken. Few users of the health care system would give up the advances of medical technology that are the hallmark of modern health care. Yet it is because of these very developments, and the fragmentation often associated with such care, that many people long for the modern version of the "old family doctor." That doctor—although lacking know-how in today's more sophisticated treatment technology—tended to many diverse physical and emotional needs.

There are numerous competing, and at times conflicting, definitions of primary care, and some of these will be reviewed in this chapter. A number of themes run through the definitions to be considered. One relates to efforts to provide continuous care by concerned providers who have the knowledge and empathy to respond to physical and emotional concerns. From this perspective, many of the primary care thrusts may be characterized as efforts to develop the contemporary counterpart of the old-fashioned family doctor. Another important theme is the emphasis on serving those populations previously underserved, such as the poor and those who live in isolated rural areas. Important also is the attention that is paid to the psychosocial components of illness and to the consumers' role in planning and participating in health care delivery.

Many approaches to developing and expanding primary care have evolved. These include building new organizational structures for delivering care, attending to training practitioners in this mode of delivery, and clarifying the functions of various primary health care providers. In this chapter emphasis is on identifying the various components of primary care and on social work's role in this aspect of health care delivery.

WHAT IS PRIMARY CARE?

Primary care can be viewed as a "concept which transcends the professional domains of the various health professions and calls for smooth collaboration among the several disciplines if a whole person approach to health service delivery is to be 'realized'" (Miller, 1983, p. 2). Another way of viewing primary care is by distinguishing it from other levels of care by the function performed, the organizational structures in which it is carried out, and the tasks performed by various providers. Ell and Morrison (1981) propose that primary care functions as a point of entry, screening, and "routing point" for the rest of the personal health care system. The range of health services thought essential for prevention, care of "common illnesses," and "stabilizing" human support needed by patients and their families around the troubles that surface in relation to health problems are included as primary care functions. Also important is the view that primary care includes assumption of responsibility for the continuing management and coordination of personal health care services. The following definition offered by Ell and Morrison (1981) is echoed by many others (for example, Lloyd, 1977; Miller, 1983; Woodward, 1983).

> The hallmarks of primary care are that it is accessible, continuous, comprehensive and coordinated in that the geographical, scheduling and financial barriers to its use are minimized; that it is provided over many years by the same source; that it is attentive to psychosocial as well as physical aspects of illness; and that it involves cooperation and communication among health care providers (p. 35S).

Miller and others identify primary care with ambulatory care, while Woodward focuses much of his discussion on alternative primary health care provider models. Davis (1983) emphasizes the relationship between the growth in primary care services, legislation that has facilitated increased access to underserved populations (for example, Medicare and Medicaid), and federal support of training for those primary care providers who serve in underserved areas.

An important definition is offered by the World Health Organization:

> Primary health care is essential health care based on practical, scientifically sound and socially acceptable methods and technology made universally accessible to individuals and families in the community through their full participation and at a cost that the community and country can afford to maintain at every stage of their development in the spirit of self-reliance and self-determination. It forms an integral part both of the country's health system, of which it is the central function and main focus, and of the overall social and economic development of the community. It is the first level of contact of individuals, the family and the community with the National Health System bringing health care as close as possible to where people live and work, and constitutes the first element of a continuing health care process (European Seminar, 1983, p. 67).

Vuori (1983) of the World Health Organization suggests that primary care can be understood as a philosophy, an approach or strategy, a level of care, and a set of activities. At a philosophical level, primary care seeks to put into operation basic principles of social justice, equality, and individual responsibility for health. As a strategy for enhancing health and health care delivery, primary care encompasses diverse activities and concepts ranging from efforts to enhance accessibility of care and legislative reforms, to recognition of the role of other sectors of the society—housing, employment, education—in health and illness. As a set of activities, primary care focuses on treatment of common dis-

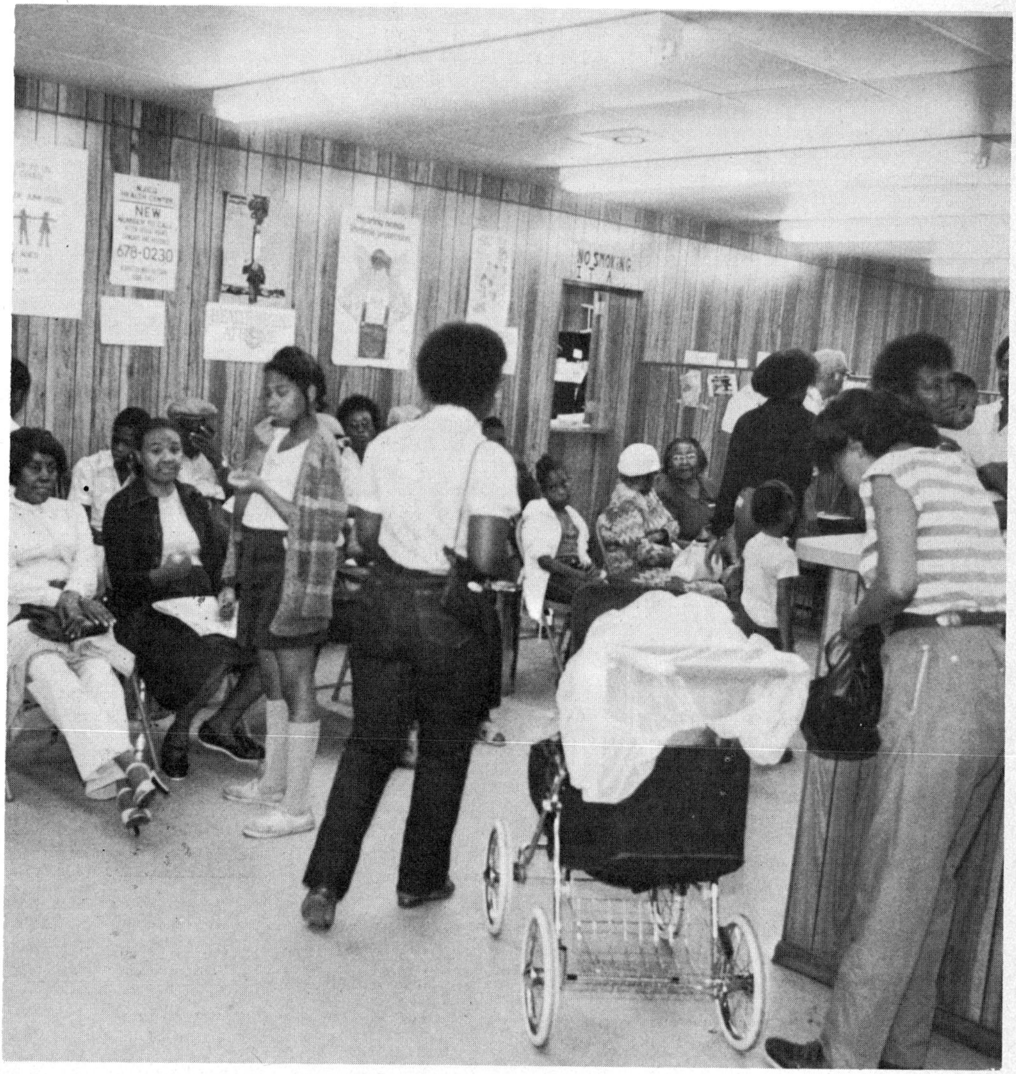

eases and health education, including prevention. Attention to psychosocial components of illness is considered an intrinsic component of primary care.

By now, the reader who is not familiar with the primary care literature may well be asking: "How come you have not yet told me what primary care is?" The reader who has raised such a question is astute and correct in discerning that the definitions presented to this point do not help in providing a clear-cut image of what is meant by *primary care*.

The reasons for the lack of clarity are many. The primary care movement was triggered by a number of forces that have already been touched on and will be briefly recapitulated here. With the numerical decline of the family physician, the ascendancy of the hospital, and the proliferation of specialists, more and more people became concerned about the fact, for example, that one physician tends to women during birth and another cares for newborns. If their eyes bother them, people are sent to an ophthamologist; and if they need surgery, it remains to be determined whether a general or specialized surgeon is required. Therefore some aspects of primary care represent an attempt to minimize the type of fragmentation triggered by the growth of specialized, technology-intensive care.

Also of importance is the growing recognition that health services for the poor are lacking in many respects. Many poor, rural areas have limited if any health care delivery systems. Urban clinics are crowded, dreary places where people spend hours waiting to be seen. Physicians usually "donate" their services—in exchange for the privilege of admitting their private patients. Here people are often shuffled from one clinic to another with little effort to coordinate their medical and psychosocial needs.

In many respects, then, primary care may be said to represent an effort to bring health care to the underserved.

The psychosocial components of illness are being increasingly recognized. Many health problems seen by physicians do not have a clear-cut biological basis. Although it is difficult to obtain an accurate assessment, some suggest that as many as 60% to 70% of the problems presented to many health care providers fall in this category. Clearly, the traditional biomedical models (Chapter 3) have not provided the conceptual underpinning and practice technology needed to respond to people who somaticize emotional complaints and to help those who are at risk for a variety of health problems because of the conditions of their lives. Pediatricians, general internists, family practitioners, and psychiatrists are considered the physicians most likely to encounter people whose psychosocial problems are implicated in the etiology of illness, as well as in its management.

These medical practitioners have been thought to need additional training to enable them to transcend the confines of the medical model in their day-to-day patient management for treatment of "common diseases and injuries." These are common ailments often intertwined with emotional problems, or poverty, or other negative effects of the stresses of daily living. Importantly, it was increasingly recognized that the services of a multidisciplinary group of health professionals were needed—and would be cost-effective—if the goals of primary care were to be achieved.

In short, primary care has many components. For these reasons, it is difficult to define in clear-cut terms. Its essential features revolve around efforts to provide health care for many of the common, though frequent health problems encountered and to provide that care in a holistic manner sensitive to the emotional and social contexts in which people live. A multidisciplinary approach is considered desirable. Continuity of care from the same group of professionals is important to avoid the fragmentation so often associated with specialized care. Primary care providers, then, need to be skilled in determining when they can manage a problem on their own and when they might more appropriately refer people to specialists. These specialists include both physicians and other service providers. The primary care concept is not limited in its application to any one social class, for the need for integrated care knows no class boundaries. However, in its development the primary care concept has been particularly useful in bringing care to those groups in the society that had been most underserved.

Primary care is an emerging concept of care designed to counteract some of the more depersonalizing, fragmented elements of health care that have been described elsewhere in this book (see particularly Chapters 1 and 5). Concretely, primary medical care is mainly provided by family physicians, pediatricians, and some internists. In its ideal form it is multidisciplinary and holistic, with considerable attention paid to efforts to refer appropriately to specialists when needed. A number of new organizational forms have been developed in the attempts to translate the concept into action. These include, but are not limited to, health maintenance organizations, community health centers, family practice residency programs, and family practice as a medical specialty. In all of these, diverse professionals function.

To implement the primary care concept it was necessary to give considerable thought and resources to translate primary care goals into reality. New providers and new approaches to training providers were needed. In response to these and related developments, federal policy began in the 1960s and 1970s to support expanded training for primary care. Experimentation with a number of primary care models was encouraged by several legislative thrusts.

Expanded training for primary care

In seeking to expand training for primary care providers, a number of approaches have been used. One has focused on efforts to train a "new type" of provider. These include new programs to upgrade and change the nature of training for family medicine (formerly termed *general practice*), to train nurses as primary care practitioners, and to educate a category of personnel known as physicians' assistants. All of these efforts are intended to increase the pool of primary care providers, which have been in short supply. In addition, these providers are to become knowledgeable and skilled in providing comprehensive, psychosocially oriented care. As these and other programs have proliferated, it has quickly become clear that each of the "new" professions involved in primary care, as well as those who are retooling, have to define functions that transcend and expand their traditional roles.

The efforts to train a new "breed" of family physicians illustrate the kinds of issues encountered in efforts to incorporate psychosocial factors. As will

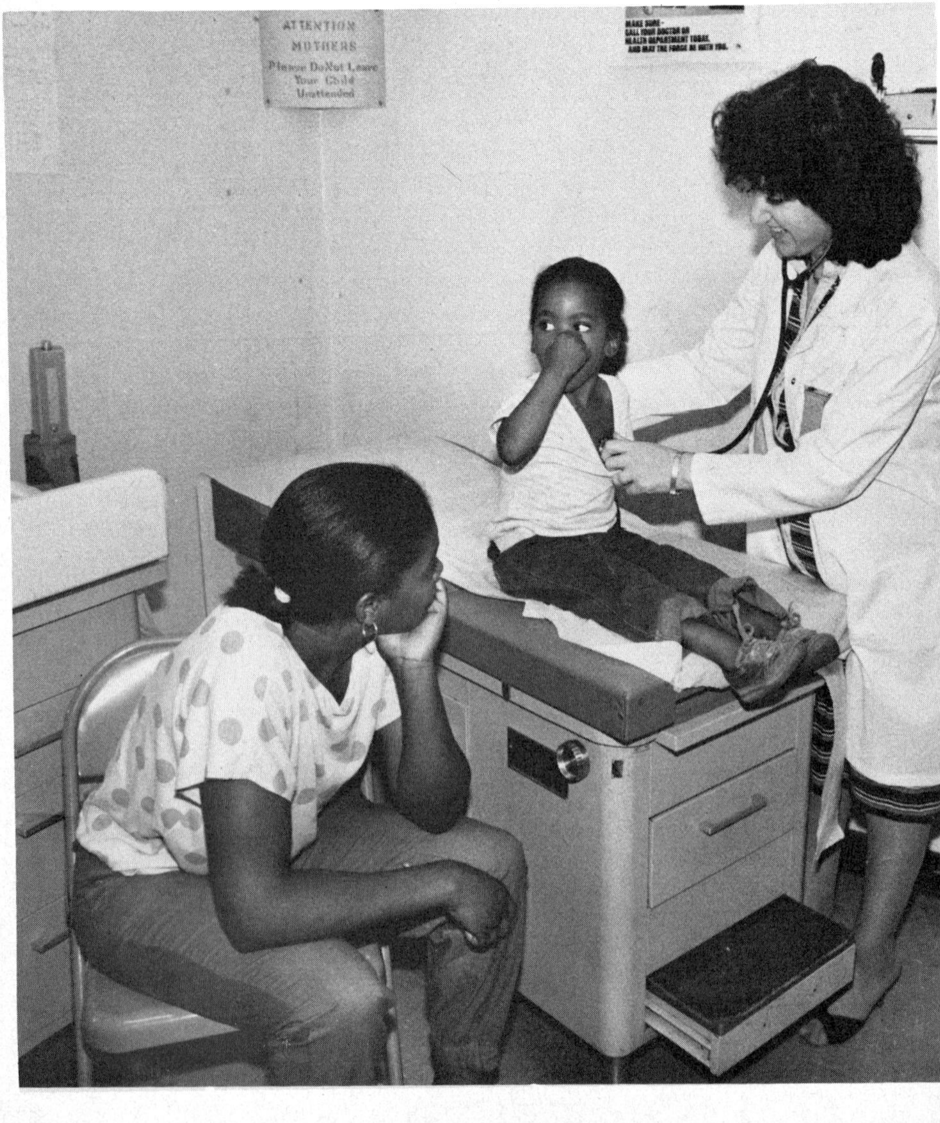

become evident, these have bearing on how social workers fit into the primary care scheme.

Family medicine: a "new" primary care specialty. In 1969 the Council on Medical Education of the American Medical Association approved family medicine as a specialty. Unlike its predecessor, general practice, this new specialty now requires 3 years of residency training following graduation from medical school.

Education in the "behavioral sciences" is an integral and required component of training for family practice. Despite variations in substance and style of behavioral science education, most programs include instruction focused on (1) acquisition of basic knowledge in the behavioral sciences; (2) communication, interactional, and interviewing skills; (3) approaches designed to enhance physician self-awareness and sensitive use of self in interaction with patients; and (4) knowledge and use of community resources.

Curry and Grant (1973), reviewing the "Essentials for Residency Training in Family Practice" as developed by the Department of Graduate Medical Education of the American Medical Association in 1968, suggest that the family physician:

1. Is oriented to the whole patient and practices both scientific and humanistic medicine
2. Is the first physician with whom many patients have contact and provides a means of entry into the health system
3. Evaluates patients' total health needs, providing that medical care within his or her sphere of competence; refers where indicated; and maintains continuity of care
4. Assumes responsibility for patients' total health care within the context of community and family
5. Plans the health management of the entire family

An elaboration of these guidelines suggests that family physicians function in (1) a patient care role, (2) a coordinating role, and (3) a community role. The first involves them in habilitation, rehabilitation, preventive medicine, and advocacy. The second focuses on their role as leaders of the health team. The third stresses knowledge, use, and improvement of community resources involved in meeting existing and future health needs. In all of these the family physician's collaboration with diverse medical and nonmedical specialists is stressed, as is knowledge of patients' families, their histories, and psychological concerns. Curry and Grant (1973) contend that "much of the effectiveness of the family physician comes from his utilization of the behavioral sciences . . . Expertise in this area is a requirement of the new family practice literature" (p. 48).

Such training is carried out in family practice residency programs. Most are hospital affiliated, although many have separate facilities, set off from the main hospital. They serve diverse population groups and aim to provide long-term, holistic care (Schlesinger, 1982).

Review of the functions ascribed to the family physician by Curry and Grant (1973) begins to specify and concretize the image of primary care envisioned by some. The material just reviewed suggests that family physicians have broad patient care aims that include many of the functions traditionally carried out by social workers. These are wide in scope and in keeping with the spectrum of views of primary care presented earlier.

Other primary care medical specialists. When family physicians, internists, and pediatricians are counted as primary care physicians (*Health, United States,* 1981) they account for 38% of all practicing physicians. Of the primary care group, 38% are family physicians or general practitioners, 44% are internists, and the rest are pediatricians (*Health, United States,* 1982).

The extent to which these physicians conform to the guidelines for family medicine reviewed previously varies considerably. The other medical specialties, especially those focused on primary care, have also begun to incorporate psychosocial learning into their curriculums.

Nursing has paid increasing attention to related issues. A review of the offerings as gleaned from catalogues of nursing schools points to this. Here, too, it is often difficult to distinguish certain components from those offered at schools of social work. Nurses learn counseling and outreach skills and often become involved in linking people with community resources. The similarity between components of the role of the public health nurse and those of the health care social worker is frequently noted.

• • •

Efforts to understand and clarify the social work role in primary care must derive from understanding of the increasing attention other disciplines aim to pay to psychosocial issues. These providers work together in a variety of primary care settings. Before considering how these providers collaborate with each other, especially with social workers, a number of the major primary care models are reviewed. This will give the reader a sense of the complexity and diversity of the settings in which primary care is rendered.

Primary care models

Health maintenance organizations (Chapter 2). According to the Department of Health and Human Services (*Health, United States,* 1981) health maintenance organizations (HMOs) are "organized systems of health care; providing comprehensive services for enrolled members for a fixed, prepaid annual fee" (p. 75). People usually become eligible to enroll in an HMO through their place of employment. Though inpatient services and those of non-primary care providers are part of the HMO concept, these prepaid health plans are usually included in discussions of primary care. The definition suggests that there is a focus on comprehensive care, though how they are organized varies. In many HMOs a variety of providers, including social workers, practice under "one roof" or in a group practice model. The physicians are usually salaried. In others, like "individual practice associations" (IPAs), physician members retain their private practices and see their HMO patients along with their fee-for-service patients. In this model the HMO concept is carried into a traditional type of private medical practice setting. Interdisciplinary collaboration is likely to be minimal.

The HMO concept was enthusiastically supported by the Department of Health, Education and Welfare in the 1970s. By 1980 enrollment in HMOs represented about 5% of those people who have health insurance coverage. By 1983, 11.6 million people received their care in health maintenance organizations. All but one American city with a population of over 1 million people has an HMO (*The New York Times,* July 31, 1983).

There was, in the past, considerable optimism about the HMO model. It was expected that prepaid, comprehensive care would be available at reduced costs. One major source of optimism was that the fee-for-service system would not intrude on the patient's decisions about care needed, thus making comprehensive and preventive services readily available to those enrolled.

As noted earlier, HMOs are primarily geared for working people who have the option of enrolling in a plan, if available in their communities, via the health insurance schemes that are part of employee benefit packages. More recent legislation makes it possible for those eligible for Medicare to enroll; the Medicaid program allows states to contract with HMOs to provide care for the poor. Luft (1982) reviewed a number of these programs. Several factors pertinent to the present discussion emerge. One of the ways in which HMOs have managed to hold costs below those of the private sector is by tight scheduling and keeping unbroken appointments to a minimum. Some studies found that people of lower socioeconomic status are more likely than middle class persons to use emergency or walk-in services and less likely to adhere to strict appointment schedules. This had led some to question whether HMOs are geared to provide the type of service that some low-income persons find comfortable. For these and related reasons some have compared the HMO utilization patterns of low-income and middle-class consumers. Research suggests that health status rather than socioeconomic level seems to be the major determinant of use. Luft's analysis (1982) leads him to believe that HMOs have managed to serve the poor adequately; the HMO emphasis on constraining costs appears not to have had major adverse impacts on the care received by this population group. There is, however, some contrary evidence. In some instances, marketing practices designed to enroll people eligible under medical coverage sought to enroll only "healthy" individuals, while advising those with ongoing health problems to stay in the fee-for-service system.

Whether social work can contribute to retaining high-quality care and keeping costs down in HMOs is an important area for inquiry.

Family practice residency programs. The major reason for the existence of family practice residency programs has already been discussed. A range of ambulatory services is provided. With few exceptions they tend to be multidisciplinary; 25% to 30% use social workers in a teaching and/or a service role (Hess, 1982; Hookey, 1978). This is discussed further in later sections of this chapter.

Community health centers. Woodward (1983) describes a number of programs, many initially set up as demonstration projects by the Office of Economic Opportunity and later on by the Bureau of Community Health services in the Department of Health and Human Services. Between 1975 and 1979 the number of projects increased from 204 to 632. In the same period the number of people served grew from 1.3 to 3.75 million.

> These primary care projects brought together a wide range of social and health services within their organizations. A capacity was built to serve the medically underserved areas in our country (Woodward, 1983, p. 56).

Seven types of programs are identified: (1) neighborhood health centers; (2) family health centers; (3) community health networks; (4) rural health initiatives; (5) migrant health centers; (6) urban health centers; and (7) hospital-affiliated primary care centers. Though each has a somewhat distinct delivery approach, team practice is characteristic of all. In some, consumers or community boards play a governance role. This feature contributes to their capacity to affect health legislation.

Involving consumers in making decisions about how health care is rendered and in efforts to effect legislative reform is in keeping with the World Health Organization concept of primary care. The financial incentives available increased the move of primary care physicans into underserved areas. This was an extremely important development, as these areas had long suffered extreme physician shortages.

Woodward (1983) suggests that these primary care models have "served as a change agent within the system, creating shifts in medical career choices, interdisciplinary service arrangements, and interests in ambulatory care . . ." (p. 62). Yet current funding restrictions are a threat to the continued expansion of this type of service. Woodward sees an enlarged role for social work—"the discipline most involved with integration of services" and "sustaining the primary care model" (p. 62).

Many community health centers combine the delivery of basic medical and related services with programs designed to meet a variety of other needs for services. During the 1960s and 1970s it was not uncommon to combine political action with health service delivery. The spirit of these early centers, which reflected the integral relationship between health, social policy, and other areas of life, is still found in some centers currently operating. Social work students and practioners are strongly encouraged to visit some dynamic, multidisciplinary, multifunction community health centers. Such visits can provide a vivid demonstration of this primary care model in action.

Though health services are the nub and core of one such center in a New Jersey ghetto (North Jersey Community Action), those who planned and manage the center are well aware of the integral relationship between health and other service needs. And so, under one roof and jointly administered are sophisticated medical and dental services, a children's day-care center, and a senior citizens' program. This program provides the opportunity for employment of senior citizens as home health aides. Recognizing the difficulty (already noted earlier) that some poor people have in adhering to rigid appointment systems, two types of scheduling mechanisms are operative. There is the regular appointment system and a drop-in service. Those who just drop in come to know that unless they have emergency problems they may have to wait—but they will be served. The halls of this center are lined with posters that alert people to the need for preventive health behavior. For example, there are reminders about hypertension screening, Pap smears, and programs to help people stop smoking. These posters are intermingled with those announcing various community development and political action thrusts. Though people often must wait to be seen and the halls are crowded with clambering children, pregnant women, and the elderly, an excitement and a sense of warmth prevail.

In Denver, my visits to a series of neighborhood health centers that serve large segments of the Hispanic community revealed a similar "esprit de corps." How has, and how can, social work make a contribution to these various primary care arrangements? A number of efforts to conceptualize and describe that role are reviewed here.

SOCIAL WORK'S ROLE

In assessing social work's participation in primary care and the potential for expanding the profession's role in primary care delivery systems a number of questions arise:

1. What is the boundary and distinction between the social worker's role and that of other providers in a system that, by definition, seeks to provide holistic, comprehensive care?
2. Given the wide range of medical and social problems people bring to health centers, which people receiving primary care require social work services (Ell and Morrison, 1981)?
3. What, if any, new, expanded, or adapted skills, different from those now used in more traditional settings, are required of the primary care social worker?

Dana (1983), Ell and Morrison (1981), and others suggest that many of the answers to these questions have yet to evolve. Research into the social work role in the education of family practitioners and reports of innovative projects begin to provide some insight.

The extent of social work participation in primary care

Hard data on the number of social workers involved are difficult to obtain. According to Hookey (1978) 1000 social workers were attached to 300 primary care clinics and medical groups. A 1976 study (Grinnell) reported that 600 social workers are attached to family medicine teaching programs. My more recent work (Schlesinger, 1982) suggests that the number has dropped substantially.* There are reports of social workers attached to the private offices of pediatricians and family practitioners. The social work role in HMOs appears not to have expanded in line with Bracht's optimistic projection (1978). He had suggested that social workers were vital to obtaining the HMO goals of health maintenance and promotion. Clearly this is a new field that calls for more extensive development, research, and conceptualization by social workers.

Boundary issues

My exploration into "Doctor/Social Worker Collaboration in Family Medicine Training" (Schlesinger, 1982) was prompted by the following question: If the new breed of family practitioner described by Curry and Grant (1973) carries out the patient care, coordinating community, advocacy roles envisioned, how does this affect the social work role vis à vis that segment of primary care in which family practitioners are involved? This initial question generated a further set of questions focused on the viability of the projected objectives for family practice. These related to the fact that family practitioners, like other physicians, are trained in medical schools where the biomedical model continues to be the primary basis for education. Given this, questions can be raised about whether subsequent residency training, with an emphasis on holistic, psychosocial care, would alter the basic dispositions likely to be acquired in medical school. Closely related are questions that stem from the fact that family physicians have relatively low status vis à vis more prestigious specialties. This low status, it seemed, might intensify efforts to master the "hard facts of medicine" at the expense of psychosocial issues.

A review of the British and American literature on the collaboration of family physicians and social workers suggests that these kinds of issues surface repeatedly. Wales (1978) contends that physicians who incorporate the newer biosocial models into their practice "run the risk of lowered prestige, scorn and belittlement usually associated with the soft sciences." Schroeder (1983) looks forward "to a day when primary care is felt to be as intellectually demanding as the intensive care unit, when physicians will find psychosocial problems as exciting and challenging as biomedical ones [and will] . . . respect the ability of non physician providers . . ." (p. 74). Though the British "GP" and social workers have collaborated for some time, problems in communication and boundary issues arise (for example, Clare and Corney, 1982; Schlesinger, 1982; Steel, 1979; Williams and Clare, 1982).

Preliminary data from a national study in which social workers and the directors of family practice programs that include social workers on the staff

*This apparent drop may be an artifact of the data collection methods used.

were surveyed about these and related issues are instructive with respect to the boundary issue. The first addresses questions on how social workers and physicians view the effect of contemporary medical education on efforts to highlight the role of psychosocial factors in patient management. Though the social workers' and medical directors' responses varied somewhat, at least 80% of both groups agreed with the view that (1) the biomedical orientation of medical education is a deterrent to incorporating psychosocial factors into patient management and (2) if family practitioners want to be recognized as competent by the larger medical community, their knowledge of biomedical factors is much more important than attention to psychosocial concern. The second view focused on responses to a series of case vignettes on whether the situations described should be handled by the family physician, a social worker, a psychiatrist, or some other mental health specialist. The situations described ranged from problems involving bizarre schizophrenic behavior to the difficulties some patients with hypertension have in complying with medical regimens, to situations calling for advocacy in respect to entitlement for benefits. The findings illustrate the boundary issues as they relate to medical dominance and the tendencies for professionals to designate most tasks to their own profession (Kane, 1975). Social workers were highly likely to view themselves as capable of handling psychiatric problems, a perception not shared by most of the physicians queried. Though physicians recognized the difficulty they have in incorporating psychosocial factors into patient management they nevertheless thought physicians should manage many of the problems presented.

One disturbing finding—from a social worker's perspective—was the fact that more physicians than social workers thought that social workers should deal with a situation in which efforts to alter legislation or regulations about health care provision were clearly called for. Hess' study (1982) of the practice patterns of social workers in family medicine programs sheds light on this finding. Hess notes that social workers in family practice tend to have a traditional therapeutic focus. Ell and Morrison (1981) suggest that social work's lack of consensus concerning its role in primary care has precluded meaningful professional participation in developing policies and appropriate organizational models.

Dana's comments (1983) may shed light on these and related findings. She suggests that the pressure to demonstrate how important social work is in primary care has deflected attention from efforts to explore and expand the role. Her comments suggest that the boundary issue might be more readily resolved if social workers were to truly embrace those components of the primary care model that focus on policy, provision, and changes in the health care delivery system.

> It would be easy to designate the biomedical model as the principal agent of social work's limitation in taking full advantage of the opportunity that the

> concept of primary health care provides for the optimum expression of social work values, knowledge and skills . . . [and to ask instead what] prevents their going beyond the role of clinical problem solvers? (p. 157)

A number of social work training models in primary care (for example, Austrian, 1983; Etrog, 1983) are exciting and innovative and begin to expand on traditional conceptions. Though there is considerable emphasis on clinical concerns there is a preventive perspective. In an interesting paper (unsigned, 1982) the author proposes some mechanisms for enhancing social work's public health role in primary care. The use of data collection systems to identify high-risk populations, the identification of community agencies accountable for specific high-risk populations, and the negotiation of agreements between primary care programs and other programs are proposed as ways by which the planning role can be emphasized.

Such a role can be played by workers who undertake planning as their primary assignment, or by those who have multifunction assignments.

Mr. Brown

In working with depressed patients routinely assigned to him in his clinical role in the family practice residency program, Mr. Brown, the social worker, noted that many of them were "displaced homemakers"—that is, middle-aged women who were recently divorced or separated.

Though most suffered acute clinical depression that required a combination of medication and psychotherapy, they also asked for help in developing skills that would aid them in their search for jobs. Woman after woman recounted how years of devotion to family and housework had left her bereft of any marketable skills. Most had come to the center complaining of somatic symptoms; depression had emerged as a common feature in helping them to understand frequent unexplainable headaches, stomachaches, and other problems with no discernable organic base.

Mr. Brown, in consultation with the director of the program, family practice residents, and other staff, invited the women to meet as a group around their common financial concerns and their need for vocational training. Together they recognized that their feelings of depression were related to feeling abandoned, inadequate, and without sufficient resources.

As he helped them to share their feelings, he also made contacts for them at local vocational schools and community colleges. A number sought training and were able to find jobs. Several special programs were developed as a result. In considering these experiences with the medical staff, review of records revealed that many of the women were able to cut back on their use of antidepressant medications.

Slowly the staff of this family practice center began to identify other groups in need of similar services. Next, the center staff—with Mr. Brown taking the lead—decided to tackle the collective problems of the middle-aged children of the elderly. Mr. Brown advocated for respite services for this group of people, who were having many somatic symptoms that appeared related to the strain of caring for their elderly parents.

These exciting developments had many spin-offs. Not only did Mr.

Brown become increasingly attuned to providing multilevel services for populations at risk, but the family practice residents became more and more attuned to these issues in their own practice. Many began to consult Mr. Brown about how they might do something other than give medication to people whose problems clearly had social origins.

As the physicians began to incorporate these matters into their own clinical practice, Mr. Brown began to wonder whether the physicians were beginning to act like social workers. On reflection, he realized that, given the center's mandate, some of this was an inevitable, though positive development. The physicians' main emphasis remained the medical management of patients—now enhanced with new insight. Mr. Brown continued to find other patient groups needing a variety of socially oriented services targeted to their particular needs.

This discussion of boundary issues points to a number of factors that consistently arise for social work in primary care settings, whether family practice programs, neighborhood health centers, or others. It is clear that other providers, such as nurses and physicians, view themselves as playing a clinical role in respect to psychosocial factors. This includes attention to a broad range of mental health problems. When all disciplines are attentive to these kinds of concerns, overlapping of roles is bound to occur. If social workers jealously guard their presumed clinical prerogatives, interdisciplinary conflicts will be intensified and other needs neglected. Social workers can, however, play a unique consulting and educational role in respect to clinical issues. Data from the study of doctor/social worker collaboration point to the importance of this role. Though many physicians have confidence in their own ability to deal with psychosocial issues, they nevertheless are eager to sharpen their skills in interviewing, in developing self-awareness, and in making targeted psychosocial assessments. Social workers function in an educational capacity because of their skills in this area. As illustrated, the social worker's efforts often help physicians to recognize their need for enhanced skills.

Those primary care settings that serve many poor people also often serve people of diverse ethnic memberships. Social workers can play an active role here, and many have developed exciting programs that pay special attention to the health and illness behaviors of diverse ethnic groups. These educational and consultative efforts can enhance the care rendered by all providers, a goal of primary care.

For many primary care providers, especially physicians, a major question revolves around when to refer to another discipline. That holds true in respect to medical as well as psychosocial problems they consider to be beyond their domain or expertise. The data presented earlier suggest that social workers who have responsibility for educating physicians concerning these matters need to develop mechanisms to help physicians and others determine at what point referral to social workers is indicated.

Despite the lofty goals expounded by the American Medical Association (that physicians take a lot of nontraditional roles), there is little evidence that many are adept at the skillful use of community resources or interested in playing an active role as advocates. If social workers in primary care come to value the coordinating, advocacy, and outreach roles more than they do at present, other primary care professionals are more likely to recognize their importance. Coordination and integration of services have always been key social work roles. As resources for primary care shrink, tasks in addition to clinical services assume even greater importance. The same is true in respect to policy formulation.

Clearly, if primary care social workers want to expand their roles, a narrow, traditional clinical base is insufficient for enhancing and sharpening social work's role. That role always seeks to integrate understanding of unique individuals and the impact of the social context and resource deficits on them. Primary care, perhaps more than other areas of health care social work, provides a unique opportunity and challenge to carry on and refine those long-standing social work traditions epitomized by the work of Jane Addams and Bertha Reynolds, among others. That is, to practice in a manner congruent with individual need and attention to systemic deficit. This has long been a professional mandate unique to social work. Such a stance is likely to generate excitement and respect for the social worker's role in this sector of health care practice.

Proposed directions

In addition to the basic thrust just suggested, a number of other proposals for enhancing social work practice in primary care need to be considered. Ell and Morrison (1981) point out that the primary care social worker is a generalist who requires a knowledge base "unique in its breadth." They identify the need for extensive knowledge of patterns of health and illness, health policy, and populations at risk for special difficulty. Particularly important are the social worker's efforts to develop resources and to become skillful in the use and building of supportive community networks. The latter is of special significance.

Earlier it was noted that many community health centers are in the isolated rural areas or inner city ghettos. Those sites provide a unique opportunity to identify or help build community-based networks around such health problems as control of hypertension. Etrog (1983) demonstrated how social workers can help groups of adolescents to enhance preventive health behavior. Ethnic groups and the natural networks that emerge out of ethnically based institutions like churches are important sources. Such networks can provide important positive feedback that can serve to reduce stressors. At the same time, economic deprivation or isolation (as with the elderly) hampers their capacity to draw on indigenous coping skills. Thus resource development is an integral component of work with indigenous networks. Schlesinger and Devore (1981) have identified a number of factors to facilitate such efforts. These include efforts to (1) build on those factors that enhance group pride (language, history, and ethnic rituals) and (2) facilitate the spontaneous caretaking traditions of indigenous networks (sharing food, making child care arrangements, and giving advice to the emotionally troubled). These networks, both informal and institutionalized via the church or benevolent societies, can be used as sites for intervention with mental health problems. Many minorities, the aged, and the less educated find it more acceptable to deal with mental health problems on their own turf than in formally organized health care settings. The efforts of groups based in the work place or the community center are often fruitful.

Ell and Morrison (1981) suggest that "what distinguishes the client seen by a social worker in primary care from the person seen in a traditional social work agency is the 'medicalization' of the presenting problem" (p. 37S). Problems as diverse as those connected to somatic stress-related symptoms, loneliness, poverty, and marital strife are brought to many primary care centers. Social workers need to become particularly skillful in their efforts, both with staff and with patients, as they participate in the process of identifying the social source of problems. Much of the primary care movement derives from the fact that "people" do not compartmentalize their problems in terms of the specialized niches built by providers. Thus medical care no more suffices to solve tension-related headaches than it does severe marital problems. That neither social work nor other primary care providers have yet developed targeted approaches that strike a fine balance between medical and social care is patently clear. Yet primary care promises the opportunity of combining clinical skill, interdisciplinary practice, community-based work, and planning efforts on behalf of population groups with a great variety of problems.

Research

Coulton (1983) has reviewed a vast research literature that relates to social work functions in primary care. Three questions informed the review:

1. What are the relationships between psychological, social, and physiological health and the use of primary care?
2. What are the advantages and disadvantages of various primary care models?
3. What are the effects of psychosocial interventions delivered in primary care settings?

The review answered some questions but, as might be expected, identified many issues calling for further inquiry. Essentially Coulton proposes that "there is a strong and consistent connection between the presence of psychosocial problems and the use of primary care" (p. 223). This suggests that specialists in psychosocial problems must participate in primary care. However, the issue of who those specialists are needs further study.

These findings do not provide ready guidelines for the social work role. The areas of needed expertise and interventive thrust suggested by Ell and Morrison (1981) are essential for primary care practice. All that they have identified is, in my view, essential for all of health care social work practice. Much of this book has been devoted to detailing the diverse knowledge and skills base.

It remains to be seen whether subsequent experience and research will serve to identify a direct service role for primary health care social work that is substantially different from the role played in the hospital or other clinical settings. What is unique is that primary care seems to offer a singular opportunity to put into practice the essential principles for health care social work practice spelled out in Chapter 6. In primary care settings, social work operates within a framework and/or organizational structure that is usually committed to social health and experimentation. For many that represents a departure from the more traditional stances found in other settings. To take full advantage of the potential is a challenge confronting social work in primary care.

SUMMARY

This chapter has identified the basic concepts of primary care with its emphasis on comprehensive, socially oriented, continuous care. Reference to research on collaboration with physicians in primary care settings suggests that the biomedical orientation is not readily diminished.

However, the fundamental tenets of primary care provide the social worker with the opportunity to play a clinical, outreach, and policy and planning role. A public health perspective is essential. Role conflicts intensify when social workers focus their efforts on a clinical role, one that is also readily assumed by other primary health care providers.

REFERENCES

Austrian, S.G.: Developing a social work training model in primary care. In Miller, R.S., editor: Primary health care: more than medicine, Englewood Cliffs, N.J., 1983, Prentice-Hall, Inc.

Bracht, N.F.: Health maintenance organizations: a model for comprehensive health and mental health care delivery. In Bracht, N.F., editor: Social work in health care, New York, 1978, The Haworth Press.

Clare, A.W., and Corney, R.H.: Social work and primary care: problems and possibilities. In Clare, A.W., and Corney, R.H., editors: Social work and primary health care, London, 1982, Academic Press, Inc.

Coulton, C.J.: A social work perspective of research in primary care. In Miller, R.S., editor: Primary health care: more than medicine, Englewood Cliffs, N.J., 1983, Prentice-Hall, Inc.

Curry, H.B., and Grant, S.W.: Role of the family physician. In Conn, H., Rakel, R., and Johnson, T., editors: Family practice, Philadelphia, 1973, W.B. Saunders Co.

Dana, B.: Collaboration in primary care: or is it? In Miller, R.S., editor: Primary health care: more than medicine, Englewood Cliffs, N.J., 1983, Prentice-Hall, Inc.

Davis, K.: National policy in primary health care: past, present and future. In Miller, R.S., editor: Primary health care: more than medicine, Englewood Cliffs, N.J., 1983, Prentice-Hall, Inc.

Ell, K., and Morrison, D.R.: Primary care, Health and Social Work (suppl.) **6**(4):35S, 1981.

Epstein, L.: Helping people: the task-centered approach, St. Louis, 1980, The C.V. Mosby Co.

Etrog, N.: A primary prevention training model for adolescent health care. In Miller, R.S., editor: Primary health care: more than medicine, Englewood Cliffs, N.J., 1983, Prentice-Hall, Inc.

European Seminar on Research in Primary Health Care, WHO-EURO (Copenhagen) and The European Centre for Social Welfare Training and Research (Vienna), Vienna, 1983.

Grinnell, R.M.: The status of graduate level social workers teaching in medical schools, Social Work in Health Care **1**:317, Spring 1976.

Health, United States, DHHS Pub. No. (PHS) 82-1232, Washington, D.C., 1981, U.S. Government Printing Office.

Health, United States, DHHS Pub. No. (PHS) 83-1232, Washington, D.C., 1982, U.S. Government Printing Office.

Hess, H.: Clinical practice variations of social workers in family practice centers, Paper presented at the annual program meeting, Council on Social Work Education, New York, March 1982.

Hookey, P.: Social work in primary health care settings. In Bracht, N., editor: Social work in health care: a guide to professional practice, New York, 1978, The Haworth Press.

Kane, R.A.: Interprofessional teamwork, Manpower Monograph No. 8, Syracuse, N.Y., 1975, Syracuse University School of Social Work.

Lloyd, W.B.: Issues in primary care. The neighborhood health center, Bulletin of the New York Academy of Medicine **53**(1):120, 1977.

Luft, H.S..: Health maintenance organizations and the rationing of medical care, Milbank Memorial Fund Quarterly; Health & Society **60**(2):268, 1982.

Miller, R.S.: Primary health care: an overview. In Miller, R.S., editor: Primary health care: more than medicine, Englewood Cliffs, N.J., 1983, Prentice-Hall, Inc.

The New York Times, July 31, 1983, Sec. 3, p. 23.

Schlesinger, E.: Comparison of the British and American Experience in collaboration between social workers and physicians, unpublished data, 1982.

Schlesinger, E.: Doctor/social worker collaboration in family medicine training, Paper presented at the annual meeting, American Public Health Association, Montreal, November 1982.

Schlesinger, E., and Devore, W.: Ethnic networks: conceptual formulations and interventive strategies, Paper presented at the annual meeting, American Public Health Association, Los Angeles, November 1981.

Schroeder, S.A.: Primary care in the 1980's: a medical perspective. In Miller,

R.S., editor: Primary health care: more than medicine, Englewood Cliffs, N.J., 1983, Prentice-Hall, Inc.

Steel, R.: The general practitioner and social worker: friends or foes? Practitioner **223**(1338):744, 1979.

Unsigned: Improving prevention services through the integration of categorical programs into the primary care setting, Paper presented at the annual meeting, American Public Health Association, Montreal, November 1982.

Vuori, H.: An overview of primary health care. In European Seminar on Research in Primary Health Care, WHO-EURO (Copenhagen) and The European Centre for Social Welfare Training and Research (Vienna), Vienna, 1983.

Wales, E.: Behavioral scientist meets the practicing physician, The Journal of Family Practice vol. 6, issue 4, 1978.

Williams, P., and Clare, A.W.: Social workers in primary health care: the general practitioner's viewpoint. In Clare, A.W., and Corney, R.H., editors: Social work and primary health care, London, 1982, Academic Press, Inc.

Woodward, K.: The primary health care model. In Miller, R.S., editor: Primary health care: more than medicine, Englewood Cliffs, N.J., 1983, Prentice-Hall, Inc.

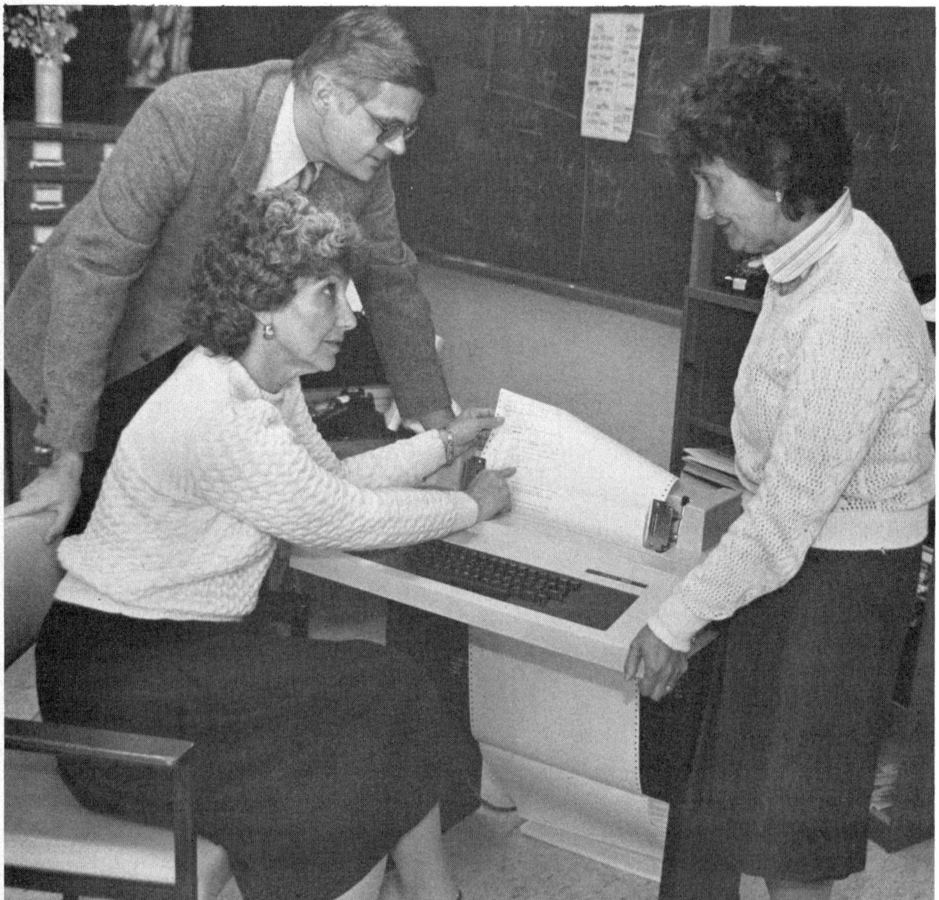

Chapter 12

Research and quality assurance

Had this book been written 15 or even 10 years ago it is doubtful that either the editors or I would have thought it appropriate, necessary, or acceptable to include a chapter on research and quality assurance in a textbook on social work practice.

For years many practitioners and students distrusted and feared research. Their distrust stemmed from the sense that examining and studying the interventive process was somehow at odds with the humanistic impulses and commitment to helping that had motivated social workers to choose that career. How could one count people's thoughts or feelings? Such counting was thought inevitably to damage the holistic, complex nature of human beings, their interactions with each other, and the process of giving help.

The fear of research and accounting for the helping process had similar sources. Many graduate students had chosen to become social workers after having had some difficulty with mathematics or the rigorous quantitative approaches required in certain segments of experimental psychology or sociology undergraduate work. After enrolling in a graduate school of social work many were dismayed or at least surprised that they were required to take research courses. They felt they had come to school to learn the skills of helping people, not to do research.

For the many years that I taught introductory graduate research courses I found that half the task involved dispelling fear and persuading students about the intricate relationship between practice skills and systematic research undertakings that contribute to more effective practice. Although many still hold this view much has changed in the intervening period. The discouraging findings of large-scale experiments designed to test social work interventive modalities (Fischer, 1973; Mullen and Dumpson, 1972) spurred efforts to find alternative means of studying practice process and outcome. Some of these newer approaches were more encouraging. For example, the work of Beck and Jones (1973) pointed to positive client assessment of the effects of social work intervention.

At the same time another set of developments was taking place. They were variously centered on increased demand for professional accountability. This demand has a variety of sources. Some are well-motivated and legitimate concerns about whether or not services included under public or voluntary auspices are truly helpful, of good quality, and delivered in a caring manner. Analogously, public bodies financing services, especially in health care, ask if these services are cost-effective, reasonably priced, and achieve desired outcomes (Rehr, 1979). Some of these questions are not well motivated. Patti (undated) suggests that certain aspects of the thrust for accountability have become "a code word to signify the antisocial welfare bias of a politically conservative administration" (p. 101). Alexander (1979) suggests that "professional accountability . . . has assumed the proportions of a national fad, the latest indoor sport for the ethical, the obsessed, and the capricious" (p. ix). These and related developments suggest that both neophyte and experienced practitioner need familiarity with some of the fundamental approaches of social work research, accountability and quality assurance, and how these have been and can be adapted to the health field.

In this chapter I will focus on identifying some of the basic concepts and strategies of research and quality assurance. I will refer to the extensive and growing literature on the subject and to my own experience as a social work educator. Much of the discussion is focused on what social workers can do in daily practice. I will begin with the assumption that the majority of readers have at some time been exposed to the fundamental tenets of social research methods. Therefore I will not concentrate on such issues as the logic of research, the approaches to hypotheses formulation and testing, or basic research design strategies. I assume the readers are familiar with these issues and therefore I will focus on those approaches that are thought to enhance the production and use of research in health care social work practice.

APPROACHES TO SOCIAL WORK RESEARCH IN HEALTH CARE

In a seminal review Coulton (1980) identifies several areas of inquiry that have clear implications for social work intervention in health care. I have selected three of the areas identified by Coulton for discussion: (1) research on social service delivery in health care, (2) the effects of such services, and (3) developments in research on social work in health care.

Social service delivery in health care

Two areas require particular emphasis: characteristics and problems of consumers and the social work role in health care, including participation in interdisciplinary endeavors, the way in which others perceive social workers, and the organization of social services.

Characteristics of consumers. Chapter 3 reviewed some of the major approaches used in identifying the process by which people determine their need for health services, particularly the services of physicians.

The impact of socioeconomic characteristics on health services use and on the degree to which discomfort is interpreted as requiring health services has been demonstrated consistently. However, some recent investigations suggest that these "structural features" have considerably less impact than do actual episodes of illness. In that discussion it was suggested that there is a need for efforts to integrate these somewhat conflicting findings into a more coherent body of propositions about the relationship between physical or emotional discomfort and service use.

A number of additional problems emerge when these considerations are applied to attempts to identify the characteristics and needs of those who use and need health care social work services. Coulton (1980) points out that decisions about who uses social services are often made by providers rather than by consumers. Recent developments in open access systems and high-risk screening procedures have not fundamentally altered that process. More of the decisions are being made by social workers than by other providers who may or may not have an accurate perception of the problems needing social work intervention. These developments offer the opportunity to raise a series of new questions. Given the situation of open access (referred to in Chapter 9), are the characteristics and needs of those who enter the health-related social service system via open access different from those who enter via more traditional referral processes? Coulton (1980) reviews studies by Altman (1965) and Glass (1977) that suggest that the use of social services was mainly related to efforts to shorten the hospital stays of those whose discharge was delayed for psychosocial reasons. Will more people become involved with social workers for emotional reasons rather than for concrete services under open access systems? Investigations suggest that this is not the case now (for example, Gentry, 1977; Stoeckle, Settler, and Davidson, 1966). Studies of the high-risk screening process and of the characteristics of people brought into social service via this mechanism are sorely needed (for example, Wolock and Schlesinger, 1983).

Such studies can be conducted in various ways. One involves using rigorous descriptive research designs in which providers in many health delivery settings are asked to respond to a series of questions about their intake procedures and the characteristics of those considered at high social risk. A more extensive and more difficult undertaking would involve surveying groups of patients discharged from hospitals within a designated time period independently of whether or not they had received social services. Such a survey could focus on their medical problems, the related psychosocial difficulties, and how these difficulties had been managed. Useful comparisons could then be made between those who did and did not receive social services and their views concerning the need and usefulness of such services. Should such a study reveal significant differences between the two groups, the findings would aid in further identifying those in need of social services. Insight into alternative ways of coping with illness-related psychosocial stresses would also be gained. Less systematic although useful approaches will be considered in the section focused on developments in research.

The social worker's role in health care. Coulton's review (1980) points out that a number of investigators have focused on the social worker's role in the health care system.

The differences between hospital social workers' view of their function and that held by other professionals have been documented. Wolock and Russell (1972) found that physicians tend to limit their requests for social work services to those of a concrete nature. Carrigan (1978) found that other health care professionals had limited expectations that social workers would initiate collaborative and planning efforts. They also expected that social workers would carry greater counseling responsibilities than they perceived them as carrying. Watt (1977) found that much of the hospital social worker's activity is related to the goals of patient care, as these are defined by physicians. This leaves limited time and opportunity to function in terms of the broader, health-oriented goals of the social worker. Wattenberg, Orr, and O'Rourke (1977) found that hospital and social work administrators agreed on the importance of the social work leadership role in the hospital. Schlesinger and Wolock (1982) found that, despite increased focus on cost control, in a 5-year period New Jersey hospital social work departments have sustained or enhanced their position with respect to departmental professionalization and involvement in hospital decision making. Work focused on social work participation in collaborative efforts was reviewed in Chapter 8.

Studies of social work practice have focused on the percent of hospital patients seen by social workers (for example, Coulton and Vielhaber, 1977) and on how workers spend their time (for example, Chernesky and Lurie, 1975–1976; Ullman and others (1971). Reviews of social work practice in nursing homes and other long-term care facilities were presented in Chapter 10. Less attention has been paid to identifying the components of the practice process as it is adapted to health settings. For example, Hollis (1973) carried out a rigorous investigation to determine if processes such as sustainment, direct influence, and ventilation were indeed characteristic of the casework process. No analogous efforts in health care social work are known to me. The efficacy of task-centered approaches to helping people deal with the coping tasks generated by long-term illness such as those described by Reid (1978) is a fruitful area for investigation.

There are limited data available to assess why health care social workers appear to spend a large amount of their time on concrete rather than emotionally centered services. Part of the answer undoubtedly lies in the fact that the need for concrete services is extensive. It is also possible, although yet undetermined, that practice processes focused on concrete needs simultaneously relieve anxiety and other emotional concerns. For example, although Hollis (1973) considered "environmental work" to be a crucial component of practice, she did not subject this process to the same kind of scrutiny as she did the emotionally focused activities.

More work is needed to further identify what it is that social workers actually do when they engage in discharge planning, refer someone to a home health facility, or review the benefits to which people are entitled under programs such as Medicaid or Medicare. Wilson (1980) has examined social workers' processed recordings of such efforts. Systematic analysis of this type of work and workers' efforts would help social workers a great deal in sharpening their skills in this area. Such analysis probably would reveal that workers are more engaged in providing support and helping people make difficult, emotionally laden decisions than they realize. As high-risk screening approaches increase it is also important to focus on strategies that help workers proceed with those clients who have not been referred. Paneth and Lipsky (1979) found that workers accustomed to operating within the traditional referral system needed help when shifting to this new mode.

Effects of health care social work services

It is unfortunate but true that to date there has been limited investigation of the effects of social work services in health care.

A few of the studies that have been done have been reviewed by Coulton. One study (Blumberg, Ely, and Kerbeshian, 1973) found that 67% of a group that had received pediatric social services found them helpful. Berkman and Rehr (1973) found that problems identified early in the hospital stay were least likely to be successfully resolved when the prognosis intensified depression or family disturbance. The positive effects of social work participation in collaborative efforts in chronic care were noted by Halstead (1976). Although these are encouraging findings, they are limited in scope. How this state of affairs might be remedied will be considered in a later section.

Developments and directions

In the earlier sections of this chapter I referred to the discouraging outcomes of large-scale experimental studies of social work intervention. "A number of creatively contrived field studies have shown that untreated groups fare as well as clients who have received social work treatment" (Fanshell, 1980, p. 13). This bleak view has been challenged, as have the research methods and assumptions on which these efforts are based. "The social work profession may have matured so that it will no longer blithely claim a capacity to transform people or eliminate problems which are rooted in pernicious social circumstances" (Fanshell, 1980, p. 13).

Recent developments have sought to identify research approaches that are more closely tied to daily, routine practice efforts and to gauge the effectiveness of practice against those goals the practitioner is attempting to achieve (Briar, 1980). A characteristic of the earlier studies is that diverse objectives for enhanced social functioning were identified by researchers, who in turn studied interventive programs to determine whether these externally defined objectives had been achieved.

Systematic experiments continue to be important. However, as was illustrated by Collins (1977), these experiments are most fruitful when the treatment variable and hypothesized outcomes are conceptualized by practitioners and are more narrowly focused. From this perspective Collins and her coworkers conducted a small-scale experiment involving a population defined as overusers of the emergency room. The client population consisted of many alcoholics, most of whom had a marginal existence. Social service goals were related to living or working arrangements and noninvolvement with alcohol. The experimental group was involved in ongoing casework services for a 5-month period and was seen at least once every 2 weeks. The control group members were seen once by the social worker and given brief service. Differences between the two groups were dramatic in terms of cost savings, keeping clinic appointments, reduction in use of emergency services, and improvement in social functioning. The last was measured using the Hunt-McVickers Client Movement Scale. Collins comments that it is "interesting to note that in this study reducing over-utilization of medical services through social services intervention was not incompatible with improved client-functioning" (p. 63).

The approaches used in this study are not overly complex and could readily be replicated or adapted to many segments of the health services sector by practitioners most likely to know the issues that require systematic inquiry. Similar approaches could be used in primary care centers to determine if there is a reduction in the tendency to "medicalize" social problems when social work intervention is used. Because hospitals are accelerating the rate of discharge, an experiment in which social workers provide intense follow-up services after discharge might help to determine whether these services are more cost effective than possible rehospitalization or other medically focused care alternatives.

Berkman and Weissman (1983) and Coulton (1980) have proposed that goal attainment scaling and single-subject designs may be approaches particularly suited to the health setting. Both of these research strategies are congruent with a practice perspective suggesting that client and worker jointly develop intervention objectives. Both approaches, described in detail by a number of writers for example, (Bloom, Butch, and Walker, 1979; Kiresuk and Sherman, 1968), make it possible to focus on clear-cut target goals and to measure small increments of change.

My students have used goal attainment scaling techniques to measure increasing proficiency in self-care skills of seriously mentally impaired young adults and reduction in acting out behavior of mentally disturbed adolescents. Berkman and Weisman (1983) suggest that the single subject design can monitor patient progress on every case to obtain continuous feedback of their intervention effects. They point out, however, that the rigors of the design process are difficult to manage in a setting where many professionals and family members converge to participate with the patient in the problem-solving process. If, for example, a patient is less anxious after a social worker has provided information about insurance coverage, it is hard to know whether the reduction in anxiety can be attributed to the worker's efforts or to others who also might have provided pertinent information.

The process by which worker and client—where possible together—identify target goals is characteristic of health care practice. They may decide together that the paraplegic client will try to overcome the fear of leaving the house in a wheelchair by trying it once weekly for a month. They will record fears, successes, and other reactions. Worker and client might rehearse the experience by anticipating the physical tasks and social reactions. The client also may agree to work on another goal, seeking work that can be done at home, by contacting prospective employers on the telephone. Review of progress by using the guidelines of the goal attainment model can begin to provide clues about the effect of social work intervention. Whether progress is made or not, workers can review their interventions with the objective of determining which strategies have and have not proved useful. It has also been pointed out that if data are carefully and consistently recorded they can be aggregated. Thus a hospital social work department might decide that goal attainment scaling would be used for all clients who are seen for a 6 month period because of difficulties with adhering to a medical regimen. Aggregated data on adherence could be compared to "outcome measures" developed for a group that had not been involved in the joint goal-setting and monitoring process.

• • •

This brief review of approaches to evaluating the outcome of health care social work intervention has focused on those that are available to every worker. The techniques are relatively easy to master and do not involve the massive allocation of funds and time required by other approaches. These other approaches are not to be minimized. Careful studies of service use patterns, organizational climate, psychosocial antecedents, and consequences of illness are but a few of the areas that call for investigation from a social work perspective.

ACCOUNTABILITY AND QUALITY ASSURANCE

The amount of social work and related literature currently devoted to accountability and quality assurance is continually proliferating. For example, the Joint Commission on Accreditation of Hospitals has devoted two issues of the *Quality Review Bulletin* (October, 1980 and a Special Edition, 1982) to varying facets of the subject. Rehr (1979) edited a most useful volume that is largely focused on health issues. The Committee on Health Quality Standards of the National Association of Social Workers (NASW) and the Joint Committee of NASW and the American Hospital Association commissioned a volume on social work quality assurance programs (Coulton, 1979). For several years, a series of conferences sponsored by the Bureau of Community Health Services and others have published their proceedings, many of which have focused on issues of quality assurance (for example, Hall and St. Denis, 1975; Jackson, 1973; Stein, Hall, and Young, 1976).

It is not possible or appropriate to attempt to do justice in this book to the creative and systematic work of so many. These efforts have their origins in the profession's growing sense that it must systematically account for and review its practices. Rehr (1979) summarizes the external forces that mandated the establishment of quality review mechanisms. These forces included the provisions in the Medicare and Medicaid legislation that those facilities that receive funds must be subject to review. The increasing cost of care and the government's role as provider of services and third-party payer "caused it to couple the concern for quality with that of cost containment" (p. 17).

Peer review was mandated because both professionals and the institutions in which they worked had shown limited inclination to monitor their work or to implement the result of evaluative efforts. The Professional Standards Review Organizations were charged with reviewing the appropriateness and quality of services to ensure proper use and maintenance of skill.

While the specific ways in which various health delivery settings and their social work components approach accountability vary, there are few that have not instituted some mechanisms for counting, describing, and monitoring the services they provide. There is, nevertheless, a substantial lack of uniformity in the procedures used (for example, Kagle, 1982). This was highlighted for me by one small effort. I asked a group of social work students assigned to diverse health settings to identify the quality assurance mechanisms currently being used in their settings. Some were able to identify the existence of regular, established peer review mechanisms and systematic procedures for recording and storing information on the types of clients served, the time spent in client contact, and social work participation in utilization review procedures, development of problem-oriented recording, and patient care audits. Some came back with blank stares; the people in their settings had only begun to think about developing procedures. Those who did find rigorous systems in place were skeptical about their utility for enhancing delivery. While many of the measures were designed to cut costs, in the students' opinions, few were coupled with concern for quality in the sense that Rehr uses that term.

This review of what may be an idiosyncratic experience is intended to point out that there may be a substantial gap between the work that is possible and what has as yet been achieved.

With these caveats as a backdrop, it is time to turn to an effort to define some of the major concepts and to call the reader's attention to some fruitful efforts.

Input, process, outcome, access

Coulton (1982) provides a framework for discussing quality assurance, suggesting that quality assurance is not associated with any particular technique, but is a concept that subsumes many methods and raises a number of questions. She defines quality assurance programs as consisting of "various procedures designed to increase the probability that the services received by clients will be adequate, appropriate and that they will be delivered in sufficient quantity" (p. 398). To carry out these functions agencies must define what are considered acceptable services (input). They must also consider issues related to beliefs concerning good practice (process) and questions of whether or not services are having the desired effects (outcome).

Input refers to the credentials of the staff members providing service. These credentials include staff educational requirements and accreditation by various accrediting and standard-setting groups. Whether or not the standards promote quality care is a question still open to empirical research. For example, an issue for health care social work is whether the quality of service provided by graduate-level social workers is superior to that of services provided by untrained or bachelor's-level workers. In 1975 Wolock compared the kind of service rendered in hospital social work departments with the proportion of graduate-level workers on the staff, focusing on the combination of concrete and counseling services rendered. Departments with high percentages of graduate workers not only provided more counseling services but also were more instrumental in securing concrete services. At the time the number of workers with bachelor's degrees in social work was too small to permit separate analysis of their work compared to those with undifferentiated bachelor of arts degrees. Systematic study of the comparative contribution of workers with bachelor's and master's degrees in social work is clearly needed.

Process studies have used the techniques of peer review and utilization review. Chernesky and Young (1979) characterize *peer review* as a process by which professionally recognized standards of care are determined and professionals monitor the quality of care given by their colleagues as evidenced in chart notations. The results are compiled, and corrective mechanisms to deal with deficiencies are developed. Those who participated in the work described by Chernesky and Young found it exciting, productive, and time consuming. This process necessarily raises questions about the reliability and validity of chart notations as an indicator of practice, how objective colleagues are in passing judgment on each other's work, and whether the process is a threatening one. These workers found that the process of participating in peer review procedures positively affected the quality of their work. Systematic attention to recording is an essential component of practice in health settings. Appendix B elaborates on this discussion and presents some models designed to facilitate documentation of social work efforts. Precise and careful recording can provide a base for identifying recurrent unmet need and the data base needed for change efforts. *Utilization review* judges if services are justified in terms of established criteria. Mandated utilization review proceedings were instrumental in identifying the fact that many hospital discharges were delayed because of psychosocial reasons and late referral to social service. Some of the groundbreaking work on high-risk screening discussed in Chapter 9 can be traced to early social work involvement with utilization review proceedings at Mount Sinai Hospital in New York City (Paneth and Lipsky, 1979).

Systematic data on how clients fare, based on adequate recording and efforts to develop resources and document their lack, can enhance social work's participation in the utilization review process. Without such data social workers are at best seen as "bleeding hearts," and at worst as bumbling, ineffectual workers who want to slow the pace and deter the efficient operations of the hospital.

Outcome studies involve a number of procedures. The direct service audit can compare the results of treatment reflected in the record with outcome criteria previously determined. For example, a social work department may develop a goal of effecting discharge to facilities congruent with client need. Review of records may indicate a repeated pattern in which the requirements of prompt discharge superseded efforts to find appropriate care. Thus many people may have gone home or to other facilities not deemed congruent with their needs. The various approaches to studying outcome that were reviewed in the discussion of social work research are useful in these kinds of efforts. For example, data gathered via goal attainment scaling (in which the goal may have been to increase the amount of times a disabled person leaves the house) can be compared with chart notations.

Access to care is one of the criteria for quality health care. High-risk clients particularly need good access. Determining if high-risk patients have programs available in a geographically convenient area at reasonable or no cost is one critical measure of access. Because of increasing conditions of scarcity "it becomes even more important that access to services be monitored" (Coulton, 1982, p. 401). Therefore social work has a particular and ongoing obligation to study the availability of care and to document, rigorously, when such care is not available.

• • •

This discussion of quality assurance mechanisms has covered only the reasons for their growth and some of the major concepts and procedures involved. Scant attention has been paid in this chapter to recording, to the political and administrative processes involved in administering quality assurance mechanisms, and to the evolving computer technology that facilitates storing and retrieving essential data. These are and have been the subjects of separate books (for example, Rehr, 1979).

Review of the massive literature referred to earlier suggests that how these programs are implemented is closely related to specific settings, organization and objectives and to the level of commitment and sophistication of those who participate in this process. I hope that these brief comments will encourage all my readers to explore the means by which they can work toward making social work practice in health care more rigorous and accountable.

SUMMARY

This chapter has focused on two main themes—research and quality assurance in health care social work. I identified a number of research areas requiring more systematic investigation. I reviewed some techniques for applied social work research as well as studies that have incorporated diverse research modalities. I emphasized those approaches that are readily learned and used by practitioners in their daily work. In the discussion of accountability and quality assurance I highlighted the factors that demand increasing attention be paid to these issues, and I identified some key concepts and strategies.

REFERENCES

Alexander, C.A.: Preface. In Rehr, H., editor: Professional accountability for social work practice, New York, 1979, Prodist.

Altman, I.: Some factors affecting hospital lengths of stay, Hospitals **39:**68, July 1965.

Beck, D.F., and Jones, M.A.: Progress on family problems: a nationwide study of clients' and counselors' views on family agency services, New York, 1973, Family Service Association of America.

Berkman, B., and Rehr, H.: Early social service case finding for hospitalized patients, Social Service Review **47:**256, June 1973.

Berkman, B., and Weissman, L.A.: Applied social work research. In Miller, R.S., and Rehr, H., editors: Social work issues in health care, Englewood Cliffs, NJ, 1983, Prentice-Hall, Inc.

Bloom, M., Butch, P., and Walker, D.: Evaluation of single interventions, Journal of Social Service Research **2**(3):301, 1979.

Blumberg, D., Ely, A., and Kerbeshian, A.: Clients' evaluation of medical social services, Social Work **20:**45, June 1975.

Briar, S.: Toward the integration of practice and research. In Fanshel, D., editor: Future of social work research, Washington, D.C., 1980, National Association of Social Workers.

Carrigan, Z.H.: Social workers in medical settings: who defines us?, Social Work in Health Care **4**(2):146, 1978.

Chernesky, R., and Lurie, A.: The functional analysis study: a first step in quality assurance, Social Work in Health Care **1:**213, Winter 1975-1976.

Chernesky, R.H., and Young, A.T.: Developing a peer review system. In Rehr, H., editor: Professional accountability for social work practice, New York, 1979, Prodist.

Collins, J.: Assessment of social services in a large health care organization: a social work administrator's perspective. In Jackson, R.C., editor: Evaluation of social work services in community health and medical care programs, DHEW Pub. No. (HSA) 77-5205, Rockville, MD, 1973, U.S. Department of Health, Education and Welfare.

Coulton, C.J.: Social work quality assurance programs: a comparative analysis, Washington, D.C., 1979, National Association of Social Workers.

Coulton, C.J.: Research on social work in health care: progress and future directions. In Fanshel, D., editor: Future of social work research, Washington, D.C., 1980, National Association of Social Workers.

Coulton, C.J.: Quality assurance for social service programs: lessons from health care, Social Work **27**(5):397, 1982.

Coulton, C., and Vielhaber, D.: Patterns of social work practice in planning for post-hospital care, Cleveland, 1977, Northeast Ohio Society for Hospital Social Work Directors.

Fanshel, D.: The future of social work research: strategies for the coming years. In Fanshel, D., editor: Future of social work research, Washington, D.C., 1980, National Association of Social Workers.

Fischer, J.: Is casework effective? a review, Social Work **18:**5, January 1973.

Glass, R.I., Mulvihill, M.N., Smith, H., Jr., Peto, R., Bucheister, D., and Stoll, B.J.: The 4 score: an index for predicting non-medical hospital days, American Journal of Public Health **67**(8):751, 1977.

Hall, W.T., and St. Denis, G.C., editors: Quality assurance in social services in health programs for mothers and children, Pittsburgh, 1975, University of Pittsburgh Press.

Halstead, L.S.: Team care in chronic illness: a critical review of the literature of the past 25 years, Archives of Physical Medicine and Rehabilitation **57**(2):507, 1976.

Hollis, H.: Casework: a psychosocial therapy, New York, 1973, Random House, Inc.

Jackson, R., editor: Evaluation of social work services in community health and medical care programs, DHEW Pub. No. (HSA) 77-5205, Rockville, Md., 1973, U.S. Department of Health, Education and Welfare.

Kiresuk, T., and Sherman, R.: Goal attainment scaling: a general method of evaluating comprehensive community health programs, Journal of Community Health **4**(6):443, 1968.

Mullen, E.J., and Dumpson, J.R., editors: Evaluation of social intervention, San Francisco, 1972, Jossey-Bass, Inc., Publishers.

Paneth, J., and Lipsky, H.: "Utilization review" and social work's role. In Rehr, H., editor: Professional accountability for social work practice, New York, 1979, Prodist.

Patti, R.: Conceptions of accountability. (mimeographed; date and source not available)

Social Work Services Joint Commission on Accreditation of Hospitals, Quality Review Bulletin, **10:** entire issue, October 1980.

Social Work review: approaches to evaluation and analysis of patient care, Quality Review Bulletin (special edition), entire issue, 1982. Joint Commission on Accreditation of Hospitals.

Rehr, H.: The climate is set for quality assurance: implications for social work. In Rehr, H., editor: Professional accountability for social work practice, New York, 1979, Prodist.

Reid, W.: The task centered system, New York, 1978, Columbia University Press.

Schlesinger, E., and Wolock, I.: Hospital social work roles and decision making, Social Work in Health Care **8**(1):59, 1982.

Stein, E., Hall, W.T., and Young, C.L., editors: Proceedings of the Working Conference on Minimum Review Criteria for Professional Social Work Practice, Pittsburgh, 1976.

Stoeckle, J., Settler, R., and Davidson, G.: Social work in a medical clinic: the nature and course of referrals to the social worker, American Journal of Public Health **56:**1570, September 1966.

Ullman, A., Goss, M.E., Davis, M.S., and Mushinski, M.: Activities, satisfactions and problems of social workers in hospital settings, Social Service Review, **45:**17, March 1971.

Watt, M.S.: Therapeutic facilitator: the role of the social worker in acute treatment hospitals in Ontario, doctoral dissertation, Los Angeles, 1977, University of California.

Wattenberg, S.H., Orr, M.M., and O'Rourke, T.W.: Comparison of opinions of social work administrators and hospital administrators toward leadership tasks, Social Work in Health Care **2**(3):295, 1977.

Wilson, S.J.: Recording guidelines for social workers, New York, 1980, The Free Press.

Wolock, I.: Hospital social work roles, unpublished data, 1975, Rutgers University School of Social Work.

Wolock, I., and Russell, H.: Physicians' views and use of social services, The Journal of Perth Amboy General Hospital **1**(4):32, 1972.

Wolock, I., and Schlesinger, E.: A study of hospital social work screening in New Jersey, Paper presented at the annual meeting of the American Public Health Association, Dallas, November 1983.

Appendixes

Appendix A*

Approaches to understanding medical information

The purpose of this appendix is to give social workers a brief introduction to the way physicians think, some familiarity with medical terminology, and an approach to learning about various diseases. It is divided in two sections. The first section briefly illustrates how physicians use the problem-oriented approach to recording information.† The second section includes the following three types of information:

1. A common disease classification system
2. A model by which physicians learn about disease processes
3. Detailed examples of the model in three disease categories: infectious diseases, cardiovascular diseases, and pulmonary disorders

The material is presented in keeping with the model by which physicians learn about the various disease entities. Most medical texts and other reference materials organize discussion of disease entities and processes in the manner used here. For each disease entity physicians learn about the disease's *pathology, etiology, epidemiology, characteristic symptoms, physical findings, treatment,* and *prognosis.*

The examples presented are intended as a guide to social workers' use of various readily available reference materials (for example, *The Merck Manual* and Frenay: *Understanding Medical Terminology*). Such reference materials are an essential part of the health care social worker's library, as is a medical dictionary. Those who work in specialized areas (for example, dialysis, psychiatry, or physical rehabilitation) need specialized reference sources, including professional journals focused on the specialty areas. Another important reference source is the *Diagnostic and Statistical Manual of Mental Disorders* (DSM-III), last revised by the American Psychiatric Association in 1980. This

* This appendix was written with the assistance of Richard S. Schlesinger, MD, DAPFP. The medical facts presented are based on his clinical experience. The following sources were consulted for factual and technical details: Petersdorf, R.G., Adams, R., Braunwald, E., Isselbacher, K., Martin, J., and Wilson, J.: *Harrison's principles of internal medicine,* ed. 10, New York, 1983, McGraw-Hill Book Co.; and *The Merck manual of diagnosis and therapy,* ed. 14, Rahway, N.J., 1982, Merck, Sharp & Dohme Research Laboratories.

† See Appendix B for examples of this approach to social work recording.

manual relies on descriptions of symptoms and signs as indicative of how patients feel and think.

The material presented in this appendix should make it easier for social workers to raise pertinent questions in their communications with physicians, nurses, and other health care personnel.

Those social workers who consistently and systematically make the effort to master this type of material will find that they can readily acquire knowledge sufficient for their purposes. The medical information gained and used to understand the impact of disease on clients must continually be integrated with the psychosocial data that forms the basis of the social worker's intervention. Medical information, when integrated with the concept of the careers of illness (Chapter 5), can provide considerable information and insight to guide the social worker's intervention.

The reader will note that where indicated, medical terms are italicized and preceded or followed by a lay definition.

THE PHYSICIAN'S APPROACH TO THE ORGANIZATION AND PRESENTATION OF MEDICAL DATA*

In recent years the problem-oriented approach to recording medical information has come into common use. Familiarly known as "SOAP," it is a way of thinking, reacting, and recording to distinguish the various components of medical information acquired and used in patient care. SOAP stands for:

*S*ubjective information obtained from the patient

*O*bjective information reflecting the physician's observations (for example, temperature, heart sounds, and laboratory findings)

*A*ssessments or diagnoses derived from the subjective and objective data

*P*lan for treatment

Another part of the problem-oriented record is the problem sheet or list; this is a work sheet. On this sheet information is entered, deleted, and noted as solved. This sheet does not necessarily become part of the record and may be rewritten when it becomes illegible. Entered on this sheet are

- Subjective problems (for example, chest pain)
- Established diagnoses (for example, a history of duodenal ulcer)
- Suspected diagnosis (for example, *R/O/MI,* standing for *R*ule *O*ut *M*yocardial *I*nfarction—heart attack)
- Psychosocial problems (for example, the patient is getting a divorce)
- Current medications
- Significant laboratory data
- Consultants, including the social worker
- Significant procedures to be undertaken

* Nurses use similar approaches. See, for example, Hanchett, E.S., R.N., Ph.D., The problem oriented system: a literature review DHEW Publication No. (HRA) 78-6, Washington, D.C., 1977, U.S. Government Printing Office.

The following example demonstrates the SOAP method of entering information that will remain a permanent part of the record. Such notes are made periodically during involvement with the patient. They are used in both ambulatory and inpatient settings.

A SOAP note

This is the fourth hospital day of a patient who was admitted with *pyelonephritis* (a kidney infection).

S Patient is "feeling better, getting hungry, worried about 16-year-old daughter alone at home unsupervised"

O T:100°, BP: $^{110}/_{70}$, pulse: 82, heart: regular, no murmurs
Lungs—clear
Abdomen—soft
Left flank tenderness decreased
White blood count 7600
Chest x-ray negative

A *Pyelonephritis* resolving

P Continue intravenous antibiotics; advance to regular diet; out of bed as tolerated; discuss situation of daughter with social worker

LEARNING ABOUT DISEASE

The following disease classification system is used in many medical texts:

- Infectious disorders
- Hematological disorders
- Cardiovascular disorders
- Pulmonary disorders
- Diseases of the urinary tract
- Diseases of the gastrointestinal tract
- Nutritional and metabolic disorders
- Endocrine disorders
- Connective tissue disorders
- Neurological disorders
- Psychiatric disorders
- Sexually transmitted diseases

The physician's model for learning about disease

Definition and pathology. The simple definition of a disease is similar to definitions usually found in the dictionary. For example, *pneumococcal pneumonia* is defined as an acute bacterial infection of the lungs caused by the *pneumococcus germ.* It is characterized clinically by an abrupt onset of fever, chest pain, cough, and bloody sputum.

Pathology is the reaction of the body to the disease and a description of how the body is affected. Thus in a textbook description of the *pathology* of *pneumococcal pneumonia,* we read that the first response of the lungs is an outpouring of *edema* fluid into the *alveoli* (simply, the lung sacs fill with body fluid). *White blood cells* (inflammatory cells) enter into this fluid accumulation; on reading a medical text the social worker will learn that this means that the lungs get filled with pus.

Etiology. *Etiology* is determining what caused the disease. Pneumococcal pneumonia is caused by *Streptococcus pneumoniae* (one of the bacteria).

Epidemiology. *Epidemiology* involves the circumstances under which the disease occurs and where and why it occurs. *Pneumococcal pneumonia* is most common in winter and early spring and is often preceded by an upper respiratory infection, but is not highly contagious. Direct transmission from one person to another is not common. Factors other than contagion play a key role in etiology. The development of pneumonia is dependent on the presence of the *pneumococcal germ,* the number of *pneumococci* present, and multiple factors in the *host* (individual) that predispose the individual to contracting the disease. Included among these factors is the state of the *immune system of the host.* The *immune system* is a person's natural response to a disease.

Symptomatology and physical findings. The symptoms of a disease are those the patient has experienced and can describe. Physical findings or signs are those that the physician can observe. For example, a complaint of feeling hot is a symptom. If a physician feels the heat of the body or records it with a thermometer, it is a sign. *Rales* in the chest (an abnormal sound heard with a stethoscope during the respiratory cycle) is an example of a physical finding. Patients with pneumonia will complain of feeling feverish and demonstrate *rales* on physical examination.

We must digress before we consider laboratory data to discuss the difference between subjective and objective findings. A subjective finding is that which patients describe to physicians (for example, "I feel tired"). An objective finding is that which physicians can see, feel, or smell.

Laboratory data. Laboratory data deal with objective findings (for example, blood tests, x-rays, or cardiograms). This information is supplied to the physicians by various laboratories. When a patient has pneumonia the laboratory will furnish the physician with the information that the number of white cells present in the patient's blood is increased. There is also a white area on the chest x-ray that is a pictorial representation of the pneumonia.

Differential diagnosis. Differential diagnosis includes all diseases that have similar subjective and objective findings. The differential diagnosis of pneumococcal pneumonia is other bacterial pneumonias, viral pneumonia, *pulmonary infarction* (blood clot in the lung), *atelectasis* (collapse of a small portion of the lung), various infections under the diaphragm, and carcinoma. Thus on the chart of a patient with pneumonia one might see under diagnosis the inscription: "pneumonia, R/O pulmonary embolus." This means the physician thinks the patient has pneumonia, although he or she could possibly have a *pulmonary embolus.* A *pulmonary embolus* refers to a clot of blood that travels to the lung, blocking an artery that supplies the lung, thus cutting the blood supply and causing *infarction*.

Treatment. Treatment is the course of action recommended by the physician. In the case of pneumonia it is bed rest, because the patient's body is worn out; fluids, because the patient is suffering excess water loss from the increased temperature; and intramuscular penicillin, which kills the pneumococcal germ. Therefore the patient is often hospitalized for this treatment.

Prognosis. Prognosis is the physician's assessment of the disease's outcome. Most patients with pneumonia would be expected to be *afebrile* (without fever) within 72 hours, out of the hospital in 1 week, and back on their feet in 2 weeks.

Examples of the physician's model for learning about disease

Infectious diseases. Infectious diseases are characterized by an invasion of the body by foreign organisms. This invasion is a necessary but not sufficient condition for the manifestation of the disease. There must also be a *morbid* response, which is a disruption of the integrity of some part of the host's bodily system.

The body can be invaded by *viruses, bacteria, parasites,* and other *microorganisms,* including *fungi.* A *virus* is a complex particle smaller than a cell. Its natural habitat is within the cell of another organism, in this case cells in the patient's body. An example of a disease induced by a virus is chickenpox. A *bacterium* is a one-celled plant. Pneumococcal pneumonia is an example of a disease caused by bacteria. Viruses cannot be eradicated by antibiotics, but bacteria can. *Parasites* can be divided into two categories: one-celled organisms such as *amoeba,* which cause *amoebic dysentery,* and many-celled organisms such as worms, which cause pinworm infestation. These invaders are capable of causing a pathological response by the body.

The example I am using to illustrate the process involved in diseases caused by infection is *infectious hepatitis,* now more precisely termed *hepatitis A.*

Infectious hepatitis (hepatitis A)

Definition and pathology. Acute infectious hepatitis is a common inflammatory liver disease caused by a virus. In an uncomplicated case the *hepatic lesion* is characterized by degeneration of the liver cells and cell death (*necrosis*). The liver is invaded by inflammatory cells. This invasion is one of the mechanisms whereby the body conquers the infection.

Etiology. Hepatitis A is caused by the hepatitis A virus.

Epidemiology. The primary method of spreading the disease is fecal-oral contact. Improper hand washing after defecation and subsequent food handling can contaminate the food, which is then consumed by others. Water and food in underdeveloped countries are frequently contaminated. Another source of infection is raw shellfish that have been contaminated by sewerage in their natural habitat.

Symptomatology and physical findings. In the *prodromal* (before development of the full disease complex) there is *anorexia* (loss of appetite), *malaise* (aches, pains, fatigue), nausea, vomiting, and fever. After the prodromal period the *icteric phase* begins (*icterus* or *jaundice* results from the absorption of *bile* by the cells of the body, producing a yellow color in the patient and dark urine). This absorption of bile is caused by the inability of the liver, because of the infection, to dispose of the bile that accumulates through the normal destruction of red blood cells. An acutely ill person will have fever and jaundice.

Laboratory data. Laboratory data include changes in the liver function tests, measured in blood samples, including elevation of *SGOT, SGPT,* and *LDH* (liver enzymes). Bile appears in the urine. Levels of *viral antigens* (substances of the virus itself) and *antibodies* (substances produced by the body in response to the invasion by the virus—part of the body's defense mechanism to destroy the virus) are elevated during the course of the disease.

Differential diagnosis. In the prodromal phase other viral infections such as *influenza* or *gastroenteritis* must be ruled out. Abdominal pain may mimic *acute cholecystitis* (gallbladder disease), pneumonia, or acute appendicitis. In the icteric phase one must consider the possibility of drug-induced or *toxic* (poisonous) *hepatitis. Infectious mononucleosis* as well as *alcoholic hepatitis* must also be ruled out in this phase.

Treatment. Because there are virtually no antiviral *agents* (medications), treatment is *supportive* (that is, maintaining good body function while the body combats the disease). Supportive measures include *antipyretic* agents (substances that reduce fever, such as aspirin), *antiemetics* (medications to stop vomiting), and *parenteral* fluids and *feeding* (parenteral means by injection—intravenously, intramuscularly, or under the skin), and bed rest. During the period of contagion isolation techniques must be instituted to prevent spreading the disease by fecal contamination.

Prognosis. The prognosis for infectious hepatitis is excellent. Recovery should be expected in approximately 6 weeks.

• • •

Thus the simple although important lesson to be learned from this example is that foreign organisms can enter the body and cause disease, and the body can mount defenses and restore the individual to good health. When the infection is caused by bacteria, antibiotics can assist the body in destroying the invading organisms.

In terms of the careers of illness model, hepatitis A is a disease of sudden onset and relatively short duration that calls for no major changes in life-style or alteration in self-image.

Cardiovascular diseases. Cardiovascular disorder is the term applied to a multitude of different diseases of the heart and blood vessels that have a wide range of etiologies. These diseases include deposition of cholesterol in the arteries, hardening of the arteries (calcification—technically known as *atherosclerosis*), diseases of unknown etiology such as high blood pressure (*essential hypertension*), diseases secondary to infection such as *cardiovascular syphilis,* streptococcal infection of the heart valves (*subacute bacterial endocarditis*), heart attack (*myocardial infarction*), and decreased blood flow to the extremities from atherosclerosis (*peripheral vascular disease*). I have selected for discussion myocardial infarction.

Myocardial infarction

Definition and pathology. A myocardial infarction (MI) is a clinical syndrome resulting from abrupt reduction in coronary flow to a segment of the heart musculature, causing heart muscle death. The coronary arteries are the source of blood supply to the heart muscle. An autopsy of a person who had a fatal heart attack would reveal that the diameter of the artery was significantly decreased by the deposition of cholesterol on the lining and a blood clot had filled the *lumen* (opening).

Etiology. Atherosclerosis of the coronary arteries is the common cause of MI. This has been associated with elevation of blood cholesterol secondary to diet, obesity, hypertension, diabetes, and heredity. It has been suggested that stress, lack of exercise, smoking, and a Type A personality are significant factors in the etiology of MI.

Epidemiology. The epidemiology of MI is complex and has been investigated extensively. The risk factors previously noted are differentially distributed, often by national origin, ethnic membership, dietary habits, and personality factors. Men are at greater risk of heart attack than premenopausal women. Social workers involved in prevention should consult the extensive literature on the epidemiology of heart disease.

Symptomatology and physical findings. The classic symptoms of patients experiencing MI are crushing chest pain radiating to the left arm, cold sweat, anxiety, and shortness of breath. Patients are restless, apprehensive, and in severe pain. The face is ashen, and the nail beds may be *cyanotic* (blue in color from poor oxygenation of the blood). Sweating is frequent and the skin is cool. Rales in the lungs may be present, indicating heart failure. The heart sounds are often distant and muffled. A *heart murmur* (an extra sound) is sometimes heard. *Auscultation* (listening with a stethoscope) of the heart may reveal a *gallop rhythm.* This gallop rhythm makes the heartbeat sound similar to a galloping horse and is indicative of *heart failure* (the impaired ability of the heart to perform its pumping function).

Laboratory data. The sine qua non of the MI is the change in the EKG or ECG (electrocardiogram) pattern. The ECG is a reflection of the electrical activity of the heart, which is disrupted by the MI. The physical pattern of an MI is *ischemia* (lack of oxygen), followed by muscle injury, and eventually *muscle necrosis* (muscle death). There are changes in the blood levels of *enzymes* normally found in muscle cells. Enzymes are substances that induce chemical change. They are usually abbreviated in the following manner: *CPK, MB fraction, SGOT,* and *LDH.* The number of white blood cells is elevated, as is the temperature.

Differential diagnosis. When diagnosing MI one must rule out *pericarditis* (inflammation of the heart lining), pulmonary embolus, lung collapse, gallbladder disease, pneumonia, and duodenal ulcer.

Treatment. Treatment of the uncomplicated MI includes bed rest and increasing the amount of oxygen available to the heart muscle. The bulk of the treatment effort is directed toward preventing complications and treating those complications when they arise. The threat of complications has been met with the proliferation of coronary care units and the emergence of *CPR* (cardiopulmonary resuscitation) and mobile cardiac ambulance services.

Cardiopulmonary arrest is treated with *CPR. Cardiac arrhythmias* (irregularities of the heart) are promptly treated with drugs, usually given intravenously, and with pacemakers. An intravenous infusion must be set up immediately so that drugs can be administered promptly. To recognize these arrythmias, cardiac monitors are attached to the patient. *Congestive heart failure* (compromise of the heart's pumping function) is treated with morphine and *diuretics,* which induce the kidneys to increase urinary output and thus decrease blood volume.

Shock, secondary to decreased heart function, is treated with drugs. Oxygen must be administered to replenish the decreased supply to the body as a whole, and the heart muscle in particular. The work of the heart is decreased by putting the patient on a light liquid diet. It is hoped that congestive heart failure will be averted by placing the patient on a low sodium diet. The pain of the MI is treated with demerol or morphine and coronary dilators such as nitroglycerin.

Long-term treatment is directed toward preventing subsequent heart attacks. Dietary changes are intended to reduce cholesterol and obesity. The cessation of smoking, exercise programs, and ultimately coronary bypass surgery are other methods of treatment.

Prognosis. The prognosis of MI must always be guarded to some degree because MI is an indicator of underlying coronary artery disease. However, prognosis can vary greatly, depending on the degree of damage, underlying disease, and reduction of risk factors.

MI is a disease for which extensive technology is used, but there is virtually no mechanism that cures the disease. The dead heart tissue heals itself by scarring. More importantly for the social worker, there is a wide range of psychosocial issues associated with MI that need attention. This disease commonly affects men in their middle years, for whom earning power is crucial.

• • •

The treatment of MI is illustrative of efforts directed toward maintaining critical body functions. This contrasts with such treatment as renal dialysis, in which a vital bodily function is performed by a mechanical device.

In terms of the careers of illness model, MI is a disease of sudden onset often requiring marked changes in life-style. These include coping with the fact that one has a chronic disease. For some this involves dramatic alteration of self-image.

Pulmonary disorders. Pulmonary disorders include the *acute respiratory distress syndrome* seen in newborns, which is a respiratory failure associated with pulmonary injury; diseases of airway obstruction, such as *chronic obstructive pulmonary disease* (*COPD*); and the pneumonias. Most of these diseases are associated with a decrease in the ability of the lungs to exchange air (that is, bring oxygen into the system and expel carbon dioxide). I have chosen *bronchial asthma* as an example of this group of diseases.

Bronchial asthma

Definition and pathology. Bronchial asthma is a form of airway obstruction that is usually reversible. Portions of the bronchial tree that allow air to pass into the lungs are narrowed by constriction of the smooth muscle lining the walls of the passages, *edema* (swelling of the tissues with fluid), and inflammation. There is excess mucus production. The lungs are voluminous and the *bronchi* (passageways) are occluded by mucus plugs.

Etiology. The underlying etiology is unknown, although heredity plays an important role. The attacks can be precipitated by allergens such as pollen, dust, irritation from pollutants in the air, infection, or the inhalation of cold air. It is generally accepted that allergy plays an important role in the etiology of bronchial asthma. The role of emotional factors is still disputed. The nature of the disease is distressing and has emotional consequences, and it is generally agreed that low oxygen levels produce anxiety. Therefore a commonsense view suggests that fighting for "the very breath of life" can produce emotional stress. Thus when one observes that an asthmatic patient is anxious, one can legitimately ask the question, "Which came first?" Between attacks patients may appear quite normal, except perhaps if they have a *barrel chest* (an increase in the diameter of the chest). Some asthmatic patients have a chronic low-grade wheeze.

Epidemiology. Asthma is evenly distributed geographically. However, the frequency of attacks is greater in areas where there is abundant foliage and high pollution levels. *Extrinsic asthma* (that which is mostly associated with allergy) appears mostly in childhood and young adulthood. The time of onset for *intrinsic asthma* (asthmatic episodes mostly triggered by infection and irritants) is usually in the middle years.

Symptomatology and physical findings. The frequency and severity of asthmatic attacks varies between individuals. An asthmatic attack is characterized by wheezing, coughing, shortness of breath, and tightness in the chest. The audible wheeze occurs during the expiratory phase of respiration.

Physical findings include audible *wheezing,* which is the high-pitched sound heard during the expiratory phase of respiration and indicates air rushing through the constricted air passageways. The patient also exhibits *tachypnea* (rapid respirations), *tachycardia* (a fast heart), and elevated blood pressure. The patient struggles for air and prefers to sit upright. *Auscultation* of the chest reveals a prolonged expiratory phase. *Cyanosis* becomes evident as the attack continues.

Laboratory data. The white blood count reveals an increase in white blood cell forms known as *eosinophils.* The sputum is tenacious, rubbery, and whitish; if infection is present it is yellow. The chest x-ray can be normal or show signs of *hyperinflation* (overinflated lungs). Arterial blood gas levels are usually measured. They show increased carbon dioxide and decreased oxygen in the blood. Pulmonary function tests measure the degree of respiratory dysfunction.

Differential diagnosis. Asthma must be differentiated from other conditions that produce respiratory difficulty, such as the *hyperventilation syndrome* (rapid respirations caused by emotional factors), heart failure, mechanical obstruction by foreign objects, or *metabolic acidosis* (the result of an acute exacerbation of metabolic diseases wherein, because of a complicated chain of events, the blood becomes acidic in nature), to which the body responds with hyperventilation.

Treatment. An acute attack is treated with bronchodilating drugs. Adrenalin is given *subcutaneously* (injected under the skin). Aminophyleine is given intravenously, and oxygen is administered. Frequently the antiinflammatory agent *cortisone* is used. Fluid administration is extremely important. Hyperventilation and fever (if infection is present) causes dehydration and leads to the production of thick, tenacious sputum. Patients must be hydrated so that fluid can enter into the thickened mucus, allowing it to be expectorated.

Between attacks chronic asthma is treated with bronchodilators. Aminophyleine-like drugs and terbutaline, among others, are given orally. *Isoproterenol aerosol* (the "inhaler" many people have seen) is another method of introducing bronchodilators. The antiinflammatory agent cortisone can be administered in a number of ways.

Long-term treatment must emphasize the avoidance of allergens and irritants. This includes maintaining a dust-free home, avoiding contact with furry animals, and reducing exposure to air pollutants. When attacks are frequent and persist over years, emotional reactions may set in. Some form of psychotherapy or counseling may help the patient cope with associated fears.

Prognosis. Prognosis is variable. Many childhood asthmatic patients outgrow their asthma in early adulthood. Bronchial asthma is a classic illustration of the interaction of heredity, environment, and possibly emotional factors.

In terms of the careers of illness model, asthma is an example of a career with slow onset that involves some life-style changes and usually has a good outcome.

Appendix B

Recording in health care social work

A number of developments have converged to give increasing importance to social work recording in health care settings. The thrust for accountability and research needs reviewed in Chapter 12 intensifies the need for clear and precise documentation of social work efforts. Interdisciplinary efforts require that the social worker's contribution become readily accessible. Using a computer for storing and retrieving information reinforces this thrust. For all these reasons considerable attention has been paid to refining and systematizing the way social workers record information. Wilson (1980) has made a major contribution in this area.

No single system is as yet available. Furthermore, recording systems need to be adapted to the particular needs of various settings. In this appendix a number of major approaches and themes are reviewed. Readers using this appendix should consider the needs of their settings and make adaptations accordingly.

THE PURPOSE OF RECORDING

The Society for Hospital Social Work Directors of the American Hospital Association (1978) has succinctly identified the purposes of social work recording. Although their comments are focused on practice in hospitals the relevance for other settings is self-evident. Fundamentally recording serves the following purposes: communication, continuity of care, comprehensive care, accountability, documentation, education, and research. The use of the social work record as an educational and research tool is self-evident.

The standards for medical record services developed by the Joint Commission on Accreditation of Hospitals (1976) is summarized as follows:

1. They function as a basis for patient care planning, continuity, and evaluation of treatment.
2. They provide documentary evidence of medical evaluation, treatment, and change in the patients' conditions while they are in the hospital or receiving ambulatory or home-based care.
3. They document communication between those practitioners ultimately responsible for the patients' care and other health professionals involved in care.

4. They serve to protect the legal interest of the patient, hospital, and practitioners.
5. They provide data for use in continuing education and research.

Communication

Because so many disciplines are involved in health care, precise communication facilitates exchange of information. Staff changes (both within the social work department and in other departments) are common occurrences. The record can forestall the disruptive effects of such changes on patient care.

Continuity of care and comprehensive care

Because problems are often diverse and of a medical and psychosocial nature, the social worker's recording plays a major role in keeping other disciplines informed of psychosocial needs and plans for continuing care.

Accountability

The record forms the basis for many of the activities related to quality assurance and accountability reviewed in Chapter 12. It is used in peer review proceedings. "Professional Standards Review Organizations and utilization review committees require documentation of patients' psychosocial problems, treatment plans, and expected outcome within a given time frame" (American Hospital Association, 1978, p. 4).

Documentation

The record may be used as evidence in legal proceedings (particularly in the areas of child abuse, adoption, commitment, guardianship, discharge planning, and transfer to other facilities). Licensing and regulatory and accrediting agencies may review records as a basis for determining whether their various standards are being met.

HOW TO RECORD

The American Hospital Association (1978) states that a recording format consistent with the hospital's medical record system needs to be developed. Social work entries should be an integral part of the patient's record. The style of recording (for example, whether the problem-oriented format is to be used) and whether additional separate social work records are to be maintained will be discussed next as separate issues. Whatever recording format is agreed on, social workers need to consider (1) why information was gathered, (2) from whom, (3) when, and (4) by what method. Distinctions should be made between those facts reported or observed and those that represent an assessment. Plans that are developed, discharge notes, and outcome statements are essential parts of the record.

The problem-oriented recording method

The basic dimensions of this approach, initially developed by Weed (1969), were outlined in Appendix A. Kane (1974) proposes an adaptation for the social work record. The SOAP format can be applied to social work recording in a manner not unlike that used by physicians, as illustrated in Appendix A. The social worker also develops a problem list. This list and subsequent entries should be devoid of jargon, focusing instead on clear statements of problems and behaviors. The list can be corrective for the older "rambling, chronological style of recording in which original problems can be lost or forgotten" (Kane, 1974, p. 415). The problem list, complete with dates on which problems were identified, might list the following information for a patient requiring discharge planning:

1. Patient, a 75-year-old widow with hip fracture, needs care following discharge.
2. Patient is eligible for 100 hours of Medicare-financed home health care.
3. Patient is agitated and fearful about returning home alone.
4. Patient worries about being a burden to her daughter.

All the problems noted in the list involve discharge needs and the patient's concerns and needs for care. A SOAP note, appropriately dated following the social worker's second interview with the patient, might look as follows:

Subjective: Patient is very upset about her hip fracture and the accompanying pain and worries about what will happen to her.

Objective: Dr. Jones, chief orthopedist, says patient needs a 3-week hospital stay. Following this she will need supervised home care because of her limited mobility.

Assessment: The worker believes this patient is reacting with levels of concern appropriate to her present condition and anticipated future needs.

Plan

1. Contact daughter to review her mother's needs with her.
2. Alert home health agency to patient's needs and ascertain ability to provide care.
3. See patient frequently for supportive discussion to advise her of her options and involve her in planning for her own care.

Repeated entries would indicate any progress in locating resources, the daughter's readiness to be involved in providing care, and any changes in the patient's emotional response.

As the social worker makes these chart entries, he or she will be communicating not only with the patient and her daughter but also with physicians, nurses, and others. Importantly, he or she will be reviewing the record and noting the entries made by others. Both the problem list and SOAP method facilitate the worker's efforts with the patient. Other modes of structured recording can be used. Some of these are reviewed by Young (1979). Whatever format is agreed on, the entry should include the reason for involvement with the client, the worker's and client's assessment of the problem, indications of collaboration with others, the goals and contracted activities agreed on, and the outcome and/or plan.

Separate social work records

In its publication on documentation the American Hospital Association (1978) suggested that working notes for planning, research, and educational purposes may be maintained separately in the social work department. The association pointed out that these records are subject to subpoena should legal action arise. Correspondence, or at least a brief account of disclosures to third parties, should be filed in the medical record.

Confidentiality

Confidentiality is of major concern to social workers. The issue is touched on by the Joint Commission on Accreditation of Hospitals, in the code of Ethics of the National Association of Social Workers, and in "A Patient's Bill of Rights" developed by the American Hospital Association.

Critical distinctions between confidentiality and privileged communication should be made. *Confidentiality* is "an agreement or trust that information obtained by the social worker from or about the patient will not be disclosed without the patient's consent to another person not involved in that confidential relationship" (American Hospital Association, 1978, p. 9). *Privileged communication* is a confidential communication protected from disclosure by law. In some states social work clients have this privilege.

Hospitals have defined policies on the disclosure of information that require the patient's consent. These policies include written reports to community agencies. However, certain information (for example, child abuse) must be reported.

REFERENCES

American Hospital Association, Documentation by social workers in medical records, Chicago, 1978, Society for Hospital Social Work Directors.

Joint Commission on accreditation of hospitals: Accreditation manual for hospitals, Chicago, 1976, The Commission.

Kane, R.A.: Look to the record: the problem-oriented record can be used, Social Work **19:**412, July, 1974.

Weed, L.L.: Medical records, medical education, and patient care: the problem-oriented record as a basic tool, Cleveland, 1969, The Press of Case Western Reserve University.

Wilson, S.J.: Recording guidelines for social workers, New York, 1980, The Free Press.

Young, A.: The chart notation. In Rehr, H., editor: Professional accountability for social work practice, New York, 1979, Prodist.

Appendix C

High-risk criteria

Throughout this book and especially in Chapter 9 I have referred to the important development of high-risk screening. This process involves social workers in identifying those health care clients thought to be at particular psychosocial risk because of the health problems for which they are obtaining care. Considerable effort has gone into refining the criteria since these mechanisms for identifying clients thought to be in particular need of social work services were first initiated. This effort still continues; however, no single set of criteria has been developed.

Coulton (1979) points out that these criteria are still in different stages of implementation. She also presents some examples of "general access" criteria. Schlesinger and Wolock (1982) found relatively little uniformity in criteria used in different hospitals, although most of the hospitals queried had developed some guidelines for screening in their own institutions. For these reasons it is not possible to present a list of high-risk criteria with universal applicability. However, it is possible to give the reader some sense of the populations and health problems that often fall into the high-risk category. Two lists are presented that derive from review of Coulton's work (1979), other sources on quality assurance, and Schlesinger and Wolock's work (1982). One list is organized by population characteristics and the other by health problem areas.

High-risk population characteristics

1. Elderly with no known relatives at the same address
2. People without relatives and who are unable to provide information
3. People transferred to a hospital from a nursing home
4. Any adult who is unable to care for himself or herself and/or has no known adequate social and financial support
5. People frequently readmitted to hospitals
6. People whose families are unable to help with their major illness

High-risk health problem areas

1. Accident victims
2. Abused or neglected children
3. Newborns who are premature or have known birth defects
4. People with severe life-threatening illnesses such as

a. Various disabling cancers
b. Conditions requiring heart surgery
c. Stroke
d. Amputation
e. End-stage renal disease
f. Burns
g. Sight-threatening eye disorders
h. Terminal illness

5. People with psychiatric disturbances, including those who have threatened to make or have made suicide attempts, or those who are assaultive or violent
6. Rape victims
7. Victims of battering, such as abused spouses, and other victims of violence

A review of these lists readily suggests that they will be expanded or contracted depending on the services provided by a facility and the social work resources available.

REFERENCES

Coulton, C.J.: Social work quality assurance programs: a comparative analysis, Washington, D. C., 1979, National Association of Social Workers.

Schlesinger, E., and Wolock, I.: Hospital social work roles and decision making, Social Work in Health Care **8**(1):59, 1982.

Appendix D

Guide for developing a community profile*

In Chapter 6 I discussed extensively the importance of understanding the community context in which health care facilities are located and where service is rendered. This appendix is intended to help the individual worker or health care setting develop such an understanding. It is presented in the belief that systematic attention to population distribution, employment levels, health status, and access to care can enhance health care social work practice in the terms considered in this book. The reader will note that attention is paid to the nature of the health services systems, their relationship to other social services, and the availability of informal and formal community care systems for long-term care. The links between the particular health facility and the larger community are important.

This profile of the community can be developed by use of census data, publications developed by local community organizations, the health care facility, planning boards, and discussions and interviews with community leaders and members.

Identification of community

1. Name and local designation (for example, "Watts," "Little Italy")
2. Type of government

Geography and transportation

1. Urban/rural/suburban
2. Location near the following:
   a. Highways
   b. Bus routes
   c. Railroads
   d. Truck routes
   e. Airports

Identity of the community

1. Distinctive characteristics (for example, a well-known univer-

*Adapted from Devore, W., and Schlesinger, E.: Ethnic-sensitive social work practice, St. Louis, 1981, The C.V. Mosby Co., pp. 267-270; Dinerman, M.: Course outline for social work practice in health care, New Brunswick, N.J., 1981, The School of Social Work, Rutgers University.

sity town, a wealthy community, a community with great disparities of wealth and poverty)
2. Unique history

Population characteristics

1. Total size of population
2. Breakdown by
    a. Age
    b. Sex
    c. Minority groups
    d. Other ethnic groups
    e. Religious affiliation
3. Educational level
    a. Median for total adult population
    b. Median for women
    c. Median for each of the major ethnic and minority groups
4. Major shifts in the population composition over the past 5 to 10 years (for example, migration of minority groups, departure of a sizable number of people in any one population group)
    a. Major urban renewal or other redevelopment efforts

Employment and income characteristics

1. Employment status
    a. Major sources and types for total adult population
    b. Major sources for women
    c. Major sources for each of the major ethnic and minority groups
2. Median income
3. Income characteristics below poverty level
4. Type of public welfare system (for example, state or county jurisdictions; state involved in Medicaid program)

Educational facilities

1. Types of schools available
2. Bilingual programs in schools
3. Minority and ethnic group members on the staffs or school boards
4. School administrators aware of the particular problems and strengths of minority and ethnic group members
5. Promotion in schools of cultural awareness and sensitivity programs

The health care system

1. Major health facilities in the community (for example, a major university teaching hospital, a network of primary care centers, well-developed home health services, functioning folk healers)

Gaps in the health care system

1. Major gaps (for example, shortage of primary care providers and mental health facilities, no community-based, long-term care facilities)

Other health and welfare resources

1. Important resources available
   a. Recreational and leisure-time facilities
   b. Social agencies
2. Bilingual staff members
3. Adequate representation of minority and ethnic group members on the staffs of hospitals and social agencies
4. Development of cultural awareness and sensitivity programs
5. Prevailing formal and informal community networks:
   a. Swapping networks for exchange of resources
   b. Church-supported health and welfare groups
   c. Ethnic-based lodges, fraternities, benevolent societies
   d. Union-sponsored health and welfare facilities
   e. Self-help groups of people with special problems (for example, alcoholic or physically handicapped patients)

Health agency's relationship to the community

1. Is the agency well-known and respected?
2. Is the agency viewed as a place to which people can readily turn?
3. Is the agency involved in the community (for example, by representation on various community boards; used as a resource by schools, churches, and others)?

Health agency's linkage with other health and social service systems

1. Are referral and linkage mechanisms with other providers well developed at the formal level (for example, well-routinized, well-functioning relationships with hospitals, home health facilities, nursing homes)?
2. Are informal networks between facilities well developed?
3. Does the facility become involved with community-wide, health and prevention activities (for example, health fairs, screening for hypertension)?

Special problems and assets

1. What are the major social problems (for example, prevalent health problems, housing, school)?
2. Is there a particular concern with crime, delinquency, and underemployment?
3. Are there particular intergroup tensions? Are there efforts for intergroup coalition?

Assessment of the community

1. What are some of the major problems of this community?
2. Does this community have a positive identity or loyalty you can describe?
3. What are the major strengths and weaknesses of the health and welfare community?
4. What are the major gaps in services?

Index

Q

R

S